IMMUNOREGULATION

IMMUNOREGULATION

Edited by

N. FABRIS
Italian National Institute on Aging
Ancona, Italy

E. GARACI
Institute of Microbiology
Rome, Italy

JOHN HADDEN
University of South Florida Medical College
Tampa, Florida

and

N. A. MITCHISON
University College
London, England

PLENUM PRESS • NEW YORK AND LONDON

Library of Congress Cataloging in Publication Data

Workshop on Immunoregulation (1981: Urbino, Italy)
   Immunoregulation.

   "Proceedings of a Workshop on Immunoregulation, held July 8–10, 1981, at Urbino, Italy"—Verso t.p.
   Bibliography: p.
   Includes index.
   1. Immune response—Regulation—Congresses. I. Fabris, N. II. Title. [DNLM: 1. Allergy and immunology—Congresses. QW 504 W9265i 1981]
   QR186 W67 1981   616.07′9   83-4777

ISBN-13: 978-1-4684-4549-7   e-ISBN-13: 978-1-4684-4547-3
DOI: 10.1007/978-1-4684-4547-3

Proceedings of a Workshop on Immunoregulation,
held July 8–10, 1981, at Urbino, Italy

© 1983 Plenum Press, New York
Softcover reprint of the hardcover 1st edition 1983
A Division of Plenum Publishing Corporation
233 Spring Street, New York, N.Y. 10013

PREFACE

Immunoregulation is one of the areas which has witnessed the most explosive advances of immunology during the past decade. It is in this area that the current view of the immune system has arisen and developed. There is indeed little doubt that immune reactions are primarily determined by messages which are generated within the immune system and passed among different types of immunologic cells. This cell communication not only determines the type, intensity and duration of the response after perturbation of the immune system by exogenous antigens, but it is also essential for preventing autoimmune reactions and their clinical consequences.

In order to assure a perfect balance within the enormous complexity of the immune system, it is not surprising that multiple self-regulatory mechanisms are organized at different levels, such as antibody feedback, idiotypic-anti-idiotypic responses, suppressor and helper T cells, lymphokine signals and genetic requirements.

A number of observations in recent years have, however, demonstrated that consistent contributions to the immunological homeostasis are given also by signals generated outside of the immune system, namely, in the central and autonomous nervous system as well as in the endocrine apparatus.

Furthermore, the interactions between the immune system and the other body homestatic mechanisms seem to be bidirectional: if immunological cells may be targets of neuroendocrinological factors, immunological products seem in turn to contribute to the neuroendocrine homeostasis.

Such a sophisticated network of neuroendocrine-immune interactions, which should take into account also the existence of
thymic humoral factors, is becoming more and more complex and
leading frequently to contradictory and confusing findings, particularly when one moves to human pathology from experimental models.

It was from these convictions and from the believe that the
immunoregulation field will deserve in the future an even greater
expansion than in the past, that the idea of a symposium, in which
a group of friends could very informally exchange ideas, discuss
difficulties, analyze past and recent findings and outline future
research aims, was born. The meeting was held in Urbino in the
summer of 1981 and the efforts of the participants are presented
in this volume. The diversification of the contributions, ranging
from the genetic control of the immune response to its modulation
by psychological conditioning, gives a comprehensive view of the
field and raises a great number of questions.

If further work will be undertaken with the aim to give
insight to some of the questions raised in the areas developed
here, then the objective of this volume will have been achieved.

N.Fabris
E.Garaci

ACKNOWLEDGEMENTS

The editors gratefully acknowledge the financial assistance
of Italian National Research Council and of Italian Education
Ministery; special thanks are extended to Sogesta S.p.A., Urbino,
for the marvellous place and organization provided to the meeting.

Thanks are also due to the staff of I.N.R.C.A. Research
Department, Ancona, and of Institute of Microbiology, University
of Rome, for the invaluable assistance during the meeting.

CONTENTS

CONTENTS

IgV$_H$ AND MHC-RESTRICTED REGULATORY

CIRCUIT IN THE IMMUNE RESPONSE

Tada, T., Suzuki, G., Abe, R.,
Kumagai, Y., Hiramatsu, K. and Miyatani, S.

Department of Immunology, Faculty of Medicine
University of Tokyo , Tokyo , Japan

1. INTRODUCTION

The term "immune circuit" has been used to designate a train process of regulatory cell interactions in which the initial input such as antigenic stimulation activates a consecutive series of lymphoid cells finally producing an output which neutralizes the input signal. Thus, it is supposed that antigenic stimulation induces antibody formation, but at the same time it does activate a series of cells that finally suppress the antibody formation. Such an internal regulatory system is maintained by selective interactions between one cell type and the other which are restricted by mutual recognition of polymorphic structures expressed on partner cells.

One of the restricting elements has been determined to be the products of major histocompatibility complex (MHC). With the well known rigid restrictions observed in the interaction between the cytotoxic T cell and target cells, and macrophage and T cells, we are aware that some of the regulatory pathways are restricted by MHC genes. Our own previous experiments indicated that the suppression of antibody response is mediated by a soluble product (antigen-specific T cell factor, TsF) made by Lyt-2^+3^+ T cell that carries determinants coded for by genes in the I-J subregion of murine MHC. TsF was found to act on Lyt-$1^+,2^+,3^+$ T cells that

1

also carry an I-J subregion gene product of the same haplotype origin (I-J restriction). In the presence of such Lyt-1$^+$,2$^+$,3$^+$ T cells which have accepted TsF, it is induced a new suppressor effector T cell with Lyt-2$^+$,3$^+$ phenotype. This cell type acts on Lyt-1$^+$ helper T cells to diminish their helper effect. It is as yet undetermined whether this I-J restricted interaction is due to the presence of anti-I-J receptors in the responding cell type or to the complementary interactions between different I-J subregion products among the member T cells (reviewed by Tada and Okumura, 1979).

Recently, the work from Benacerraf's group presented evidence that the idiotype and anti-idiotype interaction is the major restricting element of the suppressor circuit (reviewed by Germain, 1980). In their experiment, the idiotypic suppressor inducer cell of Lyt-1$^+$ phenotype induces anti-idiotypic Lyt-2$^+$,3$^+$ suppressor T cell (Ts$_2$) which finally activates the anti-idiotypic T cell of Lyt-1$^+$, I-J$^+$ phenotype. A similar type of idiotype- and MHC-restricted suppressor pathway has also been reported by Eardley et al. (1979). Such a tedious process which is inherent to the immune system is probably of importance in amplifying the initial sign to induce an output large enough for neutralizing the input. Thus, the immune system is viewed as a net composed of a variety of cells recognizing different MHC products and idiotypes with which circuitry is maintained among the constituent cells.

With the above considerations in mind, antigen-specific T cell factors, which have restricted effects in the suppression and augmentation of the antibody responses, would give an unique opportunity to examine the devices by which they recognize the second cell type to be activated. We shall briefly review our recent observations on immunoglobulin variable region (V$_H$) and MHC expressions on T cell factors, and will discuss the significance of these polymorphic structures in the immunological circuit.

2. IgV$_H$-RESTRICTED PATHWAY IN THE SUPPRESSOR CIRCUIT

During the last few years, increasing evidence suggests that immunoglobulin V region is involved in the antigen-binding site of T cell factors. Ben-Neriah et al. (1978a,b) were successful in making rabbit antibodies reactive with framework structures of variable region of heavy and light chains of M315 myeloma protein (anti-V_H and anti-V_L). These antibodies were able to react virtually with all V_H and V but not with other candidate antigens of immunoglobulin, and therefore are good probes to examine the structure of antigen-binding site. By the use of these antibodies, we were able to show that semipurified antigen-binding T cells and the suppressor factor (TsF) from them carry determinants detectable with anti-V_H but not with anti-V_L (Tada et al., 1980). This coincided with findings that some T cells carry V_H or V_L (Lonai et al., 1980; Eichmann et al., 1980) and that isolated T cell receptor is reactive with anti-V_H but not with anti-V_L (Cramer et al., 1980). In addition, it was confirmed that helper and suppressor factors, produced by T cell hybrids made by fusion between functional T cells and an enzyme-deficient thymoma cell line, BW5147, were reactive with anti-V_H (Eshhar et al., 1980, Lonai et al.,1980, Tada et al., 1980). We ourselves tested anti-V_H antisera independently provided by Dr. D. Givol and Dr. H. Eisen, and found that both anti-V_H were able to react with TsF specific for keyhole limpet hemocyanin (KLH)- and 4-hydroxy-3-nitrophenyl acetyl(NP). The presence of V_L framework is not completely ruled out,since the anti-V_L antibodies can react only with the framework of $V\lambda_2$. We can just mention that these anti-V_L antisera could not remove TsF specific for NP, the antigen which preferentially induces primary antibodies with light chain of λ_2 type.

Several attempts have been made to detect idiotypic markers on T cell factors. Germain et al. (1979) showed that TsF specific for GAT carried a major cross-reactive idiotype shared with anti-GAT antibodies. The idiotype positive TsF was found to activate anti-idiotypic T cells (Sy et al., 1979). Many other investigators looked for idiotypes which are linked to immunoglobulin allotype genes on suppressor T cells and their hybridomas. These include p-azobenzen arsonate (ABA), NP and phosphoril choline (PC), and all the results confirmed the linkage of idiotype on T cell factors to Ig allotype loci (Bach et al., 1979; Pacifico and Capra, 1980; Minami, et al., 1981; Kontiainen et al., 1981; Tada et al., 1981; Kishimoto et al., 1981). Since these idiotypic expressions are known to be linked to Ig gene clusters, it is likely that the antigen-binding receptors of T cells are encoded by IgV_H genes.

A noteworthy example is the Igh^b allotype-linked idiotype (NP^b) which is expressed on NP-specific T cells. We have examined the presence of the NP^b idiotype among the NP-binding T cells from

B10.BR (Igh^b , H-2^k) mice and hybridoma cell lines derived from
them. Mice were immunized with NP coupled to gelatin and syngeneic
mouse Ig. The T cell fraction of NP-primed spleen cells was
incubated in Petri dishes coated with NP-bovine serum albumin, and
NP-binding T cells were recovered by washing dishes with cold
medium (Taniguchi and Miller, 1978). By fluorescence staining with
various anti-idiotypic reagents, it was found that a portion of
such NP-binding T cells carry major cross-reactive idiotypes of
NP^b. In general 5 to 10% of recovered T cells were stained with
guinea pig anti-NP^b, and the majority of them carried an idiotype
detectable by a monoclonal anti-idiotype antibody (Ac38) which was
kindly provided by Drs. Michael Reth and Klaus Rajewsky. Similar
percentages of cells were stained with xenogeneic anti-V$_H$, while
none of the monoclonal and conventional anti-allotype antibodies
reacted with them. The expression of NP^b idiotype on NP-binding T
cells was found to be linked to Igh-1^b allele by examination of
different strains.

The NP-binding T cells thus obtained were suppressor T cells,
since the cells as well as their extracts (TsF) could suppress the
secondary anti-NP but not anti-DNP antibody response "in vitro",
and were unable to help the NP-specific B cells in the presence or
absence of other T cells. The NP^b idiotype was found exclusively
on Lyt-2$^+$,3$^+$ T cells.

Hybridoma cell lines were established by fusion of NP-binding
T cells from B10.BR strain and an enzyme deficient thymoma cell
line of AKR origin, BW5147. One of the hybrid, 7C3-13, expressed
an NP^b idiotype detectable by conventional guinea pig anti-NP^b by
the fluorescence activated cell sorter (FACS) analysis. The
staining with anti-idiotype was inhibitable by 10^{-7} M of a cross-
reactive hapten, NIP (4-hydroxy-5-iodo-3-nitrophenyl acetyl) ami-
nocaproic acid, while 10^{-5}M NP-aminocaproic acid was necessary for
a partial inhibition, indicating that the NP-binding receptor has
the well known property of the primary anti-NP antibodies termed
heteroclicity. The cell line also expressed an I-J^k determinant.
Isolated receptor molecules from this cell line exhibited a
similar heteroclicity which was determined by the haptenated phage
inhibition test (kindly performed Dr. M. Cramer).
In addition, Kumagai (unpublished) was successful in photoaffinity
labelling of NP-binding site of hybridoma cells using N^{125}IP-
-arylazide. The separation and biochemical analysis of NP-binding,
idiotype positive molecules of T cells are in progress.

The cell free extract from NP-binding T cells as well as
7C3-13 hybridoma had a characteristic suppressor activity in the
in vitro secondary anti-NP antibody response of NP-KLH-primed
spleen cells, which showed interesting IgV_H and/or MHC restriction. In brief, anti-NP antibody response of C57BL/6 (H-2^b,
Igh-1^b) spleen cells was suppressed by TsF derived from C3H.SW
(H-2^b, Igh-1^j), B10.BR (H-2^k, Igh-1^b) and CWB (H-2^b, Igh-1^b) but
not from C3H (H-2^k, Igh-1^j) and Balb/c (H-2^d, Igh-1^a). This indicates that in order to suppress the anti-NP antibody response of
C57BL/6 mouse, either H-2 or Igh-allotype matching is necessary.
In addition, the expression of NP^b idiotype among the produced
anti-NP antibodies was suppressed only when Igh-allotype is
identical between TsF and responding cells.

This was further substantiated by experiments using idiotype-
bearing TsF from 7C3-13 hybridoma. We cocultured CB.20 (H-2^d,
Igh-1^b) B cells and syngeneic CB.20 T cells or IgV_H congenic

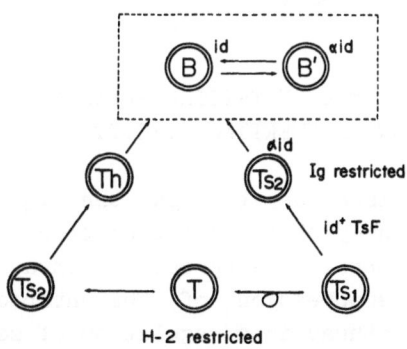

Fig.1. H-2 and IgV_H restricted pathways in the suppression of
       antibody response. The upper compartment is the network
       among B cells by mutual recognition of Ig idiotype. This
       compartment will be disturbed by a helper signal delivered
       by Th (either antigen-specific or nonspecific helper T
       cell). Ts , which produces antigen-specific id$^+$, I-J$^+$ TsF,
       on the one hand activated antigen-nonspecific second set
       of suppressor T cell (Ts$_2$ in the left) by an MHC-
       -restricted pathway, while on the other hand utilizes
       anti-idiotypic T cells (Ts$_2$ in the right) as the effector
       of suppression. The latter pathway is IgV_H restricted (see
       text).

BAB/14 (H-2^b , Igh-1^b , but the V_H gene cluster came from Igh-1^a
strain) T cells, and TsF from 7C3-13 was added to the culture.
In the latter combination, BAB/14 T cells do not share the same V.
genes with 7C3-13 which derived from B10.BR, while CB.20 T cells
have the same V_H gene set to B10.BR. The results were as follows:
1) in the combination of CB.20 B and T cells, it was found a
significant suppression of both total and idiotype positive
anti-NP PFC, and 2) the same TsF was unable to suppress the
response mounted by CB.20 B cells and BAB/14 T cells. The results
indicate that the V_H gene identity between T cells and TsF but not
between B cells and TsF is required for the effective suppression,
and that TsF can suppress the idiotype expression of responding B
cells via the activation of second cell type which is probably
anti-idiotypic T cell.

These results imply that 1) TsF carries NP^b idiotype primarily
controlled by allotype-linked V_H genes, 2) the idiotype positive
receptor has a similar heteroclicity to that observed with anti-NP
antibody molecules, and 3) such an idiotype positive TsF activates
the anti-idiotypic T cells that finally control the idiotype
expression of anti-NP antibodies.

3. IMPLICATIONS FOR THE MHC RESTRICTED PATHWAY
IN THE SUPPRESSOR AND AUGMENTING CIRCUIT

The question arises as to how the V_H-restricted pathway
relates to the previously observed MHC-restricted suppression. Our
view is that MHC-restricted suppressor pathway is concerned with
the major over-all suppression of the antibody response, while
idiotype-restricted pathway is a regulation of selected population
of B cells carrying certain idiotypes. Fig. 1 illustrates two
pathways in the suppression of B cell response, the interplay of
which is important for the regulation of the magnitude and quality
of the response.

What, then, is the nature of MHC restriction in the regulatory circuit? The questions can be specifically asked whether
there is any particular mechanism involving the heterogeneity of
MHC products on interacting T cells and factors, and what the role
of such products is in the selective activation of consecutive
cells in the circuit.

In order to answer these questions we have recently developed a number of monoclonal antibodies reacting with I region-
-coded determinants on suppressor and augmenting T cells and their
hybridoma cell lines. By the conventional combinations of I region
incompatible congenic strains, i.e., B10.A(3R) and B10.A(5R), and
A.TH and A.TL, and by fusing the immunized spleen cells with
myeloma cell line, we were able to produce several monoclonal
antibodies detecting the I region products exclusively expressed
on T cells but not on B cells. These monoclonals now can
distinguish the molecules expressed on TsF producer, TsF acceptor,
subsets of helper T cells (Th_1 and Th_2), augmenting T cell (Ta)
and probably the helper for cytotoxic T cell (Hiramatsu et al.,
1981, Kurata et al., in preparation). Of interest is that these
monoclonals do not react with conventional Ia antigens on B cells
and macrophages (class II antigen, Klein et al., 1981).
By serological analyses, we were able to demonstrate considerable
heterogeneity of I region products expressed on functionally
different subsets of T cells. Preliminary biochemical studies of
the products with these monoclonals revealed that the I region
products on TsF and TaF are entirely different molecules from
known B cell Ia antigens, and that they are uniquely expressed on
some but not all T cells. The loci coding for such T cell-specific
Ia molecules were unambigously mapped in I-A and I-J subregions.

These results suggest that Ia antigens on functional T cells
in the regulatory circuit are distinct from known B cell Ia
antigens (class II) regardless of the same subregion assignments,
and that the heterogeneity of such molecules is involved in the
restricted interactions among the member T cells. It is further
suggested that there are multiple loci within I region that code
for a family of molecules on fuctionally different T cell subsets
for their mutual recognition. Since the boundaries of I-A, I-J and
I-E/C subregions have been only arbitrary assigned by the occurrence of some recombinant mice, it is possible that there are
multiple I region loci exclusively expressed on T cells tandemly
lined along the MHC chromosomal segment. It also urges us to
reconsider the organization and function of I region loci in a
manner opposite to the over-simplification made by Klein et al.
(1981) to incorporate a new multigene family. We would thus
propose a new category of I region molecules expressed only on T
cells ("class III" antigens), although biochemical definition will
be forthcoming. Since it has been well documented that the
identity of I-A or I-J subregion between TaF or TsF and responding

cells is required for the effective enhancement or suppression of responses (Tada et al., 1977), such unique I region products on T cells (class III antigens) should be responsible for the restricted cell interactions in the regulatory circuit.

4. CONCLUSION

We have examined two restricting elements in the regulatory circuit, i.e., IgV_H and T cell-specific I region gene products. Both of them are extremely heterogeneous molecules coded for by multigene families. Of particular interest for us is the nature of I region gene products expressed only on functional T cell subsets. Their heterogeneity and polymorphism in association with IgV_H products are suitable devices for the cell to recognize the second partner cell, thus activating MHC- and IgV_H-restricted cellular circuit.

Our hypothesis for the restricted cell interaction is summarized as follows. Let us assume that the antigen-receptors of all T cells have an essentially similar prototype which is composed of such T cell-specific I region gene products and V_H-related structures. The ligand-binding site is probably encoded by a V_H gene though the constant structure is as yet undetermined.
The second structure is the allelic product of one of the T cell I region loci which are tandemly lined in the MHC region. Since the number of known alleles in K, D and Ia loci are less than 100 for each, the selection of one or more T cell I region genes in conjunction with V_H product would be able to explain the genetic restrictions in cell interactions. With the future biochemical and functional studies of T cell I region loci and their products, it seems feasible to us that the I region is involved in the antigen-receptor of T cells as originally hypothesized by Benacerraf and McDevitt (1972).

REFERENCES

Bach, B.A., Greene, M.I., Benacerraf, B., and Nisonoff, A., 1979, Mechanisms of regulation of cell-mediated immunity. IV. Azobenzene-arsonate-specific suppressor factor(s) bear cross--reactive idiotypic determinants the expression of which is linked to the heavy-chain allotype linkage group of genes,

J. Exp. Med. 149:1084

Benacerraf, B., and McDevitt, H.O., 1972, Histocompatibility-linked immune response gene, _Science_ 175:273.

Ben-Neriah, Y., Lonai, P., Gawish, M., and Givol, D.,1978a, Preparation and characterization of antibodies to the λ chain variable region (V_λ) of mouse immunoglobulins, _Eur. J. Immunol._, 8:792.

Ben-Neriah, Y., Wuilmart, C.,, Lonai, P., and Givol, D., 1978b, Preparation and characterization of anti-framework antibodies to the heavy chain variable region (V_H) of mouse immunoglobulins, _Eur. J. Immunol._, 8:797

Cramer, M., Krawinkel, U., Melchers, I., Imanishi-Kari, T., Ben-Neriah, Y., Givol, D., and Rajewzky, K., 1979, Isolated hapten-binding receptors of sensitized lymphocytes. IV. Expression of immunoglobulin variable regions in (4-hydroxy--3-nitrophenyl)acetyl (NP)-specific receptors isolated from murine B and T lymphocytes, _Eur. J. Immunol._, 9:332.

Eardley, D.D., Shen, F.W., Cantor, H., and Gershon, R.K., 1979, Genetic control of immunoregulatory circuits. Genes linked to the Ig locus govern communication between regulatory T-cell sets, _J. Exp. Med._, 150:44.

Eichmann, K., Ben-Neriah, Y., Helzelberger, D., Polke, C., Givol, D., and Lonai, P., 1980, Correlated expression of VH framework and VH idiotypic determinants on T helper cells and on functionally undefined T cells binding group A Streptococcal carbohydrate, _Eur. J. Immunol._, 10:105.

Eshhar, Z., Apte, R.N., Lowy, I., Ben-Neriah, Y., Govil, D., and Mozes, E., 1980, T cell hybridoma bearing heavy chain variable region determinants producing (T,G)-A--L specific helper factor, _Nature_, 286:270.

Germain, R.N., 1980, Antigen-specific T cell suppressor factors: Mode of action, _Lymphokine report_, 1:7.

Germain,. R.N., Ju,S-T., Kipps, T.J., Benacerraf, B. and Dorf, M.E., 1979, Shared idiotypic determinants on antibodies and T-cell-derived suppressor factor specific for the random terpolymer L-Glutamic acid-L-alanine-L-tyrosine, _J. Exp. Med._, 149:613.

Hiramatsu, K., Ochi, A., Miyatani, S., Segawa, A., Tada, T., 1981, Monoclonal antibodies specific for I region determinants uniquely expressed on T cells with helper and augmenting functions, _Nature_, submitted.

Kishimoto, T., Suemura, M., Sugimura, K., Okada, M., Nakanishi, K., and Yamamura, K., 1981, Characterizations of T cell-

-derived immunoregulatory molecules from murine or human T
hybridomas, in "Lymphokine Reports, Vol. 5: A Forum for Non-
-Antibody Lymphocyte Products," M. Feldmann, ed., Academic
Press, New York, in press.

Klein, J., Juretic, A., Barevanis, C.N., and Nogy, Z.A., 1981,
The traditional and a new version of the mouse H-2 complex,
Nature, 291:455.

Kontiainen, S., Culbert, E.F., Cecka, M., Simpson, E., MaKenzie,
I.F.C., and Feldmann, M., 1981, T cell hybridomas producing
hapten specific suppressor factors, Immunology, in press.

Lonai, P., ben-Neriah, Y., Steinman, K., and Givol, D., 1978,
Selective participation of immunoglobulin V region and major
histocompatibility complex products in antigen binding by T
cells, Eur. J. Immunol., 8:827.

Lonai,P., Puri, J., and Hammerling G., 1981, H-2 restricted antigen
binding by a hybridoma clone that produces antigen-specific
helper factor, Proc. Natl. Acad. Sci., USA, 78:549.

Minami, M., Okuda, K., Furusawa, S., Benacerraf, B., and Dorf,
M.E., 1981, Analysis of T cell hybridomas. I. Characteriza-
tion of H-2 and Igh restricted monoclonal suppressor factors,
J. Exp. Med., in press.

Pacifico, A., and Capra, J.D., 1980, T cell hybrids with arsonate
specificity. I. Initial characterization of antigen-specific
T cell products that bear a cross-reactive idiotype and
determinants encoded by the murine major histocompatibility
complex, J. Exp. Med., 152:1289.

Sy, M-S.., Dietz, M.H., Germain, R.N., Benacerraf, B., and Greene,
M.I., 1980, Antigen and receptor driven regulatory mechanisms,
IV. Idiotype bearing I-J$^+$ suppressor T cell factors (TsF)
induce second order suppressor T cells (Ts$_2$) which express
anti:idiotypic receptors, J. Exp. Med., 151:1183.

Tada, T., Taniguchi, M., and David, C.S. ,1977, Suppressive and
enhancing T cell factors as I region gene products: properties and the subregion assignment, Cold Spring Harbor Symp.
Quant. Biol., 41:119.

Tada, T., Takemori, T., Okumura, K., Nonaka, M., and Tokuhisa, T.,
1978, Two distinct types of helper T cells involved in the
secondary antibody response: independent and synergistic
effects of Ia$^-$ and Ia$^+$ helper T cells, J. Exp. Med., 147:446.

Tada, T., and Okumura, K., 1979, The role of antigen-specific T
cell factors in the immune response, Adv. Immunol., 28:1.

Tada, T., Hayakawa, K., Okumura, K., and Taniguchi, M.,1980,
Coexistence of variable region of immunoglobulin heavy chain

and I region gene products on antigen-specific suppressor T
cells and suppressor T cell factor - a minimal model of functional antigen receptor of T cells, Molec. Immunol., 17:867.

Tada, T., Suzuki, G., and Hiramatsu, K., 1981, Some comments on
the antigen-receptors expressed on functional T cell hybridomas. in "Lymphokine Reports, Vol. 5: A Forum for Non-Antibody Lymphocyte Products," M. Feldmann, ed., Academic Press, New
York, in press.

Taniguchi, M., and Miller, J.F.A.P., 1978, Specific suppressive
factors produced by hybridomas derived from the fusion of
enriched suppressor T cells and a T lymphoma line, J. Exp.
Med., 148:373.

SUBPOPULATIONS OF HUMAN LYMPHOCYTES AND THEIR

ALTERATIONS IN IMMUNODEFICIENCY DISEASES

Max D. Cooper, Toru Abo, Willem A. Kamps,
Patricia L. Haber and Charles M. Balch

The Cellular Immunobiology Unit of the Tumor Inst.
Depts. of Pediatrics, Surgery and Microbiology, and
The Comprehensive Cancer Center, University of
Alabama in Birmingham, Alabama 35294, U.S.A.

1. INTRODUCTION

The two major lines of immunocompetent cells, T and B cells, are thought to derive from a common lymphoid precursor or more directly from the multipotent hemopoietic stem cell. For both T and B cells, it is clear that special inductive microenvironments play important roles in the initiation of their separate differentiation pathways. The epithelial thymus serves both as a generation site for T cells and as a source of hormones that can modulate proliferation and function of T cells even after they enter the circulation to migrate through peripheral lymphoid tissues. The inductive micro-environments for the B cell pathway in mammals are not as sharply delineated, and these change during development. The fetal liver is an early site of B cell generation, and bone marrow assumes this function later. Much has been learned about the details of the development and differentiation of functionally diverse subpopulations of T and B cells in recent years, and practical markers are now available for the study of these processes in humans.

In this article we will outline the normal development of T and B cell subpopulations, and some of the developmental defects

13

seen in individuals with immunodeficiency diseases. In addition we will briefly discuss the development of the natural killer (NK) cell, the most recently recognized member of the host defense system.

2. DEVELOPMENT OF T CELLS

A useful differentiation scheme for human T cells has been proposed by Reinherz and Schlossman (1980) based on data obtained using a panel of monoclonal antibodies to T cell surface antigens. This model, with slight modification, is shown in Fig. 1.

A small subpopulation (ca 10%) of thymocytes express both the T9 and T10 antigens (Reinherz et al., 1980). Though these serve as useful markers for immature thymocytes located in the thymic cortex, they are not exclusive to these cells. The T9 antigen has recently been identified as the transferrin receptor (composed of 2 disulfide-linked glycosylated polypeptide chains of approx. 90,000 daltons each) which is expressed by cycling immature cells of many lineages (Trowbridge et al., 1981; Sutherland et al.,

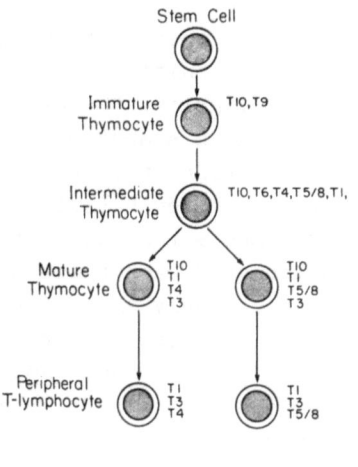

Fig. 1. Hypotetical model of human T cell differentiation outlined by the expression of cell surface antigens detected by a panel of monoclonal antibodies. Modification from the original proposed by Reinherz and Schlossman (1980).

1981). The T10 antigen may also be expressed by NK cells in the blood.

In the ensuing stages of differentiation, thymocytes lose the transferrin receptor and begin to express several other differentiation antigens on their cell surface. These include T6, the human counterpart of the mouse TL antigen, which is expressed only during intrathymic stages of T cell differentiation. Other antigens acquired in the thymus continue to be expressed by mature T cells after they enter the circulation. T1, T4, T5 and T8 are examples of the latter category of T cell antigens. They are expressed on 65-80 per cent of all thymocytes even in fetuses as young as 11 weeks of gestational age (Kamps and Cooper, unpublished). T3 appears to be acquired later, as it is expressed by a relatively small subpopulation of thymocytes (ca 40%) and all of the circulating T cells.

An additional important feature of this intrathymic differentiation process is the preferential loss of the T5 and T8 antigens by maturing T cells that acquire helper or inducer functions and the loss of T4 antigen by T cells that acquire suppressor and cytotoxic capabilities. Thus, mature Th cells exhibit the phenotype $T1^+ T3^+ T4^+$, and Ts/c cells are $T1^+ T3^+ T5^+$ $T8^+$.

It is noteworthy that cells bearing the T1, T3, T5 and T8 antigens do not 'appear in the bone marrow and liver until around the 13th week of gestation (Kamps and Cooper, unpublished). Since the bone marrow is an important source of stem cells, this observation provides strong support for the idea that expression of these antigens is induced in the thymic environment.

3. T CELL DIFFERENTIATION DEFECTS IN INFANTS
   WITH SEVERE COMBINED IMMUNODEFICIENCY (SCID)

Defects involving four different levels in the T cell differentiation pathway have been defined in six SCID patients whose circulating lymphocytes were examined using this panel of monoclonal antibodies (Reinherz et al., 1981; Edwards et al., 1981). In one, no lymphocytes bearing any of the thymus acquired T cell antigens were detected in the circulation. Two infants with SCID had abundant $T9^+ T10^+$ lymphocytes in peripheral blood samples,

but these were negative for the T3, T4, T6 and T8 antigens. Two
other SCID patients had circulating lymphocytes with the intrathymic phenotype T3$^+$ T4$^+$ T8$^+$ T10$^+$; interestingly, the T6 antigen was
not expressed. The circulating T cells in the sixth SCID patient
expressed the Ts/c phenotype T3$^+$ T5$^+$; he had a striking paucity of
cells expressing the T3$^+$ T4$^+$ helper phenotype.

4. CIRCULATING T CELLS IN INDIVIDUALS WITH
CONGENITAL THYMIC DYSPLASIA (DIGEORGE SYNDROME)

This syndrome is attributed to unknown influences that
compromise the development of the thymus and parathyroid glands
from the third and fourth pharyngeal pouches and of the outflow
tract of the heart and aortic arch. Usually a small, but histolo-
gically normal, thymus can be located with difficulty in an
ectopic position (Lischner, 1972). In keeping with this finding,
reduced numbers of circulating T cells are usually present in
affected individuals. In five such individuals, the circulating T
cells were phenotypically normal, but the T4$^+$:T8$^+$ ratio was 5.2
±1.5 as compared with 1.9 ± 0.3 for normal controls (Reinherz et
al., 1981).

5. DEVELOPMENT OF B CELLS

The first recognizable cells of the B lineage, called pre-B
cells, express μ heavy chains at a cytoplasmic level only
(reviewed by Osmond, 1980; Cooper, 1981). Large cycling pre-B
cells are derived from immunoglobulin negative precursors in the
liver of fetuses during the ninth week of gestation. They give
rise to small post-mitotic pre-B cells that also lack light
chains. Small pre-B cells are the immediated precursors of B
lymphocytes that express complete IgM molecules on their surface.
By the twelfth week of gestation, some of the sIgM$^+$ members of
emerging B cell clones begin to express another immunoglobulin
class, IgG, IgA, or IgE, and for a time in their life history B
cells express surface IgD molecules as well (Gathings et al.,
1977). This pattern of generation of B cell isotype diversity is
illustrated in Fig. 2, and is discussed in detail elsewhere
(Cooper et al., 1980).

The process of B cell generation continues in the bone marrow throughout life so that newly formed B lymphocytes are constantly being seeded into the circulation, from which they migrate into the B cell compartments in spleen, lymph nodes and other peripheral lymphoid tissues.

6. DEVELOPMENTAL DEFECTS IN B CELL DIFFERENTIATION

Immunoglobulin deficiency diseases may be associated with 'blocks' at one of several levels in the B cell differentiation pathway (reviewed by Cooper and Lawton, 1979). Differentiation is apparently aborted at a stem cell level in many of the infants with SCID, older individuals with thymoma and acquired agammaglobulinemia, and in a few individuals with other forms of late onset panhypogammaglobulinemia, since bone marrow samples from these patients lack both pre-B and B cells. A later differentiation arrest is seen in boys with X-linked agammaglobulinemia. They have normal numbers of bone marrow pre-B cells but few of these proceed to the sIgM⁺ cell stage in differentiation (Pearl et al., 1978). The small number of B cells that are formed appear normal; they may give rise to a surprisingly large plasma cell progeny in some cases.

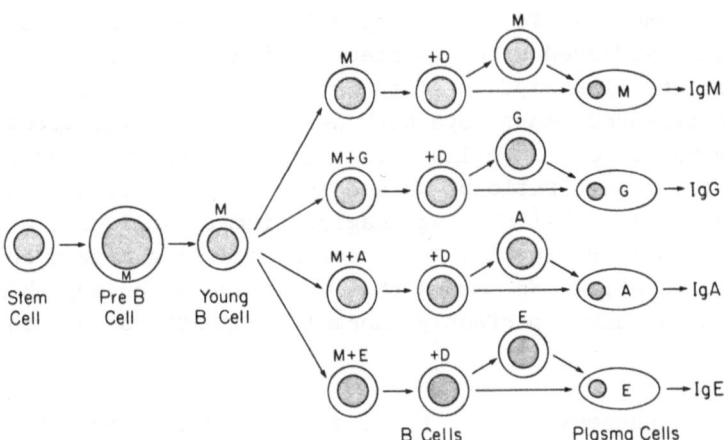

Fig. 2. Model of the generation of isotype diversity during the life history of a hypothetical B cell clone.

Most of the late onset forms of panhypogammaglobulinemia usually included in the diagnostic category of common varied immunodeficiency, feature a late arrest in B cell differentiation (Cooper et al., 1971; Grey et al., 1971). Affected individuals have normal numbers of circulating B lymphocytes and these may respond to stimulation by antigen with proliferation but fail to differentiate normally into mature plasma cells. Usually B cells of all isotypes can be found in these patients.

In boys with the X-linked form of dysgammaglobulinemia featured by high levels of IgM and low or absent IgG and IgA B lymphocytes expressing IgM and IgD are present in normal numbers but IgG and IgA B cells are missing (Schwaber et al. 1978; our unpublished observations). Thus their defect would appear to be in regulation of the heavy chain isotype switch process. In contrast, individuals with isolated IgA deficiency have IgA B cells but most of the IgA B cells are of the immature phenotype characterized by expression of sIgM and sIgD as well (Conley and Cooper, 1981). Most of the IgA B cells in the circulation of normal individuals older than one year of age no longer express IgM and IgD.

7. DISTRIBUTION OF T CELL SUBSETS IN IMMUNOGLOBULIN DEFICIENCY SYNDROMES

Monoclonal antibodies to T cell antigens have recently been used to enumerate T cell subpopulations in the circulation of individuals affected with a variety of immunoglobulin deficiencies (Reinherz et al., 1981; Aiuti, personal communication). As it might be expected, most boys with X-linked agammaglobulinemia have normal numbers of T cells (Fig. 3). As a group, they exhibit a relatively normal ratio of Th and Ts/c subpopulations. Occasional individuals with X-linked agammaglobulinemia will have a reversal of the normal ratio of $T4^+:T5^+$ cells, and some have a relatively high T4/T5 ratio. We assume that these are secondary aberrations since others have perfectly normal proportions of the T cell subsets.

Normal numbers of T cells and a normal distribution of $T4^+$ and $T5^+$ cells are the rule in individuals with isolated IgA deficiency.

By contrast, individuals with the late onset forms of pan-hypogammaglobulinemia often have significant imbalances in their subpopulations of T subsets, despite having normal total numbers of T cells. As a group, these patients, have reduced numbers of $T3^+$ $T4^+$ cells and a significant increase in $T3^+$ $T5^+$ cells (Fig.3). This observation is in keeping with previous evidence of increased suppressor T cell activity in such patients (reviewed by Waldmann and Broder, 1979).

Unusual distribution patterns of T cell subpopulations in selected panhypogammaglobulinemic patients with B cells are especially informative. One 17 year old boy with panhypogammaglobulinemia had low numbers of $T3^+$ $T4^+$ cells and very high levels of $T3^+$ $T5^+$ cells that suppressed differentiation of his brother's cells in PWM cultures (Reinherz et al.,1979). Activation of the expanded population of suppressor T cells was also suggested by their expression of HLA-DR (Ia) antigen.

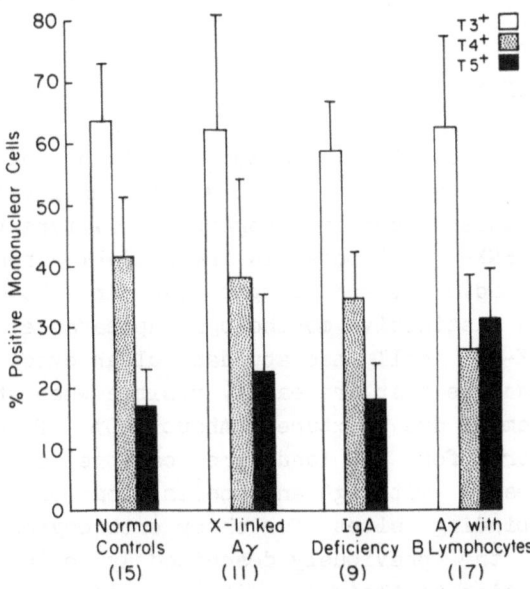

Fig. 3. Analysis of the distribution patterns of T cell subsets in primary antibody deficiency diseases. Adapted from the data of Reinherz et al. (1981).

A complete absence of T4+ cells was seen in a 10 year old girl with panhypogammaglobulinemia and B lymphocytes. She had normal numbers of T cells, all of which expressed T3 and T5 antigens (Reinherz et al., 1981).

Another individual with panhypogammaglobulinemia and B cells deserves special mention. This boy was perfectly well until 10 years of age when he developed chronic active hepatitis. Four months into this illness, we noted that he was panhypogammaglobulinemic (IgM 15, IgA 13 and IgG 96 mg/dl). No plasma cells were seen in his liver, that otherwise displayed the histologic features typical of chronic active hepatitis. Analysis of his circulating T cells revealed a complete reversal of the T4:T8 ratio (1:3.7). The most notable feature of this boy's illness was the onset of normal immunoglobulin synthesis along with remission of the hepatitis following treatment with high doses of prednisone (our unpublished observations). This may have been due to a selective effect of steroids on suppressor T cells (Bradley and Mishell, 1981). In any event, it is a remarkable example of hormonal influence on the regulation of the immune system.

8. DEVELOPMENT OF NK CELLS

The recent production of a monoclonal antibody (HNK-1) to an antigen expressed by human NK cells provides a valuable tool for the study of this recently recognized cell type (Abo and Balch, 1981). The HNK-1 antibody is selectively reactive with a population of medium sized lymphocytes in blood that have NK activity and a distinctive morphologic appearance. Unlike T and B cells, the HNK-1+ cell has abundant clear cytoplasm containing azurophilic granules that are easily visible when stained with the May-Grumwald-Giemsa dye mixture. About 90% of the HNK-1+ cells express receptors for IgG and are capable of lysing chicken erythrocytes coated with IgG antibodies. Some of the HNK-1+ cells have exposed binding sites for sheep erthrocytes, and thus were included among the previously described Ty cells (Grossi et al., 1978). In addition to their capacity to spontaneously lyse target K562 tumor cells, HNK-1+ cells can lyse IgG coated chicken erythrocytes.

In tracing the development of HNK-1+ cells, we noted their presence in small numbers in hemopoietic tissues of human fetuses

12-14 weeks of gestational age (Abo et al., 1981). For unknown reasons, however, the HNK-1$^+$ population of cells does not expand greatly until after birth. HNK-1$^+$ cells account for less than 1% of the mononuclear blood cells in newborns, an average of 5% in children under 15, around 12% in individuals aged 15 to 30, and 22% in adults beyond the age of 30 years. This age related increase in the frequency of circulating HNK-1$^+$ cells correlates with a parallel rise in NK and K cell activities.

HNK-1$^+$ cells migrate preferentially to the spleen where they constitute approximately 15% of the mononuclear cells. By contrast they account for less than 1% of the cells in thymus, lymph node and bone marrow, although they are probably derived from bone marrow stem cells (Abo and Balch, 1981).

One particularly interesting feature of the distribution of HNK-1$^+$ cells in the context of this conference is the signi- ficantly higher frequencies of these cells that we noted in blood samples from males as compared with those from female donors of all ages (Abo et al., 1981). Significantly higher values for NK cell activity have also been noted for males of all ages (H. Pross, personal communication). This may relate to the suppressive effect of estrogen on NK cell maturation (Seaman et al., 1979). This would appear to be another point at which hormonal control may be exerted on the host defense system.

Interferon has been shown to induce heightened activity of NK cells in lysing tumor cell targets (Djeu et al.,1979),and there is evidence that T cell growth factor can enhance the growth of NK cells (Kuribayashi et al., 1981). Thus a variety of humoral factors, some hormonal and other produced by immunocompetent cells, may regulate the NK cell population which may play an important role in eliminating tumors and virus infected cells (reviewed by Herberman, 1981; Roder et al., 1981).

9. DEVELOPMENTAL DEFECTS IN NK CELLS

A dramatic reduction in NK cell activity has been found in individuals with the Chediak-Higashi Syndrome (Roder et al., 1980) and in homozygous beige mice with a comparable gene defect (Roder et al., 1979). Since normal numbers of their blood mononuclear cells bind to the target tumor cells, it was postulated that NK cells are present in affected individuals but are functionally impaired (Roder et al., 1981). In support of this idea, we have recently observed normal numbers of HNK-1$^+$ cells in a boy with Chediak-Higashi Syndrome. His functionally defective NK cells were characterized by the presence of a single large granule in their cytoplasm rather that the multiple small granules seen in normal NK cells (Abo, T., unpublished). Thus, it seems likely that the functional abnormality in the Golgi endoplasmic reticulum lysosome (GERL) unit is responsible for the cytolytic defect in this genetic disease (White and Clawson, 1979).

We could not find any HNK-1$^+$ cells in a baby with reticular dysgenesia, a stem disorder allowing for normal erythrocyte and platelet production but not for normal development of the other types of blood cells. It is likely that other developmental defects affecting NK cell development and function will be found, and the study of these "experiments of nature" may provide greater insight into the regulation of this pathway of differentiation.

ACKNOWLEDGEMENTS

We thank Ann Brookshire for help in preparing this paper. Studies in our laboratories were supported by NIH grants CA 16673, 5M01-RR32 and March of Dimes, Birth Defects Foundation 1-608.

REFERENCES

Abo, T., and Balch, C.M., 1981, A differentiation antigen of human NK and K cells identified by a monoclonal antibody (HNK-1), J. Immunol., in press.
Abo, T., Cooper, M.D., and Balch, C.M., 1981, Postnatal expansion of the NK and K cell population in humans as a function of age and sex, Nature,submitted.
Bradley, L.M., and Mishell, R.I., 1981, Differential effects of glucocorticosteroids on the functions of helper and suppressor T lymphocytes, Proc. Natl. Acad. Sci. USA., 78:3155.
Conley, M.D., and Cooper, M.D., 1981, Immature phenotype of IgA B cells in IgA deficient individuals, N. Engl.J. Med., in press.
Cooper, M.D., 1981, Pre-B cells: Normal and abnormal development, J. Clin. Immunol., 1:81.
Cooper, M.D., Lawton, A.R., and Kincade,P.W., 1971, Agammaglobuli-

nemia with B lymphocytes: Specific defect of plasma cell diffe-
    rentiation, Lancet, ii:791.
Cooper, M.D., Lawton,A.R., Preud'homme, J.L., and Seligmann, M.,
    1979, Primary antibody deficiencies, in "Immune Deficiency,"
    M.D. Cooper, A.R. Lawton, P.A. Miescher and H.J. Muller-
    -Eberhard, eds., Springer-Verlag, New York, p. 31.
Cooper, M.D., Kearney, J.F., Gathings, W.E.,and Lawton, A.R., 1980,
    Effects of anti-Ig antibodies on the development and differen-
    tiation of B cells, Immunol. Rev., 52:29.
Djeu, J.Y., Heinbaugh, J.A., Holder, H.T., and Herberman, R.B.,
    1979, Augmentation of mouse natural killer cell activity by
    interferon and interferon inducers, J. Immunol., 122:175.
Edwards, K.M., Cooper, M.D., Lawton, A.R.Sanders, D.S., and Wright,
    P.F., 1981, Severe combined immunodeficiency associated with
    absent T4 helper cells, J. Pediatr., submitted.
Gathings, W.E., Lawton, A.R., and Cooper M.D., 1977, Immunofluore-
    scent studies of the development of pre-B cells, B lymphocytes
    and immunoglobulin isotype diversity in humans, Eur. J. Immu-
    nol., 7:804.
Grewy, H.M., Rabellino, E., and Pirofsky, B., 1971, Immunoglobulins
    on the surface of lymphocytes. IV. Distribution in hypogamma-
    globulinemia, cellular immunodeficiency and chronic lymphatic
    leukemia, J. Clin. Invest., 50:2368.
Grossi, C.E.,, Webb, S.R., Zicca, A., Lydyard, P.M., Moretta, L.,
    Mingari, M.C., and Cooper, M.D., 1978, Morphological and histo-
    chemical analyses of two human T-cell subpopulations bearing
    receptors for IgM or IgG, J. Exp. Med., 147:1405.
Kuribayashi, K., Gillis, S., Kern, D.E., and Henney, C.S., 1981,
    Murine NK cell cultures: Effects of interleukin-2 and interfe-
    ron on cell growth and cytotoxic reactivity, J. Immunol.,
    126:2321.
Lischner, H.W., 1972, DiGeorge Syndrome(s), J. Pediatr., 81:1042.
Osmond, D.G., 1980, Production and differentiation of B lymphocytes
    in the bone marrow, in "Immunoglobulin Genes and B Cell Diffe-
    rentiation," J.R. Battisto and K.L. Wright, eds., Elsevier/
    /North-Holland, New York, p. 135.
Pearl, E.R., Vogler, L.B., Okos, A.J., Crist, W.M., Lawton, A.R.,
    and Cooper, M.D., 1978, B lymphocyte precursors in human bone
    marrow. An analysis of normal individuals and patients with
    antibody deficiency states, J. Immunol., 20:1169.
Reinherz, E.L., Rubenstein, A., Geha, R. Strelkauska, A.J., Rosen,
    F.S., and Schlossman, S.F., 1979, Abnormalities of immunoregu-
    latory T cells in disorders of immune function, N. Engl. J.

Med., 301:1018.

Reinherz, E.L., and Schlossman, S.F., 1980, Current concepts in immunology. Regulation of the immune response-inducer and suppressor T lymphocyte subsets in human beings, N. Engl. J. Med., 303:370.

Reinherz, E.L. Kung, P.C., Goldstein, G., Levey, R.H., and Schlossman, S.F., 1980, Discrete stages of human intrathymic differentiation: Analysis of normal thymocytes and leukemic lymphoblasts of T-cell lineage, Proc. Natl. Acad. Sci., USA, 77:1588.

Reinherz, E.L., Cooper, M.D., Schlossman S.F., and Rosen,F.S., 1981, Abnormalities of T cell maturation and regulation in human beings with immunodeficiency disorders, J. Clin. Invest., in press.

Roder, J., and Duwe, A., 1979, The beige mutation in the mouse selectively impairs natural killer cell function, Nature, 278:451.

Roder, J.C., Haliotis, T., Klein, M., Korec, S., Jett, J.R., Ortaldo, J., Herberman R. B., Katz, P., and Fauci, A.S., 1980, A new immunodeficiency disorder in humans involving NK cells, Nature, 284:553.

Roder, J.C., Karre, K., and Kiessling, R.1981, Natural killer cells, Prog. Allergy, 28:66.

Seaman, W.E., Merigan, T.C., and Talal, N.,1979, Natural killing in estrogen-treated mice responds poorly to poly-I-C despite normal stimulation of circulating interferon, J. Immunol., 123:2903.

Schwaber, J., Lazarus, H., and Rosen, F.S.,1978, Restricted classes of immunoglobulin produced by a lymphoid line from a patient with agammaglobulinemia, Proc. Natl. Acad. Sci., USA, 75:2421.

Sutherland, R., Delia, D., Schneider, C. Newman, R., Kemshead, J., and Greaves, M., 1981, Proc. Natl. Acad. Sci., USA, in press.

Trowbridge, I.,S., and Omary, M.B., 1981, Human cell surface glycoprotein related to cell proliferation is the receptor for transferrin, Proc. Natl. Acad. Sci., USA., 78:3030.

Waldmann, T.A., and Broder, S., 1979, T cell disorders in primary immunodeficiency diseases, in: "Immune Deficiency," M.D.Cooper, A.R. Lawton, P.A. Miescher, and H.J. Mueller-Eberhard, eds., Springer-Verlag, New York, p. 5.

White, J.G., and Clawson, C.C., 1979, The Chediak-Higashi Syndrome: Microtubules in monocytes and lymphocytes, Amer. J. Hematol., 7:349.

T-CELL INDEPENDENT ACTIVATION OF HUMAN B CELLS BY ANTI-Ig

ANTIBODIES AND PROTEIN A-CONTAINING STAPHYLOCOCCI

M. Ricci, S. Romagnani, Grazia M. Giudizi,
F. Almerigogna, Roberta Biagiotti, G.F. Del Prete
and E. Maggi.

Clinical Immunology, University of Florence
Policlinico di Careggi, Viale Morgagni
50134 Firenze (Italy)

1. INTRODUCTION

The agents to be considered as polyclonal activators of human B cells (PBA) can be distinguished in two categories: the first category includes antibodies against B cell surface components, such as anti-immunoglobulin (Ig) antibodies (Chiorazzi et al., 1980) and the second one comprises of some micro-organisms, such as Ebstein-Barr virus (Tosato et al., 1980), Staphylococcus aureus (Forsgren et al., 1976), Haemophilus influenzae (Banck and Forsgren, 1978), etc.

The "in vitro" polyclonal activation of human B lymphocytes can result in cell proliferation and/or differentiation or maturation, characterized by Ig production and secretion. Certainly, two of the most important problems related to polyclonal activation of human B cells concern: (1) the characterization of B cell subpopulations involved in the primary activation, (2) the nature of PBA receptors on B cell surface and the mechanisms of activation.

We have studied the polyclonal activation of human B cells employing Staphylococcus aureus bacteria of the Cowan I strain

(Cowan Staph) as the principal stimulant. The mitogenic activity of these bacteria has been compared with that of Staphylococcal protein A (SpA) and with the effect of F(ab')$_2$ fragments of antibodies against Ig determinants.

2. COWAN STAPH IS A T-CELL INDEPENDENT POLYCLONAL B CELL ACTIVATOR (PBA)

In initial experiments, it was found that human purified T cells from either tonsil or peripheral blood (PB) origin are unable to respond in vitro to Cowan Staph, whereas the response of purified B lymphocytes was greater than that of the unfractionated population. When increasing concentrations of autologous T lymphocytes were added to highly purified B cells from tonsil, there was no increase of the proliferative response to Cowan Staph. In contrast, a marked response to PHA could be restored (Romagnani et al., 1978).

Ig production induced by Cowan Staph on human lymphocytes, like B cell proliferation, is also probably a T-cell independent phenomenon. In fact, purified B cells of PB were unable to produce Ig in cultures stimulated with pokeweed mitogen (PWM), but released noticeable amounts of either IgM or IgG in the presence of Cowan Staph. The addition of T lymphocytes to B-cell rich fractions did not induce any significant increase of the amount of IgM and IgG released into the supernatant of Cowan Staph--stimulated cultures (Romagnani et al., 1980a). These results were supported by experiments in which umbilical cord blood lymphocytes were stimulated with PWM and Cowan Staph. As expected, no Ig production was seen in supernatants of cultures stimulated with PWM, whereas a significant amount of IgM was found in the supernatants of Cowan Staph-stimulated cultures from 6 out of 9 newborns (Romagnani et al., 1980a).

3. REACTIVITY OF PROTEIN A WITH HUMAN B CELLS

In another series of experiments the proliferative response of human lymphocytes to Cowan Staph was compared with the response induced on the same cells by soluble SpA and SpA coupled to Sepharose beads (SpA-Seph). SpA-Seph, like Cowan Staph, activated purified tonsillar B cells, but it was unable to induce prolife-

ration of highly purified T lymphocytes. In contrast, soluble SpA
was unable to activate highly purified tonsillar B cells, but it
was very active on unfractionated lymphocytes and still able to
stimulate purified T cells, even though at a significantly lesser
degree than unfractionated polulations (Romagnani et al., 1978).
These data suggest that SpA present on the bacterial surface is
responsible for the mitogenic activity of Cowan Staph and, when
presented to human lymphocytes on an insoluble matrix, it acts as
a selective T-cell independent B-cell mitogen.

In order to investigate better the nature of human lymphocytes able to react with SpA, we also tested the ability of different subpopulations of tonsil or PB lymphocytes to form rosettes
with human erythrocytes coated with SpA (SpA-HRBC). A significant
proportion of tonsil lymphocytes and a small proportion of PB
lymphocytes formed rosettes with SpA-HRBC. SpA-rosette forming
cells were found in purified suspensions of T lymphocytes, whereas
the number of SpA-rosette forming cells was significantly increased in cell suspensions depleted of E-rosette forming cells.
Depletion of surface Ig (sIg) bearing cells abolished the ability
of non-T cell suspensions to form rosettes with SpA-HRBC (Romagnani et al., 1980b). These data confirm that human lymphocytes
capable to reacting with SpA when presented to cells on an insoluble matrix are B lymphocytes.

Further experiments were carried out in order to test the
capacity of IgM-bearing and IgM-lacking B cells to bind to SpA.
The subsets of B cells were separated by positive or negative
selection by rosetting with HRBC coated with immunosorbent-
-purified anti-IgM, anti-IgG or anti-IgA antibodies. The data
obtained supported that a proportion of IgM-bearing B cells binds
to SpA; IgM-lacking B cells able to react with SpA are mainly
IgG-bearing cells (Ricci et al., 1981). This conclusion was also
supported by results obtained by studying the SpA reactivity of
lymphocytes from patients with chronic lymphocytic leukemia (CLL).
Lymphocytes from ten out of seventeen patients with CLL were
unable to form rosettes with SpA-HRBC, whereas most lymphocytes of
seven patients reacted with SpA. Cells from six of these seven
patients had sIgM and sIgD; lymphocytes from one patient had sIgG.
The membrane components reacting with SpA were not passively
absorbed, but actively synthesized by CLL, as shown by experiments
with proteolytic enzymes. In addition, the binding to SpA was
clearly independent of the type of light chains of sIg (Romagnani
et al., 1981a).

4. NATURE OF THE MEMBRANE COMPONENTS OF
HUMAN B CELLS REACTING WITH SPA

To investigate the nature of membrane components of B lymphocytes capable of reacting with SpA, we tried to inhibit the
binding of SpA to cells by incubation in capping conditions with
$F(ab')_2$ fragments of antibodies against human Ig or non-Ig surface
antigens. Incubation of tonsillar B cells with $F(ab')_2$ fragments
of antibodies against the Fab region of human IgG virtually
abolished the ability of these cells to react with SpA-HRBC,
whereas incubation with $F(ab')_2$ fragments of antibodies against β_2
-microglobulin had no effect. A significant reduction of the
number of rosettes formed by B cells with SpA-HRBC could be
observed after incubation with $F(ab')_2$ fragments of antibodies
against or γ chain. The inhibition of SpA rosetting by anti-μ
chain antibodies could be obtained with either antibodies prepared
in rabbit or monoclonal antibodies (Romagnani et al., 1981b).

5. HUMAN B CELL ACTIVATION BY COWAN
STAPH AND ANTI-Ig ANTIBODIES

The ability of distinct subpopulations of human B cells to
proliferate "in vitro" in the presence of Cowan Staph was then
investigated. After depletion of cells capable of forming rosettes
with SpA-HRBC the cell proliferation induced by Cowan Staph was
virtually abolished. Depletion of IgM-IgD-bearing cells resulted
in a strong reduction of the proliferative response; after
depletion of Ig-bearing cells there was a lower effect on the
Cowan Staph-induced proliferation (Romagnani et al., 1980d). These
data indicate that the binding of SpA to human lymphocytes is
critical for the cell proliferation induced by Cowan Staph. They
also suggest that human B cells capable of reacting with SpA and
which are induced to proliferate by Cowan Staph are mainly
IgM-IgD-bearing lymphocytes.

In another series of experiments the mitogenic activity of
Cowan Staph on unfractionated, IgM-bearing and IgM-deficient
tonsillar B cells was compared with the mitogenic activity of
$F(ab')_2$ fragments of anti-μ chain antibodies. Both reagents were
able to activate purified human B cells and still more human B
cells enriched for IgM-bearing lymphocytes, whereas they were
poorly mitogenic for IgM-deficient human B cells. The effect of

addition in culture of monovalent Fab fragments of antibodies
against human μ chain was also investigated. Monovalent Fab fragments of anti-μ antibodies were unable to activate human B cells
but induced a complete inhibition of the proliferative response
induced by F(ab')$_2$ fragments of anti-μ antibodies.
Moreover, the addition of monovalent Fab fragments of anti-
antibodies to the cultures consistently resulted in a partial
inhibition of the Cowan Staph-induced B cell proliferation
(Romagnani et al., 1981b). These data indicate that B cells which
proliferate in the presence of Cowan Staph are mainly IgM-bearing
lymphocytes and suggest that the binding of SpA to sIgM is
probably critical in the triggering of the proliferative response.

We could also show that Cowan Staph are able to induce a
proliferative response by cells from some patients with CLL. Cowan
Staph-induced proliferation was related to the ability of leukemic
lymphocytes to react with SpA-HRBC. This observation allowed us to
better investigate the mechanisms by which Cowan Staph is capable
of inducing B cell proliferation. In fact, PB lymphocytes from
patients with CLL were not induced to proliferate by anti-Ig
antibodies, but showed a proliferative response after stimulation
with Cowan Staph. The Cowan Staph-induced proliferative response
of cells of the patients B.B. (whose PB lymphocytes had sIgG) was
strongly reduced by the addition in culture of F(ab')$_2$ fragments
of either anti-Fab or anti-γ chain antibodies, whereas it was not
affected by the presence of F(ab')$_2$ of anti-μ chain antibodies. In
contrast, the Cowan Staph-induced proliferation of cells from
patient C.P. (whose PB lymphocytes had sIgM and sIgD) was strongly
reduced by the addition to the cultures of F(ab')$_2$ fragments of
either anti-Fab or anti-μ chain antibodies, but it was not
significantly altered by the presence of anti-γ chain antibodies
(Romagnani et al., 1981c). These data suggest that an interaction
between SpA present on the bacterial cell wall and sIg of both IgM
and IgG classes plays an important role in the triggering of the
Cowan Staph-induced proliferative response of leukemic B lymphocytes.

6. NATURE OF THE SPA-REACTIVE REGION OF SURFACE IMMUNOGLOBULINS

Another series of experiments was performed in order to study
the nature of sIg region responsible for the interaction with SpA
and, therefore, for the induction of the polyclonal proliferative

Table 1. Protein A-reactivity of serum and cell surface
monoclonal IgM.

	No.of Cases	SPA-Reactivity
CLL Lymphocytes (with sIgM or sIgM and sIgD)	37	14 (37%)[a]
Waldenstrom's Macroglobulins	13	5 (38%)[b]

[a]More than 50% PB lymphocytes formed rosettes with SpA-HRBC.
[b]Purified macroglobulins were retained by a SpA-Seph column.

response of human B cells. Recently, it has been shown that human serum IgG can react with SpA by both Fc and Fab region, whereas rabbit serum IgG shows Fc-, but not Fab-reactivity (Inganas et al, 1980). In addition, it was found that the Fab region of IgG capable of binding to SpA is also present in a proportion of human serum IgM, IgA (Inganas, 1981). Thus, two kinds of reactions between Ig and SpA should be considered: the classical interaction with Fc and an alternative one with a structure located in the $F(ab')_2$ region of different Ig classes. Also taking into account these data, we tested the ability of Ig from different species to inhibit the Cowan Staph-induced proliferative response. The addition of human and guinea pig IgG to the cultures abolished the proliferative response induced by Cowan Staph, whereas the addition of rabbit IgG, as well as IgG from horse, ox and goat had little or no effect (Romagnani et al., 1981b). These results suggest that the B cell activating property of SpA is not related to the classical Fc binding. Indeed, the addition to the cultures of isolated $F(ab')_2$ fragments prepared by pepsin digestion from normal human IgG resulted in a complete inhibition of the proliferative response to Cowan Staph at concentrations equal or lower than those of the undigested IgG molecules. The inhibitory activity of $F(ab')_2$ fragments could be completely removed by absorption on a column of SpA-Seph and it was recovered in the material eluted from the column by 1M acetic acid (Romagnani et al., 1981b).

In further experiments, the ability of monoclonal IgM prepared

Table 2. Protein A-reactivity of a monoclonal IgM and its
         $F(ab')_2$ fragment.

Monoclonal IgM (P.E.)	Percent of Binding			
	Anti-μ[a]	Anti-γ[a]	Anti-F(ab')$_2$[a]	SPA[a]
Undigested	21.9	1.4	9.0	21.7
$F(ab')_2\mu$[b]	1.0		27.5	8.4

[a] labelled with ^{125}I.
[b] obtained by pepsin digestion for 2.5 h at 37°C and purified
by gel filtration on sephadex G-100 and Sephadex G-150.

from different donors to inhibit the Cowan Staph-induced B cell
proliferation was investigated. For this purpose, we examined
preliminarly the capacity of 13 monoclonal IgMs to bind to
SpA-Seph and we found that five bound to SpA-Seph, whereas the
other eight did not (Table 1). It is noteworthy that the
percentage of SpA-reactive monoclonal serum IgM (38%) is similar
to that of CLL, whose PB lymphocytes had been found able to form
rosettes with SpA-HRBC (37%).

The addition to the cultures of normal B cells of a
SpA-reactive monoclonal IgM consistently resulted in a marked
reduction of the Cowan Staph-induced proliferative response. In
contrast, the addition to the cultures of two SpA-unreactive
monoclonal IgM did not show any inhibitory activity on the
responsiveness of B cells to Cowan Staph (Romagnani et al.,
1981b).

We are now trying to elucidate the nature of the SpA-binding
region of monoclonal IgM responsible for the inhibitory activity
of the Cowan Staph-induced B cell proliferation. In preliminary
experiments we found that $F(ab')_2$ fragments, obtained by pepsin
digestion from a SpA-reactive monoclonal IgM, still maintained the
ability to react with SpA, even though at a lesser extent than
undigested IgM molecules (Table 2).

7. CONCLUDING REMARKS

The results reported in this paper indicate that: (1) the mitogenic activity of Cowan Staph on human B cells is due to an interaction of SpA present on the bacterial cell wall with surface IgM and IgG (and perhaps immunoglobulins of other classes); (2) the reactivity of SpA with the F(ab')$_2$ part of sIg of different classes rather than the classical Fc - SpA reactivity is probably responsible for the mitogenicity of Cowan Staph; (3) this means that there is a direct participation of Ig receptors in the B cell activation induced by certain nonspecific stimulants, that is that in certain circumstances the sIg molecule itself can be the PBA-receptor; (4) moreover, since the F(ab')$_2$ reactivity of SpA does not correlate with light chain type, allotypes or idiotypes, it may be suggested that an interaction between SpA and certain structure of framework regions of heavy variable domains is responsible for the mitogenic activity of Cowan Staph on human B cells. The meaning of this pathway of reactivity is at the present unknown.

REFERENCES

Banck, G., and Forgren, A., 1978, Many bacterial species are mitogenic for human blood B lymphocytes, Scand. J. Immunol., 8:347.

Chiorazzi, N., Fu, S.M., and Kunkel, H.G.,1980, Stimulation of human B lymphocytes by antibodies to IgM and to IgG. Functional evidence for the expression of IgG on B lymphocyte surface membranes, Clin. Immunol. Immunopathol., 15:301.

Forsgren, A., Svedjelund, A., and Wigzell, H., 1976, Lymphocyte stimulation by protein A of Staphylococcus aureus, Eur. J. Immunol., 6: 207.

Inganas, M., Johansson, S.G.O., and Bennich, H.H.,1980, Interaction of human polyclonal IgE and IgG from different species with protein A from Staphylococcus aureus: demonstration of protein A reactive sites located in the F(ab')$_2$ fragments of human IgG, Scand. J. Immunol., 12:23.

Inganas, M., 1981, Comparison of mechanisms of interaction between protein A from Staphylococcus aureus and human monoclonal IgG, IgA and IgM in relation to the classical Fc$_\gamma$ and the alternative F(ab')$_2$ protein A interaction, Scand. J. Immunol., 13:343.

Ricci, M., Romagnani, S., Giudizi, M.G., Almerigogna, F., Biagiotti,

R., Del Prete, G.F., and Maggi, E., 1981, Mechanisms of human
B cell activation by Staphylococcus aureus, in: "Human B cell
activation," A.S. Fauci, ed.,Raven Press, New York,in press.

Romagnani, S., Amadori, A., Giudizi, M.G., Biagiotti, R., Maggi, E.
and Ricci, M., 1978, Different mitogenic activity of soluble
and insoluble Staphylococcus protein A (SpA), Immunology,
35:471.

Romagnani, S., Del Prete, G.F., Maggi, E., Falagiani, P., and Ricci,
M., 1980a, T-cell independence of immunoglobulin synthesis by
human peripheral blood lymphocytes stimulated with SpA-contai-
ning Staphylococci, Immunology, 41: 921.

Romagnani, S., Giudizi, M.G., Almerigogna, F., and Ricci, M., 1980b,
Interaction of Staphyloccal protein A with membrane components
of IgM- and/or IgD-bearing lymphocytes from human tonsil, J.
Immunol., 124:1620.

Romagnani, S., Almerigogna, F., Giudizi, M.G., and Ricci, M., 1980c,
Rosette formation with protein A-coated erythrocytes: a method
for detecting both IgG-bearing cells and another subset of human peripheral blood lymphocytes, J. Immunol. Meth., 33: 11.

Romagnani, S., Giudizi, M.G., Almerigogna, F. Nicoletti, P.L., and
Ricci, M., 1980d, Protein A of Staphylococcus aureus is mitogenic for IgG-bearing, but also for a subpopulation of IgM- and/
/or IgD-bearing human lymphocytes, Immunology, 39:417.

Romagnani, S., Giudizi, M.G., Almerigogna, F., Biagiotti, R., Belle-
si, G., Bernardi, F., and Ricci, M., 1981 a, Protein A reactivity of IgM- and IgD-bearing lymphocytes from some patients
with chronic lymphocytic leukemia, Clin. Immunol. Immunopathol.,
19:139.

Romagnani, S., Giudizi, M.G., Biagiotti,R., Almerigogna, F.,Maggi,
E., Del Prete, G.F., and Ricci, M., 1981b, Surface immunoglobulins are involved in the interaction of protein A with human
B cells and in the triggering of B cell proliferation induced
by protein A-containing Staphyloccus aureus, J. Immunol.,
in press.

Romagnani, S., Giudizi, M.G., Biagiotti, R., Almerigogna, F., Del
Prete, G.F., Maggi, E., and Ricci, M., 1981c, Protein A-reactivity of lymphocytes from some patients with chronic lymphocytic leukemia mediated by an interaction with the $F(ab')_2$ region
of surface immunoglobulins, Scand. J. Immunol., in press.

Tosato,G., Magrath, I.T., Koski, I.R., Dooley, N.J. and Blaese, R.
M., 1980, B cell differentiation and immunoregulatory T cell
function in human cord blood lymphocytes, J. Clin. Invest.,
66:383.

THE RISE AND FALL OF THE ANTIGEN BRIDGE

N.A. Mitchison

Imperial Cancer Research Fund, Tumour Immunol. Unit
Department of Zoology, University College, London
Gower Street, London WC1E 6BT, U.K.

The antigen bridge as a mechanism of interaction between T and B cells has had a good run. An early example may be found in Mitchison, Rajewsky and Taylor (1970) and an up-to-date one in Eichmann (1980). The essential feature remains the same throughout, that a molecule of antigen joins the T cell receptor one side to the B cell receptor on the other. What is added in the more recent versions is an I-A/E molecule and a receptor for it, which have to be added in order to conform with the rules of dual recognition by T cells. The purpose of this paper is to discuss an alternative model of the interaction, which omits this bridge.
At the end of the day one may feel that the difference is more apparent than real, but an important point of principle is involved. The theme which is developed here has already been described in outline in a workshop summary (Pernis and Mitchison, 1980). Its discussion in that workshop reflected principally the ideas of H.M. Grey, K. Hannestad, and W.E. Paul, and it is referred to in the published summary as a revolution in under standing of the function of regulatory T cells.

The alternative model of T-B interaction is illustrated in Fig.1. First the B cell binds antigen via its surface immunoglobulin. Next, the antigen is processed in a step which involves denaturing and possibly cleavage. The antigen then associates with I-A/E molecules on the cell surface, where it is recognized by activated T helper cells. At this stage the regulatory signal is transmitted to the B cell. Macrophages or dendritic cells are normally required as antigen-presenting cells to an earlier stage in order to activate the regulatory T cell. In this process an antigen bridge between the T and B cell receptors does not form, and the B cell receptor's sole function is to sponge up antigen. Nor is there any scope in this model for an antigen-specific T cell factor capable of acting upon B cells, as illustrated in Mitchison, Rajewsky and Taylor (1970) and as demonstrated in vitro by M. Feldmann and others (vide M. Feldmann's contribution to this volume).

It must be emphasized that the issue between the alternative models has not yet been settled, and that, while the newer model accommodates well the data cited in this article, there are other data which fit less well. The controversy is likely to run on for a while, until more is known about the molecular capabilities of B cells.

The evidence in favour of this model may briefly be summarized as follows. First, B cells can readily recognize intact pro-

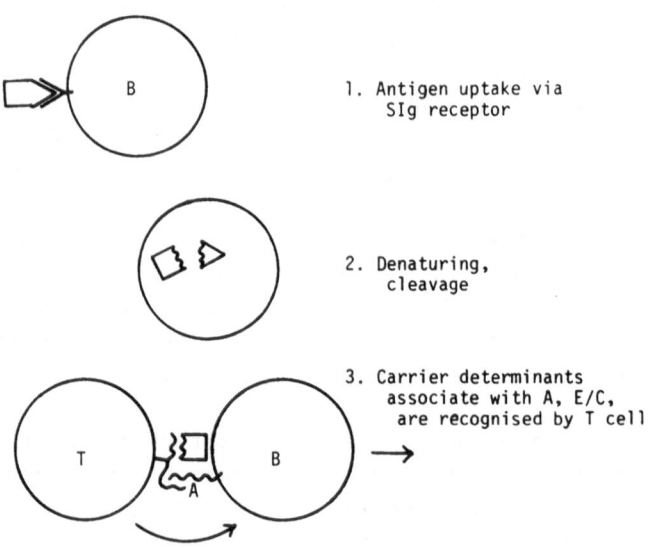

1. Antigen uptake via SIg receptor

2. Denaturing, cleavage

3. Carrier determinants associate with A, E/C, are recognised by T cell

Note: no antigen-bridge, no antigen-specific helper factor

Fig. 1. Obligatory antigen-processing in the alternative model of T-B interaction.

teins, and are well able to distinguish between reactive and denatured forms of the same globular protein. T cells on the other
hand seem unable to recognize conformational determinants present
only in native proteins (Jorgensen and Hannestad, 1979; Corradin
et al., 1979; Chesnut et al., 1980). The bridge theory can cope
with this information only by postulating a partially denatured
state for globular antigens, which is hard to envisage. Secondly,
there is direct evidence that B cells can serve as antigen-presenting cells based on the greater activity of rabbit anti-mouse Ig
as compared with normal rabbit Ig as an inducer of mouse T cell
proliferation (Chesnut and Grey, 1981). This is compatible with
the idea that any antigen which binds to the B cell receptor will
be presented effectively to T cells. Thirdly, it has long been
known that antigens which cannot be processed do not stimulate T
cells: witness the ineffectiveness of D-polypeptides as carriers
of hapten as compared with similar L-polypeptides (Katz et al.,
1971).

If we accept this model, at least provisionally, certain
consequences follow. One concerns antigenic determinants normally
present on the surface of the B cell itself. An example of these
would be the determinants present on the immunoglobulin receptors
specific for idiotype, allotype, and isotype. All of these are
believed to represent targets for regulatory T cells. Another
example would be histocompatibility antigens present on B cells
in experimental systems where they serve as targets of regulatory T cells. It is hard to believe in such cases that the B
cell normally and continuously processes its own receptors:
for one thing, this would imply that such receptors would
turn over rapidly, for another this should saturate the I-A/E
association sites, and for a third it would be extraordinarily
wasteful. Accordingly one might expect that those regulatory T
cells which look at such determinants would operate on principles
different from those of other T cells, and might require neither
processed antigen nor an I-A/E association. One would thus be
postulating two classes of T cell receptors, one directed at
classical foreign antigens, and the other at B cell receptors
as antigens. This dichotomy fits well with proposals now being
made about the nature of idiotype-specific T cells. These are
claimed indeed to lack I-A/E restriction (Bottomley, 1981; Janeway
et al., 1981).

How far does this dichotomy extend through T cells?

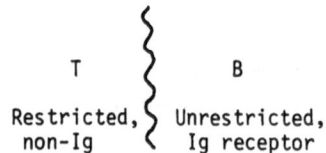

T   B

Restricted,   Unrestricted,
non-Ig   Ig receptor

Fig. 2. The Renaissance world.

Figs. 2 and 3 expresses a view about this. In the Renaissance Pope
Alexander VI divided the world between Spain and Portugal, and for
a while the world of lymphocytes seemed equally to divide between
T and B cells. But in the modern world we may have to accept that
some helper T cells are not restricted by products of the major
histocompatibility complex, and if so the old clear division
breaks down. As illustrated in Fig. 3, B cells have never convincingly been shown to be restricted by the MHC.
Cytotoxic (Tc) cells appear always to be so restricted. Helper
(Th) cells may well include a small category of unrestricted
cells, with specificities of the type described above, and therefore appear on both sides of the divide. So do suppressor (Ts)
cells, which appear in this figure mainly on the unrestricted side
for the following reasons. On the whole those of the regulatory T
cells and those of their factors which adsorb onto solid phase
antigen (i.e. antigen not associated with I-A/E molecules) are
suppressive. Thus, for example, absorption onto solid phase
antigen is currently used as a selection step in the isolation of suppressor T cell clones (Fresno et al., 1981a), and the
hapten-binding T cell receptors which can be isolated on solid
phase come from suppressor T cell populations (Krawinkel et al.,

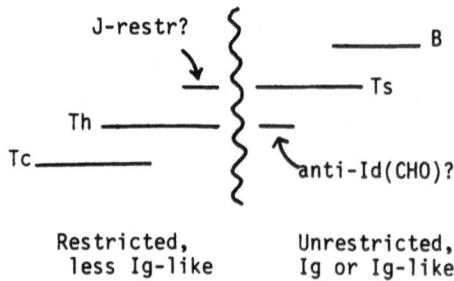

J-restr?   B

                              Ts
Th
Tc
                        anti-Id(CHO)?

Restricted,   Unrestricted,
less Ig-like   Ig or Ig-like

Fig. 3. The Modern age.

1979; Cramer and Reth, 1981). Furthermore suppressor factors do
not generally recognize MHC products in association with antigen
on their targets (Fresno et al., 1981b; Greene et al., 1979;
Taniguchi et al., 1980; Feldmann and Kontiainen, 1981), while
helper factors can do so (Andersson and Melchers, 1981; Fischer et
al., 1981).

Suppressor T cells are not here assigned entirely to the
unrestricted category for reasons which are largely philosophical
in character. If helper T cells exist on both sides of the divide,
why should no suppressors do so too? If helper cells have I-A/E to
guide them, will it not help in the organization of the immune
response to have another guidance element for suppressor cells?
The case for I-J as such an element has recently been argued
(Czitrom et al., 1981); an important point in this argument is the
evidence that certain suppressor factors, when tested "in vivo",
show restriction by I-J.

Returning for a moment to the vexed question of the MHC-re-
striction of helper factors, it is becoming increasingly clear
that a distinction has to be made between small, unactivated and
large, activated B cells as target for help. This distinction is
made forcibly in several pieces of recent work from the Basel
Institute for Immunology (Andersson and Melchers, 1981; M.H.
Julius, M. Schreier, personal communication). The interaction with
helper cells which is I-A/E restricted occurs at the initial step
involving the small B cell. After this initial activation B cells
become accessible to unrestricted helper factors.

The immunoglobulin-likeness of these receptors is a deep and
important issue, but one which at the present time must be
inconclusive, because of the paucity of molecular data. What we
know most about is the character of regulatory factors released by
T cells. Most of the hard information concerns antigen-specific
suppressor factors, a subject reviewed by M. Feldmann in this
volume. Here the case for an immunoglobulin-like molecule rests on
(i) the presence on the factors of idiotypes defined by antisera
raised against humoral antibodies, and (ii) the presence on the
factors of Ig-V-region determinants defined in the same way. It is
entirely possible that MHC-restricted receptors have a totally
different molecular structure. The major obstacle for this thesis
is the alleged presence of Ig-V-related idiotypes on carrier-specific T helper cells (Eichmann and Rajewsky, 1975; Julius et al.,

1978). Since the experiments which support this claim have been largely carried out "in vivo", using unseparated populations of lymphocytes, one can argue that the effects observed may have been obtained either via idiotype-specific helper cells, or via suppressor cells controlling the generation of helper cells.

Finally a note about the possible importance of carbohydrate antigens in idiotypic regulation. A cursory survey suggests that idiotypic control has been detected mainly in responses to antigens which elicit weak carrier-specific T helper cell activity. A good example is the A5A idiotype in the response of mice to streptococcal vaccine, a carbohydrate antigen. This suggests that the non-restricted type of helper T cell may be encouraged to join in the immune response when the more usual carrier-specific T cells are lacking.

What are the implications of this dichotomy of regulatory cells for immunoregulation at large, the subject of the present workshop? Its main effect is to strengthen the case for dividing regulatory cells into a rather large number of subsets or "parallel sets" (Mitchison, 1980). An excellent example of the kind of splitting of sets which one has in mind is provided by Tada's contribution to this workshop. Subdividing is not a new idea, and indeed it has already often been proposed that the helper and suppressor cells which fall on either side of the divide shown in Fig. 3 belong to different subsets as defined by other markers such as I-J. To the extent that the case for subdivision has been strengthened by new ideas concerning cooperation, so also has the case for regulatory circuits.
The more complex the circuit, the more scope there is for flip-flop and other integration properties. And this in turn allows more scope for the kind of higher level controls which are under discussion here. This complexity will not make it easier to pinpoint the mode of action of nervous or endocrine control agents; indeed it may make precise analysis more difficult. What is certain is that the more complex and flexible the system, the easier it becomes to imagine ways of perturbing it.

ACKNOWLEDGEMENT

I thank Martin Raff for cogently arguing much of the case put here.

REFERENCES

Andersson, J., and Melchers, F., 1981, T cell-dependent activation
    of resting B cells: requirement for both nonspecific unrestric-
    ted and antigen-specific Ia-restricted soluble factors, Proc.
    Natl. Acad. Sci., USA, 78:2497.
Bottomley, K., 1981, The influence of helper T cell subsets on B
    cells responding to T-dependent and T-independent forms of pho-
    sphorylcholine, in: "Immunoglobulin Idiotypes," (ICN-UCLA Sym-
    posia vol. XX) C. Janeway, E.E. Sercarz, H. Wigzell and C. Fred
    Fox, eds., Academic Press, New York, in press.
Chesnut, R.W. and Grey, H.M., 1981, Studies on the capacity of B
    cells to serve as antigen-presenting cells, J. Immunol.,
    126:1075.
Chesnut, R.W., Endres, R.O. and Grey, H.M., 1980, Antigen recogni-
    tion by T cells and B cells: recognition of cross-reactivity
    between native and denatured forms of globular antigens, Clin.
    Immunol. Immunopathol., 15:397.
Corradin, G., Chesnut, R.W. and Grey, H.M., 1979, Antigen degrada-
    tion by macrophages as an obligatory step in the presentation
    of antigen to T lymphocytes, Ric. Clin. Lab., 9:311.
Cramer, M. and Reth, M., 1981, Isolated hapten-specific T-cell rece-
    ptor material, in: "Immunoglobulin Idiotypes," (ICN-UCLA Sympo-
    sia, vol. XX) C. Janeway, E.E. Sercarz, H. Wigzell and C. Fred
    Fox, eds., Academic Press, New York, in press.
Czitrom, A., Mitchison, N.A. and Sunshine, G.H., 1981, I-J, F, and
    hapten conjugates: Canalisation by suppression, in: "Immunobio-
    logy of the Major Histocompatibility Complex," 7th Int. Convoc.
    Immunol., Niagara Falls, N.Y., 1980, M.B. Zaleski, C.J. Abeyou-
    nis and K. Kano, eds., S.Karger, Basel, p. 243.
Eichmann, K., 1980, Conclusion: a simple, conservative model of anti-
    gen specificity, Springer Semin. Immunopathol., 3:277.
Eichmann, K. and Rajewsky, K., 1975, Induction of T and B cell immu-
    nity by anti-idiotypic antibody, Eur. J. Immunol., 5:661.
Feldmann, M. and Kontiainen, S., 1981, The role of antigen specific
    factors in the immune response, in: "Lymphokines,", vol. 2,
    Academic Press, New York, p. 87.
Fisher, A., Zanders, E.D., Beverley, P.C.L. and Feldmann, M., 1981,
    Human long term helper lines, in: "Lymphokines," vol. 5, Aca-
    demic Press, New York, in press.
Fresno, M., Nabel, G., McVay-Boudreau, L. Furthmayer, H. and Cantor,
    H., 1981a, Antigen-specific T lymphocyte clones. I. Characteri-
    zation of a T lymphocyte clone expressing antigen-specific sup-

pressive activity, J. Exp. Med., 153:1246.

Fresno, M., McVay-Boudreau, L., Nabel, G. and Cantor, H., 1981b,
    Antigen-specific T lymphocyte clones. II. Purification and bio-
    logical characterization of an antigen-specific suppressive
    protein synthesized by cloned T cells, J. Exp. Med., 153: 1260.

Greene, M.I., Bach, B.A. and Benacerraf, B., 1979, Mechanisms of re-
    gulation of cell-mediated immunity. III. The characterization
    of azobenzenearsonate-specific suppressor T-cell-derived-sup-
    pressor factors, J. Exp. Med., 149:1069.

Janeway, C.A. Jr., Bottomley, K., Dzierzak, E.A., Eardley, D., Du-
    rum, S. and Gershon, D., 1981, The development and functions
    of immunoglobulin dependent T cells, in: "Immunoglobulin Idio-
    types," (ICN-UCLA Symposia, vol. XX) C. Janeway, E.E. Sercarz,
    H. Wigzell and C. Fred Fox, eds., Academic Press, New York,
    in press.

Jorgensen, T. and Hannestad, K., 1979, T helper lymphocytes recogni-
    ze the VL domain of the isologous mouse myeloma protein, Scand.
    J. Immunol., 50:663.

Julius, M.H., Cosenza, H. and Augustin, A.A., 1978, Evidence for
    the endogenous production of T cell receptors bearing idioty-
    pic determinants, Eur. J. Immunol.,8:484.

Katz, D.H., Davie, J.M., Paul, W.E. and Benacerraf, B., 1971, Car-
    rier function in anti-hapten antibody responses. IV. Experimen-
    tal conditions for the induction of hapten-specific tolerance
    or for the structure of hapten-specific anamnestic responses
    by "non-immunogenic hapten-polypeptide conjugates," J. Exp.
    Med., 134:201.

Krawinkel, V., Cramer, M., Melchers, I., Imanishi-Kari, T. and Ra-
    jewsky, K., 1978, Isolated hapten-binding receptors of sensiti-
    zed lymphocytes. III. Evidence for idiotypic restriction of
    T-cell receptors, J. Exp.Med., 147:1341.

Mitchison, N.A., 1980, MHC molecules as guides for T lymphocyte pa-
    rallel sets, in: "Strategies of Immune Regulation," E. E., Ser-
    carz and A.J., Cunningham, eds., Academic Press, New York,p.21.

Mitchison, N.A., Rajewsky, K., and Taylor, R.B., 1970, Cooperation
    of antigenic determinants and of cells in the induction of an-
    tibodies, in: "Developmental Aspects of Antibody Formation and
    Structure," J. Sterzl and I. Riha, eds., Academia, Prague,
    vol. 2, p. 547.

Pernis, B. and Mitchison, N.A., 1981, Workshop summary: Network con-
    trol of B cell activity, in: "Immunoglobulin Idiotypes," (ICN-
    UCLA Symposia, vol. XX), G. Janeway, E. E. Sercarz, H. Wigzell
    and C Fred Fox, eds., Academic Press, New York, in press.

Taniguchi, M., Takei, T., and Tada, T., 1980, Functional and molecular organization of an antigen-specific suppressor factor
from a T cell hybridoma, <u>Nature</u>, 283:227.

PRIMATE HELPER FACTORS:

COMMENT ON THE 'ANTIGEN BRIDGE'

Marc Feldmann

Imperial Cancer Research Fund.,Tumor Immunology Unit
Department of Zoology, University College, London

While it is ingenous to conceive of a new way of looking at
the role of the 'antigen bridge' in T-B interaction, there are
still many virtues of the formed view, which I feel is more
consistent with the bulk of experimental data. It is also appropriate to point out the difficulties of the new formulation, and
that it does not resolve any of the inherent problems of the T-B
contact models of cell cooperation.

Implicit in any direct T-B contact model of cell interaction,
be it with traditional or heretical forms of antigen bridging, is
the problem of the efficiency of T-B contact, if both T and B
cells are rare antigen specific cells occurring at frequencies of
less than 1/10 . This problem is compounded if T cell help
involves, as recent evidence suggests, not a single antigen
specific helper cell, but also others reactive to immunoglobulin,
and yet others which release non specific amplifying and differentiation signals. It makes little difference whether these
signals have to be delivered concurrently to a B cell or in
sequence, and there remains a major logistic problem of assuming
rare cells collide efficiently with each other, as it is known
that recirculation and homing of T and B cells differs markedly.
For these reasons, many workers, ourselves included, have been
moved to look for molecular messengers of T-B collaboration - T
cell factors.

Let us examine the experimental evidence supporting the h_ere-
tical form of antigen bridging. The most direct comes from the experiments of Chesnut and Grey (1981). This involves T cells primed
to rabbit Ig, and using rabbit anti mouse Ig treated B cells to
present antigen. This is an interesting preliminary experiment,
which, as the authors point out, has dubious relevance to the case
with conventional antigens. Here all the B cells were coated wiht
antigen and their receptors were capped, patched and internalised,
with digestion of the internalised complexes. The final assay was
T cell proliferation, which is only the first stage of T cell help
and correlates poorly with it. Clearly much further work is necessary before it can be said that' B cells can serve as antigen presenting cells'. Thus antigen presentation to T cells by B cells
remains to be tested, and the generation of antibody needs to be
measured, not just proliferation. It would be of interest to see
if tolerant B cells can present antigen, and also to determine
whether Fab fragments of Ig which do not rapidly cross link, cap
and internalise, are also effective.

If B cells had a major role in antigen presentation to T
cells, it would be expected that evidence of B cell handling of
antigen, its breakdown, and retention of fragments on the surface,
would be available from the ample literature on antigen handling
reported in the 1960's and 1970's. However, lymphocyte binding of
antigen has usually been reported as very transient, in the first
few minutes after the injection of some, but not all, antigens.
Later, antigen was found associated with accessory cells (reviewed
Basten and Mitchell, 1976). I feel that the presence of persisting
antigen associated with various accessory cells (dendritic cells,
dendritic follicular cells, marginal zone macrophages) implies
that these cells have a role in the process of cell interaction
leading up to B cell triggering. If we envision B cells presenting
antigen to T cells, the antigen retaining accessory cells present
in the B cell areas of the lymphoid tissues are left with only a
trivial role.

If it is accepted that T cells only recognise denatured
antigens, whereas B cells only recognise native antigens, then
there is a problem as to the form of antigen which is involved in
a classical bridge. I doubt that this is the case. T cells can

recognise   cross   reactivity   between native and denatured antigens
(Chesnut   et al., 1980; Ishizaki, 1975), and short peptides, and it
is   plausible   that T cell receptors can find these peptides within
a   native   protein,   permitting   the   bridge to exist. Clearly this
question needs further investigation.

If   it   is   proposed   that   the new form of the antigen bridge
entirely   supersedes   the   previous,   the   role of antigen specific
helper   factors   is hard to envision. Yet the experimental evidence
for   such   factors   has progressively accumulated, until now almost
20   independent   groups have studied them, in rodents and primates,
"in   vivo"   and   "in   vitro",   with   protein   or synthetic antigens
(reviewed   Feldmann et al., this   volume).   Could any of this be
reconciled   with   the   new   form   of   antigen   bridging? I can only
imagine   one   way, if the specific helper factor also possesses the
capacity to transmit the signal to activate B cells.

The   immune   system   is   known   to   possess a certain degree of
redundancy,   a   variety   of pathways for performing closely similar
tasks.   Thus   there are many Killer cells: T Killer cells, K cells,
NK   cells,   macrophage   killers,   etc. The same is true for antigen
presentation: there   are   typical macrophages, and various types of
dendritic   cells.   Perhaps   in   certain   circumstance,   where   only
minimal   antigen   degradation is required, B cells could present to
certain   types   of   T cells. Yet I am reluctant to accept any form of
direct   T-B   contact   as the only form of B cell stimulation, as it
is   possible to demonstrate that T-B contact is not necessary in so
many   instances,   and   also   because   B cell triggering even in the
presence   of   HF   also   requires   accessory cells whose function is
also   under   MHC linked Ir gene control (Howie and Feldmann, 1978).
These   latter   results   have led us to propose a unifying scheme of
lymphoid   cell   interactions, comprising of a number of units, each
unit   involving   a lymphocyte and its apropriate antigen presenting
cell.   Lymphocyte   triggering   would involve perusal of a series of
'messages'   such   as   factors   on   the   surface of the appropriate
presenting cell (reviewed Feldmann et al., 1979).

The   direct   T-B   contact   model   of   antigen   makes   a   clear
prediction,   that   B cell triggering should be possible in the
absence   of   all   accessory   cells   and   their products. I await an
experimental test of these conflicting views.

REFERENCES

Basten ,A. and Mitchell, J., 1976, Role of macrophages in T cell-
    -B cell collaboration in antibody production, in "Immunology
    of the macrophage", D.S. Nelson, ed., Academic Press, N.Y.,p. 85.
Chesnut, R.W. and Grey, H.M., 1981, Studies on the capacity of B
    cells to serve as antigen presenting cells, J. Immunol.,
    126:1075.
Chesnut, R.W., Endres, R.O. and Grey, H.M., 1980, Antigen recogni-
    tion by T and B cells: recognition of cross reactivity between
    native and denatured forms of globular antigens, Clin. Immunol.
    Immunopathol., 15:397.
Feldmann, M., Cecka, J.M., Cosenza, H, David, C.S., Erb,P., James,
    R., Howie,S., Kontiainen, S., Maurer, P, McKenzie, I., Parish,
    C.R., Rees, A., Tood, I., Torano, A., Winger, L. and Woody, J.,
    1979, On the nature of specific factors and the integration
    of their signals by macrophages, in: "T and B lymphocytes:
    Recognition and Function", F. Bach, B., Bonavida and E.
    Vitetta, eds., Academic Press, New York,p. 343.
Howie, S. and Feldmann, M., 1978, Immune response (Ir) genes
    expressed at macrophage B-lymphocyte interactions, Nature,
    273:664.
Ishizaka, K., Okudaira, H. and Kind, T.P., 1975, Immunogenic
    properties of modified antigen E. II. Ability of urea-denatured
    antigen and polypeptide chain to prime T cells specific for
    antigen, Eur. J. Immunol., 114:110.

IMMUNOREGULATION OF "IN VITRO" ANTIBODY RESPONSE

TO AZOBENZENEARSONATE (ABA)-PROTEINS

G. Doria, C. Mancini, Giovanna Agarossi,
Daniela Fioravanti, S. Vietri, and L. Adorini

CNEN-Euratom Immunogenetics Group, Laboratory of
Radiopathology, C.S.N. Casaccia, Rome, Italy

1. INTRODUCTION

The impact of exogenous antigen on the immune system activates a complex series of events which determine the onset, intensity, and duration of the antibody response. This antigen-induced perturbation of the immune system, which leads to antibody
production by B cells, involves antigen-presentation by accessory
cells and activation of immunoregulatory T cells with helper,
suppressor, or amplifier function. Idiotypes and anti-idiotypes
are major recognition structures shared by cells and soluble
factors interacting in each immunoregulatory circuit (Herzenberg
et al., 1980). The intriguing complexity of immunoregulation
stimulated the interest of several outstanding immunologists who
have produced in recent years an enormous amount of information on
a few immunoregulation system. The immune response to azobenzenearsonate (ABA) is one of these well defined systems which has
been intensively investigated "in vivo" by Nisonoff's and Benacerraf's groups, at the levels of both antibody production and
delayed-type hypersensibility (Nisonoff and Greene, 1980).

From the demonstration that injection of double hapten-conju-
gates induces hapten-specific helper (Hamaoka et al., 1975) and
suppressor T cells (Yamamoto et al., 1977; Lewis and Goodman

(1978) were able to develop an "in vivo" system to study the
immunoregulatory role of ABA-specific T cells in the anti-trinitrophenyl (TNP) antibody response of mice immunized with keyhole
limpet hemocyanin (KLH) conjugated with TNP and ABA (TNP-ABA-
-KLH). This experimental model has been modified in our laboratory
to devise an "in vitro" system that facilitates the dissection of
the network components involved in the anti-ABA immune response.
The experiments described in the two following sections illustrate
the induction and evaluation of ABA-specific helper and suppressor
T cells regulating the "in vitro" anti-TNP antibody response to
TNP-ABA-KLH.

2. ABA-SPECIFIC HELPER T CELLS

As previously described (Adorini et al., 1981), ABA-specific
helper T cells were induced in popliteal lymph nodes of (C57B1/

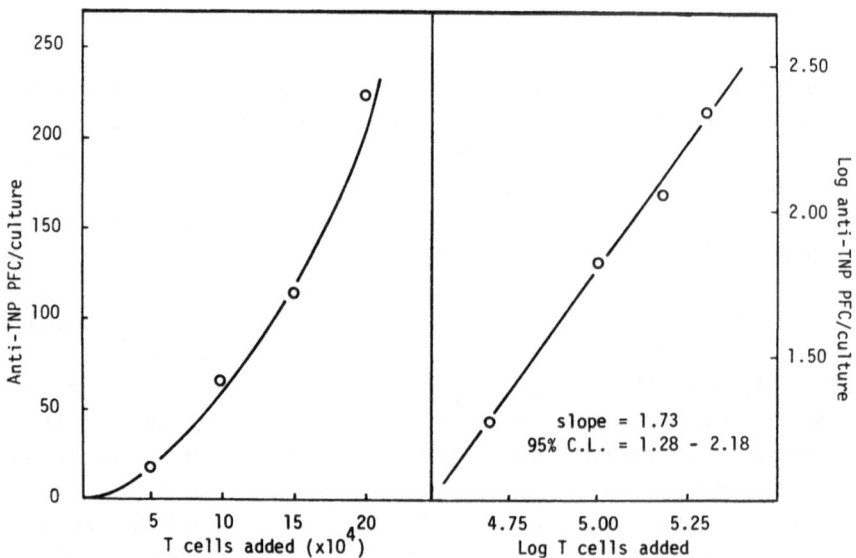

Fig. 1. Anti-TNP PFC response of 1×10^6 unprimed speen cells cultured for 5 days with 100 ng TNP-ABA-KLH and graded numbers
of T cells from ABA-KLH primed mice. The data of the left
panel fit a straight line when plotted on log-log scales in
the right panel. Slope is the regression coefficient calculated by the least-squares method and C.L. are its confi-
dence limits.

Table 1. Anti-TNP PFC response of lymph node cells from primed mice.

Lymph node cells from mice primed with	Antigen in culture	anti-TNP PFC
ABA-KLH	-	10
ABA-KLH	TNP-ABA-KLH	481
ABA-OVA	-	17
ABA-OVA	TNP-ABA-KLH	164
ABA-BGG	-	90
ABA-BGG	TNP-ABA-KLH	220

Each culture contained 10^6 cells, without or with 100 ng TNP-ABA-KLH

/10xDBA/2)F1 mice by injecting their hind footpads with ABA conjugated to KLH or to bovine gamma globulin (BGG) or to ovalbumin (OVA). Each ABA-protein conjugate was emulsified in complete Freund's adjuvant (CFA) immediately before injection.
Popliteal lymph node cells were harvested 8 days after priming and cultured for 5 days without or with TNP-ABA-KLH. The "in vitro" anti-TNP antibody responses from a typical experiment reported in Table 1 clearly show that ABA-specific helper cells can be induced by priming the mice with ABA-KLH, ABA-OVA, or ABA-BGG. The higher anti-TNP PFC response obtained with lymph node cells from ABA-KLH primed mice suggests that ABA-specific and KLH-specific helper cell populations were both cooperating with B cells in the "in vitro" anti-TNP antibody response to TNP-ABA-KLH. The coexistence of these two helper cell populations was investigated in the following experiment. T cells from ABA-KLH primed mice were enriched by positive selection on anti-mouse Ig-coated plates and cultured in graded numbers ($5-20 \times 10^6$) with a constant number (1×10^6) of unprimed syngeneic spleen cells and TNP-ABA-KLH.
As shown in Fig. 1 (left panel), after 5 days of culture the anti-TNP PFC response of the spleen cells increases with the increasing number of ABA-KLH primed T cells in a non linear manner, suggesting the existence of T cell-T cell cooperation.
Indeed, the same data in a log-log plot (right panel) fit a straight line with a regression coefficient of 1.73 which is

statistically greater than 1. According to Mosier and Coppleson
(1968), this finding suggests the existence of two interacting
helper T cells. Unpublished results from our laboratory indicate
that the ABA-specific helper T cell population may comprise two
cell subpopulation characterized by different radiosensitivities
and models of interaction with B cells.

3. ABA-SPECIFIC SUPPRESSOR T CELLS

ABA-specific suppressor T cells were induced in the spleen by
injecting (C57Bl/10xDBA/2)F1 mice i.v. with ABA-conjugated syngeneic spleen cells (ABA-SC) as described by Bach et al., (1978),
except that spleen cell donors were exposed to 2000 R before
sacrifice. Eight days after priming with $10x10^6$ ABA-SC, spleen
cells were harvested and cultured for 5 days with lymph node cells
from ABA-KLH primed mice and TNP-ABA-KLH or TNP-KLH. The results
of Table 2 show that the anti-TNP PFC response of ABA-KLH primed
cells is suppressed by the addition of cells from ABA-SC primed
mice and that suppression is ABA-specific because it requires the
presence of ABA on the carrier moiety of the immunogen. Data (not
shown) from out laboratory demonstrated that these ABA-specific
suppressor cells are T cells because they are inactivated by
treatment with monoclonal anti-Thy 1.2 and C.

Since thymic involution and the increase of auto-immunity
with aging (Walford, 1980) lead to the prediction that in old ani-

Table 2. ABA-specificity of suppressor T cells

Cells ($x10^5$) in culture from mice primed with			Anti-TNP PFC/culture	
ABA-KLH	None	ABA-SC		
9	3	–	385 ± 8^a	332 ± 7
9	–	3	176 ± 13	346 ± 7
Antigen in culture			TNP-ABA-KLH	TNP-KLH

a = Standard error

mals suppressor T cells should be fewer or less active than in young animals, experiments were carried out to induce and evaluate suppressor T cell activity in spleen cell populations from young (3-4 months) and old (20-21 months) mice. Suppressor T cells were induced by injecting young and old mice with ABA-SC ($0.5-10 \times 10^6$). Eight days later the spleen cells from these mice were cultured for 5 days with lymph node cells from ABA-KLH primed young mice and TNP-ABA-KLH. The results of Table 3 illustrate that suppression is greater and more easily induced in old than in young mice. Controls not shown demonstrated that also in old animals the induced suppressor cells are ABA-specific T cells. The increase of suppressor activity with aging is still compatible with thymic involution if the decline in number of suppressor T cell precursors or amplifiers is compensated by a greater inducibility in the old milieu. Moreover, suppressors from old animals could be more active than suppressor from young animals when tested "in vitro" on the same target cells from young mice. However, the increase in suppressor activity observed in spleen cells from old mice is not compatible with the well known increase in autoimmune diseases with aging.

This discrepancy could be dissolved by the data from the two experiments reported in Table 4. It can be seen that spleen cells from old mice injected with 10×10^6 ABA-SC are very effective in

Table 3. Induction of ABA-specific suppressor T cells in young and old mice

Cells ($\times 10^5$) in culture from mice primed with		Anti-TNP PFC/culture		
ABA-KLH	ABA-SC			
9 (3)[a]	–	475 ± 15[b]	475 ± 15	475 ± 15
9 (3)	1 (3)	355 ± 10	297 ± 4	213 ± 9
9 (3)	1 (20)	137 ± 11	152 ± 12	153 ± 7
ABA-SC injected ($\times 10^6$)		0.5	2	10

a = Numbers in parentheses indicate the age in months when mice were primed. b = Standard error.

Table 4. Effect of ABA-specific suppressor T cells from old
mice on target cells from young and old mice

Cells ($\times 10^5$) in culture from mice primed with			Anti-TNP PFC/culture	
ABA-KLH	None	ABA-SC	Exp. 1	Exp. 2
9 (4)[a]	3 (20)	–	410 ± 12[b]	357 ± 6
9 (4)	–	3 (20)	181 ± 20	123 ± 10
9 (20)	3 (20)	–	249 ± 6	303 ± 6
9 (20)	–	3 (20)	268 ± 2	273 ± 10

a = Numbers in parentheses indicate the age (month) when
mice were primed. b = Standard error.

suppressing the anti-TNP PFC response of ABA-KLH primed cells from
young but not from old mice. The loss of sensitivity to suppression with aging may reflect changes in helper T cell populations
and reactivities (Doria et al., 1980) and explain why autoreac-
tive clones are not suppressed in old animals.

4. CONCLUSION

The analysis of cellular components of the "in vitro"
antibody response to ABA-proteins has been focussed on ABA-
-specific immunoregulatory T cells. The role of idiotype-anti-
-idiotype reactions in modulating the functional network for the
ABA system is under investigation in our laboratory.
Preliminary results from "in vitro" stimulation of cells from
ABA-KLH primed A/J mice have shown that ABA-specific idiotype and
monoclonal anti-idiotype antibody play significant roles in regulating the outcome of the immune response. This molecular approach
will be extended to investigate cellular and humoral age-related
changes which may account for alterations of immunoregulatory
mechanisms during senescence.

ACKNOWLEDGMENT

The work was supported by Istituto Pasteur - Fondazione Cenci Bolognetti.

REFERENCES

Adorini, L., Pini, C., D'Agostaro, G., Di Felice, G., Mancini, C., Pozzi, L.V., Vietri, S. and Doria, G., 1981, Induction of azo-benzenearsonate (ABA)-specific helper and suppressor T cells and "in vitro" evaluation of their activities in the antibody response to T-dependent ABA-protein conjugates, J. Immunol., 127:000

Bach, B.A., Sherman, L., Benacerraf, B. and Greene, M.I., 1978, Mechanisms of cell-mediated immunity. II. Induction and suppression of delayed-type hypersensitivity to azobenzenearsona-te-coupled syngeneic cells, J. Immunol., 121:1460.

Doria, G., D'Agostaro, G. and Garavini, M., 1980, Age-dependent changes of B-cell reactivity and T cell-T cell interaction in the "in vitro" antibody response, Cell. Immunol., 53:195.

Hamaoka, T., Yamashita, T., Takami, T. and Kitagawa, M., 1975, The mechanism of tolerance induction in thymus-derived lymphocytes. I. Intracellular inactivation of hapten-reactive helper T lymphocytes by hapten-nonimmunogenic copolymer of D-amino acids, J. Exp. Med., 141:1308.

Herzenberg, L.A., Black, S.J. and Herzenberg, L.A., 1980, Regulatory circuits and antibody responses, Eur. J. Immunol., 10:1.

Lewis, J.K. and Goodman, J.W., 1978, Purification of functional, determinant-specific, idiotype-bearing murine T cells, J. Exp. Med., 148:915.

Mosier, D.E. and Coppleson, L.W., 1968, A three-cell interaction required for the induction of the primary immune response "in vitro", Proc. Natl. Acad. Sci., 61:542.

Nisonoff, A. and Greene, M.I., 1980, Regulation through idiotypic determinants of the immune response to the p-azophenylarsonate hapten in strain A mice, in: "Immunology 80," M. Fougereau and J. Dausset, eds., p. 57.

Walford, R.L., 1980, Immunology and aging, Am. J. Clin. Pathol., 74:247.

Yamamoto, H., Hamaoka, T., Yoshizawa, M., Kuroki, M. and Kitakawa,
    M., 1977, Regulatory functions of hapten-reactive helper and
    suppressor T lymphocytes. I. Detection and characterization
    of hapten-reactive suppressor T cell activity in mice immuni-
    zed with hapten-isologous protein conjugate, J. Exp.Med., 146:74.

IS THE IMMUNE SYSTEM A FUNCTIONAL IDIOTYPIC NETWORK?

J. Urbain

Université Libre de Bruxelles, Lab. of Animal
Physiology 67, rue des Chevaux
B 1640 Rhode-St-Gènese, Belgium

1. INTRODUCTION

Although supported by a lot of data it is fair to say that the idiotype network hypothesis is not universally accepted. This is partly due to the fact that many people do not talk about the same things even when they use the same words. Furthermore, different contradictory models have been put forward.

The word network implies connectedness between different elements of the immune system and idiotype network means that idiotypes are involved in clonal interactions. In a broad and clear sense, the network hypothesis states that immune regulation is partially due to signals generated within the system and more precisely, to idiotypic-antiidiotypic interactions. The idiotype network hypothesis does not claim that idiotypic interactions are the only means of interlymphocytic communication. In fact, it now appears likely that at least three kinds of connectedness are used in the immune system.
a) An antigen can bridge "idiotypic communities" which normally ignore each other when antigen is absent. Associative recognition of different epitopes, linked to the same backbone, allows transmission of signals between lymphocytes of different specificities (the Mitchisonian link).
b) T lymphocytes are "the leaders" of the immunological orchestra and they recognize as a rule, an antigen or idiotype (anti--idiotype) only in the context of membrane markers encoded by the

57

MHC. The MHC markers serve as cellular semaphores, as flags which
identify the compartment to which cell belongs. They give arrows
in the idiotypic network.
c) Idiotypic interactions can bridge lymphocytes even though
signals (positive or negative) are not transmitted via these
interactions. Signals are defined by the compartments to which
interacting lymphocytes belong. Associative recognition of MHC
markers and idiotypes govern the fate of interactions (induction
or suppression).
d) As a result of successful interactions, "factors" are released
from T cells or passed from membrane to membrane. These factors
could be parts of T cell receptors.

In fact, three main proposals were put forward to explain
regulation in the immune system.
1) The two signal theory of Bretscher and Cohen (Bretscher and
Cohn, 1970).
2) The one non specific signal hypothesis of Coutinho-Moller.
3) The idiotype network hypothesis (Jerne, 1974; for review, see
Urbain et al., 1981).

A comparative discussion of these proposals is instructive
and revealing. In their original form, they all appear to be
wrong. However, it should be stressed that some part of the truth
was correctly guessed in each proposal. Associative recognition is
indeed a crucial event in immune regulation. Immunoglobulin receptors pick up antigen and do not transmit physiological signals
(with the possible exception of immature B lymphocytes): most antigens lack an inherent triggering ability. Indiotypic interactions are used in the language of lymphocyte communication. All
these points will be discussed in detail elsewhere.

In the remaining of this paper, we shall examine some data
from our group, arguing that the immune system is a functional
idiotypic network, in the sense defined above.

2. THE NETWORK AS A LOGICAL NECESSITY

The most astonishing property of the immune system is the
diversity of the immunological repertoire. The immune system is
complete: it is able to respond even to an unpredictable antigenic
stimuli. Therefore being complete, the immune system cannot avoid

the recognition of its own elements. In other words, each immunoglobulin recognizes or is recognized idiotypically by another
immunoglobulin within the same individual. The idiotypic network
is a logical necessity, as was suggested by the genial hunch of
N.K. Jerne. The coexistence of idiotypes and auto-anti-idiotypes
has now been amply documented. The formal network is formally
proven (for review, see Urbain et al., 1981; Bona and Hiernaux,
1981).

The main question becomes: is this coexistence of significance for immunoregulation? Available data allow a positive answer
to this question. An apposite point of view has been put forward
(Cohn, 1981). The occurrence of auto-anti-idiotypic antibodies of
T helper or suppressor cells bearing auto-antiidiotypic receptors
would be due to breaking of self-tolerance (defined as negative
unresponsiveness) and would be artefacts. Since the same immunoglobulin can be both an idiotype (recognizing an antigen X) and an
anti-idiotype, such a view is inconsistent and would lead to an
empty immune system, completely paralyzed by self-tolerance, even
in the context of two signal theory.

3. THE IDIOTYPIC NETWORK AS AN EXPERIMENTAL NECESSITY

Immunologists are confronted with two main problems: the
origin of antibody diversity and the regulation of the immune
response.

The problems of regulation can be broadly divided into:
a) The selection of the repertoire available to antigen.
b) The regulation of the expression of the immunological repertoire. This second problem has been discussed in details elsewhere (see Urbain et al., 1981) and concerns the rise and fall in
antibody affinity, the class switches, the recruitment phenomena,
the idiotype dominance within one individual, the feedback loop..

The first problem stems directly from studies about idiotypes
defined "à la Oudin" (idiotypes specific for one individual and
one antigenic specificity). As a rule, different animals, when
confronted with the same antigen, synthesize different idiotypes.
Exceptions to this rule, the recurrent idiotypes, have been extensively described.

Idiotypy can "a priori" be explained in two ways:
a) idiotypes could be due to disparate genetic repertoires in different individuals. This would ensure if the immunological repertoire is built "de novo" in each individual by somatic mutations;
b) idiotypy could stem from regulatory phenomena which allow differential expression of available repertoire in different individuals. This hypothesis predicts the occurrence of many silent idiotypes whose expression is prevented by "naturally occurring suppressors" with anti-idiotypic receptors. We reasoned that induction of immunity against these suppressors would favour the expression of silent idiotypes. This was checked in the following way.

We start with a randomly chosen idiotype, isolated from a rabbit. A similar idiotype was detected in only one out of 60 other rabbits immunized with the same antigen. A second series of rabbits are immunized with Ab1 to elicit second order anti--idiotypic antibodies (Ab2). These Ab2 are then injected into a third series of rabbits which respond by the synthesis of anti--antiidiotypic antibodies (Ab3). Antigen is then given in these rabbits and the corresponding antibodies are called Ab1'.

The results are clear cut, highly reproducible and have been obtained with seven antigenic systems and two species (mice and rabbits).

Anti-idiotypic antibodies were also raised against Ab1' antibodies (Ab2') and against purified Ab3 to obtain anti-anti-anti-idiotypic antibodies (Ab4). In nearly all cases, Ab1' antibodies are idiotypically similar to Ab1. Ab3 antibodies, while they do not react with antigen, are sharing idiotypic specificities with Ab1 since Ab4 (anti-Ab3) recognizes specifically Ab1.

In a way, Ab3 looks like Ab1 and Ab4 looks like Ab2. These results have been described and discussed extensively elsewhere (Urbain et al., 1977; Cazenave, 1977; Wikler et al., 1979).

We shall limit to point out that :
a) There is no need to consider extended networks growing "ad infinitum", since fourth-order antibodies (Ab4) are strongly similar to Ab2. The diversity does not increase during the cascade immunization.

b) Most rabbits have closely related repertoire, even though they express different idiotypes when injected with the same antigen. Therefore, the total repertoire in each individual is drastically reduced by suppressive mechanisms.

c) The immune response is not due solely to antigenic selection but also to the idiotypic history of the animal. A given rabbit can learn to make antibodies of another rabbit and this learning can be transmitted by maternal immunoglobulins (Wikler et al., 1980).

d) Similar results can be obtained in mice (Cazenave et al., 1978). Furthermore, using the MOPC 460 system, it has been shown that induction of Ab3 antibodies inactivates suppressor T cells whose receptors are anti-idiotypic (anti-MOPC 460) (Bona and Paul, 1979). Therefore, in agreement with our working hypothesis, silent lymphocyte clones are not insignificant minorities but are kept under active supppressive mechanisms.

Up to now, we have considered and discussed the problems of the selection of available repertoire. The one idiotype which appears after antigenic stimulation is the one which escapes suppression. This suppression is linked to the presence of naturally occurring suppressors. It is one of the fundamental problems to unravel the mechanisms of induction of "spontaneous" suppressors. These suppressors can be counteracted by anti-anti-idiotypic antibodies (Ab3).

We can now ask the question: what about suppressors which appear during an immune response? Is it possible to get rid of this inhibitory activity? Is it possible to endow animals with an immunological memory directed against the receptors of these suppressors?

To study this question, we addressed the suppressors which predominate in the immune response against many tumors. It is known that in several tumor systems, a weak immune response is elicited. A weak cytotoxic activity (probably linked to a weak helper activity) can be demonstrated. Concomitantly or subsequently, this anti-tumor response is superseeded by suppressor T lymphocytes which enhance tumor growth. For some unknown reasons, tumors can sabotage the immune system. A few remarks are necessary before considering our data. Tumor immunologists live with the hope that tumor cells display neoantigens which could be targets for an efficient immunotherapy.

Despite some evidence, it is fair to say that no formal proof has
yet been put forward, regarding these neoantigens. While it is
obvious that the membrane of the tumor cell is altered, it could
be due to an enhanced expression of a normal membrane component.
Tumor cells could be stem cells frozen in their stem state. Stem
cells proliferate rapidly and they do so possibly because they
display on their membrane, receptors for proliferation signals. If
the regulatory mechanisms which control the expression of these
receptors are modified and if the genes coding for the receptor
are translocated near an efficient promoter, there will be continuous and enhanced production of these receptors. The weak immune
response could be directed against these self components. A strong
induction of suppressor T cells would follow to inhibit the
autoimmune process directed against the tumor cells. Some will
argue that, unlike transplantable tumor induced by virus or
chemical agents, spontaneous tumors are not immunogenic. Since the
immune system can respond in a positive or negative way, the fact
that no clear positive reaction is detected does not justify the
conclusion of non immunogenicity. After all, suppression T lymphocytes were first detected in non responder animals.

Anyway, whatever the usual weak response against some tumors
is anti-self or anti-non-self, it is worthwhile to try in the
light of network concepts to manipulate the immune system in order
to abrogate the suppressive mechanisms.

Since our previous work showed that it was possible by an
immunization cascade to elicit the synthesis of a given idiotype
and since Binz and Wigzell succeeded in inducing tolerance to
transplantation antigens by blast auto-immunization, we tried to
induce immunity against suppressors (Tilken et al., 1981). Sarcoma
T2 has been induced by methylcholanthrene. After grafting of
sarcoma cells, two waves of cytotoxic activity can be observed,
peaking at one week and 4 weeks. Between these two waves,
suppressor T lymphocytes, which inhibit cytotoxic lymphocytes, can
be detected in the spleen of tumor bearing animals. These
suppressors can be enriched, as blasts, by the sedimentation velo-
city method (1 g) (for details, see N. Schaaf-Lafontaine, 1978).
Suppressors from ten donors were purified and injected into syngeneic mice using the immunization schedule of Binz and Wigzell. The
effects of blast isoimmunization were evaluated by measuring the
weight of sarcoma T2, grafted one week after the last immunization. A statistically significant reduction of tumor growth was
found.

It is interesting to note that in a sample of 40 mice autoim-
munized with blastic suppressors, 20% of them are completely free
of tumors. Sixty per cent show a significant reduction in tumor
growth while the procedure has no effect at all in 20% of mice.

There is a wide scattering of data, as expected in such
systems. The same scattering is also observed in the experiments
of Binz-Wigzell. Recently Flood et al., (1980) have immunized
syngeneic mice with blastic helper (?) cells of regressor mice.
After such treatment, the tumor which normally regresses, is able
to grow.

What are the mechanisms which operate in mice immunized
against blastic suppressor cells and grafted with tumors? Our
working hypothesis is that suppressor T cells mixed with adjuvant
and functionally inactivated are able to stimulate helper cells.
Suppressor cells should possess two kinds of receptors: one
physiological receptor, which recognizes a self membrane marker of
T helper cells and an immunological receptor which interacts with
complementary idiotypic receptors of helper cells. As a result,
the cytotoxic potential of immunized mice is enhanced. This is in
agreement with our findings that such a protocol in the P815
system, leads to high primary responses in terms of cytotoxicity
(up to 60% of cytotoxicity). The validity of such an hypothesis is
now tested using well defined idiotypic system.

A second point relates to the fact that immunization against
suppressor does not work in 20% of mice. Understanding this
failure would allow improvement of the results. A simple idiotypic
explanation seems straightforward. Suppressor T cells, which are
used for immunization, are usually prepared from 8 to 10 donors.
Therefore, recipients are immunized with a panel of Ts_1, Ts_2, Ts_3.
Ts_8 cells (the number identifies the donor).

As a result, the immune system of the recipient responds by
the activation of anti-Ts_1, anti-Ts_2, ... anti-Ts_8 immunity. If
the tumor is grafted in a recipient which normally develops Ts_4,
the procedure will work. By contrast, if the recipient develops
Ts_{15}, after tumor challenge, there will be no immunological protection. In short, the success is critically linked to the idiotypic diversity of suppressor T cells. This point should be care-

fully studied in all experiments involving immunization with subpopulations of T cells.

4. THE IDIOTYPIC NETWORK AS A NECESSITY OF EVOLUTION

For a long time, there has been a flood of speculations about
the nature of the Generator or Diversity (GOD). Aminoacid sequencing of immunoglobulins did not solve the problems. With the
advent of nucleic acid technology, it has been possible to go
deeper inside these problems. On the basis of hybridization cuves
made in DNA excess, it was claimed that the gene number game was
over and that the number of Ig V genes was not greater than the
number of hemoglobin genes! We know now that these conclusions
were wrong. With Southern blots, genetic engineering and DNA
sequencing, a number of fascinating points has emerged:
a) These studies have revealed a strange mosaicism: the light
chain is made up of the joining of V_L, J_L, and C_L genes; the heavy
chain gene is still more fragmented and results from the combination of V_H, D_H, J_H, and C_H pieces.
b) The number of germ line pieces is fairly high: several hundreds
of V_H genes, at least 30 D segments and 4 J pieces. This provides
us with a bunch of around 50.000 germ line heavy chains and a few
thousand germ line light chains. This means that the germ line
repertoire is able to encode 10^7 to 10^8 complete immunoglobulins.
Furthermore, fluctuations are observed at the border of recombi-
nation of different pieces. The possibility of fusion between D
segments has been suggested.
c) It should be stressed that this large number of germ line genes
seems enough to cover the antigenic universe. In every case examined (levane, arsonate, NP, ...) there is always at least one
germ line gene. This could suggest that both an idiotype and its
corresponding antiidiotype are germ line encoded;
d) Aminoacid sequencing has recently revealed (especially through
the use of hybridoma) that the number of aminoacid sequence seems
still to be larger than the number of germ line genes. Variable
regions of heavy chain of IgG exhibit more diversity than the
corresponding parts of IgM. It is claimed that a process of
somatic mutations operates after the switch γ to μ (Bothwell et al.,
1981; Hood et al., 1981). This could be due to intergenic
conversion phenomena.

The functional meaning of these somatic alterations is unfortunately unknown. Are these processes involved in immunological learning, in idiotype selection? Studies by the group of Hood, do not suggest that "somatic variants" differ significantly in the affinity of their binding site for the antigen (phosporycholine...).

The real point has never been to know if there are somatic mutations or not. The number of dividing lymphocytes is such that somatic mutations occur certainly. The surprise is that these somatic mutations occur late in the development of lymphocytes (all proponents of somatic mutations have suggested that the process of somatic mutations was taking place at the level of immature lymphocytes). Fascinating experiments should tell us in the near future, whether high affinity antibodies are already present before the introduction of antigen or if they arise as somatic variants. The decrease in binding affinity (Urbain et al., 1972; Doria et al., 1972) which follows the rise in affinity should be revaluated in the light of these findings. This decrease in binding affinity has been attributed to the activation of suppressor T lymphocytes some of which are bearing anti-idiotypic receptors, complementary to the idiotypes of high affinity antibodies (for a detailed discussion, see Urbain, Wuilmart, Cazenave, 1981). In our studies, (Tasiaux et al., 1978), thanks to the use of peripheral blood lymphocytes from rabbits, it was possible to study repeatedly the same animal during the course of a normal immune response without adjuvant. Furthermore, the methods used excluded artefacts such as the detection of antigen instead of auto-anti-idiotypic receptors, since high affinity idiotypes (anti-TMV antibodies) are used to label lymphocytes from the same animal and from other rabbits immunized against TMV as controls. Moreover, the fact that auto-anti-idiotypic receptors can be detected on lymphocytes also labelled by anti- and anti-a_1, but not anti-b_4 , excludes detection of immunoglobulins absorbed via their Fc receptors. The results show an inverse relationship between the changes in antibody affinity and the level of lymphocytes bearing auto-anti-idiotypic receptors.

We can now come back to the question : what is the function of the high number germ line genes? How are they conserved during evolution? Apparently, most of them would not be used during the lifetime of one individual? How can the immune system evolve in anticipation of future needs? The solution to this dilema which has always been the crux of germ line theories is possibly the

idiotypic network. Clearly, the selection pressure due to external
antigens is insufficient to conserve all these genes. If most
immunoglobulins are indeed anti-idiotypic towards other Ig and if
these recognition phenomena are used in the regulatory circuitry,
then an internal selective pressure will allow the conservation of
a large number of germ line L genes. In other words, the immune
system is a functional idiotypic network partially encoded in the
germ line (for a detailed discussion, see Urbain et al., 1981).
The idiotypic network is the trick for information storage in
evolution and for some aspects of regulation, any immune response
being modulated by a second order immune response.

REFERENCES

Binz, H., Frischknecht, H., Wigzell, H.,1979, Some studies on
    idiotypes and antiidiotypic reactions and receptors in anti-
    -allo-MHC T cells immunity, Ann. Immunol. (Inst.Pasteur),
    130C:272.
Bona, C., Paul, W.E., 1979, Cellular basis of expression of
    idiotypes, J. Exp. Med., 149:532.
Bona, C., Hiernaux, J. 1981, Immune response: idiotype anti-idio-
    type network, CRC Crit. Rev. Immunol.. 2:33.
Bothwell, A., Paskino, M., Reth, M., Imanishi, T., Rajewsky, K.,
    Baltimore, A., 1981, Heavy-chain variable region contri-
    bution to the NP family of antibodies somatic mutation
    evident in a 2a variable region, Cell, 24:625.
Bretscher, P., Cohn, M., 1970, A theory of self-non self discri-
    mination, Science., 169:1042.
Cazenave, P.A., 1977, Idiotypic antiidiotypic regulation of anti-
    body synthesis in rabbits, Proc. Natl. Acad. Sci., USA, 74:5122.
Cohn, M. 1981, Commentary. Conversation with N.K. Jerne on Immune
    Regulation: associative versus network recognition, Cellular
    Immunology, 61:425.
Doria, G., Schiaffini, G., Garavini, H., Mancini, C., 1972, The
    rise and fall of antibody avidity at the level of single
    immunocytes, J. Immunol., 109:1245.
Flood, P., Kripke, M., Fowley, D., Schreiber, H., 1980, Suppres-
    sion of tumor rejection by autologous antiidiotypic immunity.
    Proc. Natl. Acad. Sci., USA, 77:2209.
Jerne, N.K., 1974, Towards a network theory of the immune system.
    Ann. Immunol. (Inst. Pasteur), 125C:373.
Schaaf-Lafontaine, N., 1978, Separation of lymphoid cells with

a suppression effect on the activity of cytotoxic cells in vitro during the growth of a syngeneic mouse tumor, Int. J. Cancer, 21:329.

Tasiaux, N., Leuwenkroon, R., Bruyns, C., Urbain, J., 1978, Possible occurrence and meaning of lymphocytes bearing auto-anti-idiotypic receptors during the immune response, Eur. J. Immunol., 8:464.

Tilkin, A.F., Schaaf-Lafontaine, N., Van Acker, A., Boccadoro, M., Urbain, J., 1981, Reduced tumor growth after low dose irradiation or immunization against blastic suppressor T cell, Proc. Natl. Acad. Sci., USA, 78:1809.

Urbain, J., Van Acker, A., De Vos-Cloetens, C., Urbain-Vansanten, G., 1972, Increase and decrease in binding affinity of antidodies during the immune response, Immunochemistry, 9:121.

Urbain, J., 1974, Cellular recognition and evolution, Arch. Biol., 85:139.

Urbain, J., Wikler, M., Franssen, J.D., Collignon, C., 1977, Idiotypic regulation of the immune system by the induction of antibodies against antiidotypic antibodies, Proc. Natl. Acad. Sci., USA, 74:5126.

Urbain, J., Cazenave, P.A., Wikler, M., Franssen, J.D., Mariame, B., Leo, O., 1980, Idiotypic induction and immune networks, in: "Immunology 1980", Dausset, J. and Fougereau M., eds., Acad. Press., New York, p. 81.

Urbain, J., Wuilmart, C., Cazenave, P.A.,1981, Idiotypic networks in immune regulation, Contemp. Topics in Molecular Immunology, 8:113.

Wikler, M., Franssen, J.D., Collignon, C., Leo, O., Mariame, B., Van de Walle, P., De Groote, D., Urbain, J., 1979, Idiotypic regulation of the immune system, J. Exp. Med., 150:184.

Wikler, M., Demeur, C., Dewasme, G., Urbain, J., 1980, Immunoregulatory role of maternal idiotypes. Ontogeny of immune networks, J. Exp. Med., 152:1024.

SYSTEMIC NETWORK REGULATION HYPOTHESIS:

SOME EXPERIMENTAL EVIDENCE

G.C. Andrighetto, B. Benato and G.Tridente

Chair of Immunopathology, University of Padova
Borgo Rome Hospitals, 37100, Verona, Italy

1. INTRODUCTION

The problem of antibody production and in general the internal regulation of the immune system was first focused by Jerne (1974) when he proposed a "network theory" based on internal antigenic properties of an idiotype.

Starting from Jerne's qualitative model, Hoffman (1975,1978) and Richter (1975, 1978) formulated quantitative mathematical models which focused the major role of T lymphocytes and the mimimum of anti-idiotype interactions effective for immune regulation. Moving from these observations and from recent experimental data (Wikler et al., 1979; Tilkin et al., 1981) we have attempted a systemic approach to Jerne's and Richter's theories to give a phenomenological version of immune system regulation.

The model introduces a double index symbolism which facilitates graphic representation of paratope-idiotype interactions and allows a formulation of a system of differential equations, susceptible both of mathematical and empirical challenge.

2. HYPOTHESES

2.1. Definitions of : Immune System, Network and Immune Response

a) The immune system is defined by all components and functions which lead to immune response.

b) The network indicates the functional net which operates through the immune system to regulate the immune response, via idiotype anti-idiotype recognition.

c) The immune response is comprised of normal response (NRP) and tolerance. The first leads to the antibody response and/or to cellular specific effectors, the second is an unresponsive network-induced active state.

2.2. Network Components

a) Soluble immunoglobulins (Ig) are antibody molecules with light and heavy chains. The variable portion has paratope and idiotype structures. They combine with the antigen forming immune-complexes with idiotype receptors of T and B cells and with other Ig idiotypes.

b) B lymphocytes have binding Ig receptors which are able to recognize T (Binz and Wigzell, 1976; Binz et al., 1979), B (Eichmann, 1978) and Ig (Wikler et al.,1979) idiotypes. These cells can be specifically stimulated to divide and to differentiate (Pernis, 1978) giving antibody forming elements, whose final Imorphological stage is the plasma cell. Such a cell, however, is devoided of surface Ig receptors and is involved in the network only as source of soluble Ig.

c) T lymphocytes have antigen binding receptors which are considered to be different from B receptors, at least structurally (Eichmann, 1975; Edelman, 1976; Cazenave et al., 1977). However, they are able to recognize T (Binz et al., 1979), B (Woodland and Cantor, 1978) cells and Ig (Cosenza et al., 1977) idiotypes. T cells can be stimulated to proliferate (Cosenza et al., 1977) acquiring specific T-effector functions (Binz et al., 1979).

2.3. Mode of Interaction

We consider the idiotypic identification as the principal interactive event among the network components. An idiotypic identification takes place when an element of a certain population with paratope "i" and idiotype "k" (e.g. B_{ik}) meets an element of another population whose paratope "k" can recognize the idiotype of the first, and whose idiotype is "j" (e.g. T_{kj}); in this case an interaction between the two emi-molecules is possible through the formation of a $B_{ik} T_{kj}$ complex. By convention the paratope is placed to the left of the idiotype symbol and the target (B_{ik}) is placed to the left of the recognizing element (T_{kj}). Therefore, this process of idiotypic identification can be expressed by a formal writing with two non-commutable indexes i.e. $B_{jk} \neq B_{kj}$.

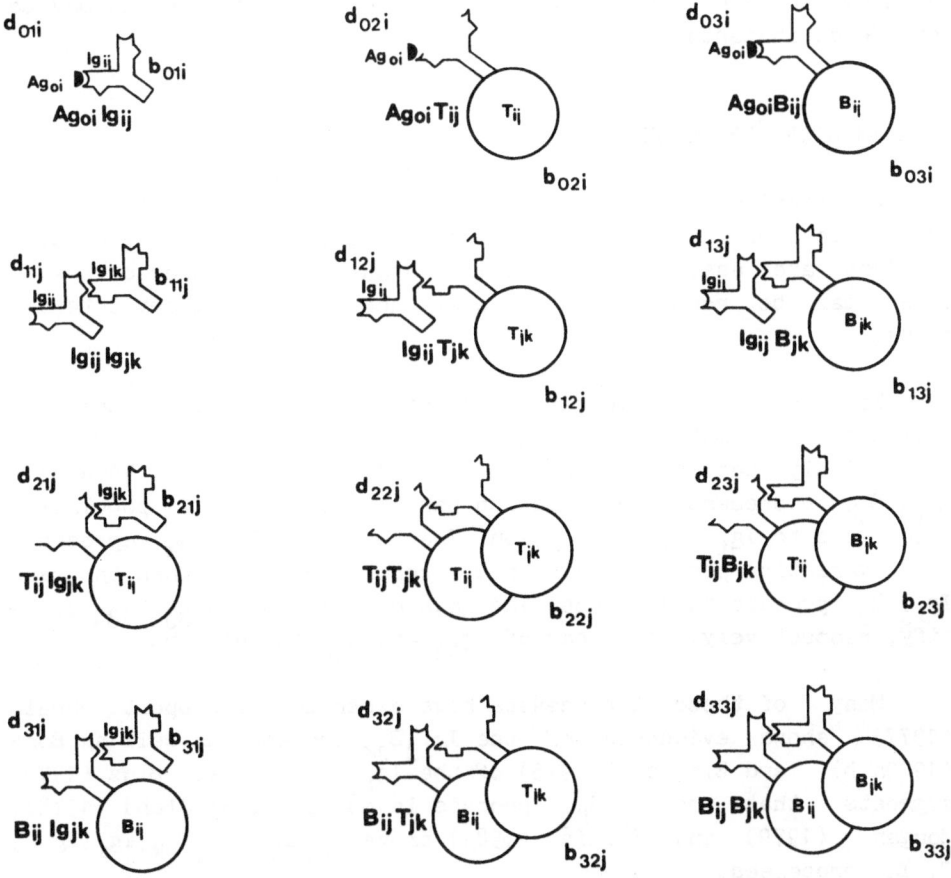

Fig. 1. Matrix arrangement of some basic elementary (binary) processes which may take place for antigen recognition and for network regulation. Although all combinations are theoretically possible, their specific weight in the network functioning may be different and is quantitable through "d" and "b" rate coefficients. The formalization of each interaction allows the writing of the relative equations (see Appendix A).

The above defined idiotype concept is functional and not structural, i.e. an idiotype exists when a paratope which recognizes it exists. So that, if the idiotype expressed by a set of elements (e.g Ig) are recognized by the same paratope expressed by another set of elements (e.g. B cells), they belong functionally to the same idiotype set.

Idiotypic identification takes place in a brief span of time compared to the operational time of the system, i.e. it may be considered instantaneous.

3. ELEMENTARY PROCESSES

We consider the elementary processes as binary interactions among receptors and/or antibody emi-molecules. Since these interactions are assumed to be as instantaneous, processes of higher order can be reduced to a temporal succession of binary interactions.

We focused 12 elementary processes (Fig. 1) and put them like elements in a matrix of 4 rows and 3 columns. If Ig_{ij} and B_{jk} are respectively the sizes of two considered populations then d_{13j} $Ig_{ij} B_{jk}$ represents the variation per time unit of Ig_{ij} population size due to $Ig_{ij}B_{jk}$ interaction. The term $b_{13j} Ig_{ij}B_{jk}$ represents the variation per time unit of B_{jk} population size, when the same $Ig_{ij} B_{jk}$ process takes place. The rate coefficients d_{13j}, b_{13j} quantify, respectively, the decay of Ig_{ij} and B_{jk} stimulation.

Many of these 12 processes have experimental support. Urbain (1977) shows evidences of the $Ig_{ij}B_{jk}$ process, as well as Bona (1979a,b) and Eichmann (1975) of the $Ig_{ij}T_{jk}$ process. Binz (1979) suggests that the $T_{jk}B_{kj}$ process is possible. Woodland (1978), Morgan (1979) and Tilkin (1981) prove $B_{ij}Ig_{jk}, B_{ij}T_{jk}, Ig_{ij}Ig_{jk}, T_{jk}T_{kj}$ processes.

4. SYSTEMIC NETWORK REGULATION HYPOTHESIS

The above mentioned results outline the possibility that the regulation of immune response may be carried out by a set of general interacting phenomena. These phenomena, limited and confronted with theoretical and empirical evidences, have to be integrated in a systematic structure. From the theoretical point of view, Richter (1978) showed that 4 "functional units of antibodies: Ab_i (i=1,2,3,4)", suppressive on the target, are sufficient to explain normal response (NRP), low zone tolerance (LZT) and high zone tolerance (HZT).

Wikler, (1979) showed that an antigen can evoke the production of 4 families of antibodies; the first Ab_1 being triggered by the antigen, the other three (Ab_2,Ab_3,Ab_4) triggered in turn by the idiotype of the previous antibody population. The idiotypical and paratopical analysis of the four populations showed that Ab_4 idiotype is similar to Ab_2; Ab_3 and Ab_1 share the same idiotype, but with different paratopes (Ab_3 does not recognize the antigen).

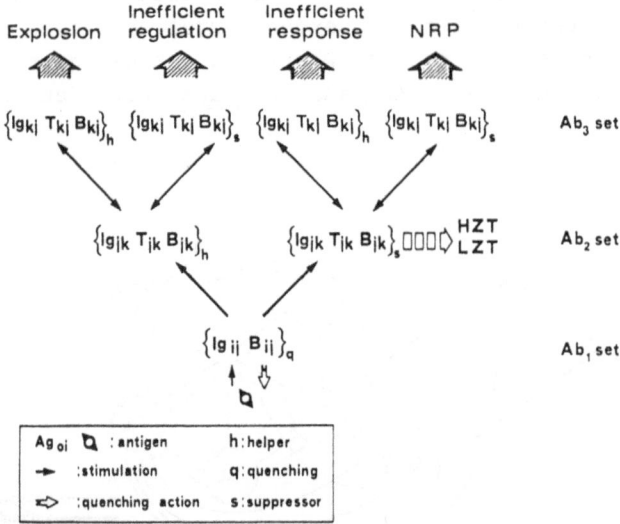

Fig. 2. Pathways of interaction among Ag, the recognizing set and the regulatory sets.
   Set 1 recognizes and reacts against Ag_{oi} (which is assumed for simplicity as T-independent and devoid of paratope) with a quenching action. The quenching set 1 triggers set 2 and eventually set 3 leading to a situation compatible with the expression of normal response (NRP) or with antigen dependent conditions of specific tolerance (LZT, HZT). This occours only when both regulation sets express suppressor activity, otherwise the network is brought to unbalanced situations of explosion, inefficient regulation or inefficient response.

Taking into account Richter's theoretical model and Wikler's experimental results, we suggest the following network model where the systemic regulation is performed by a subsequent interaction of the following sets of populations:

$$Ab_1 \quad set= Ig_{ij}, T_{ij}, B_{ij}$$

$$Ab_2 \quad set= Ig_{jk}, T_{jk}, B_{jk}$$

$$Ab_3 \quad set= Ig_{kj}, T_{kj}, B_{kj}$$

The set components are defined by general assumptions reported in 2.1. Possible interactive pathways among the proposed sets, either assigning helper or suppressor function to each regulatory set, are visualized in Fig. 2. This implies that the theoretical pathway which better fits with experimental situation of NRP, LZT, HZT, is represented by pathway where Ab_1 set has quenching activity on the antigen and Ab_2 and Ab_3 are both suppressor sets.

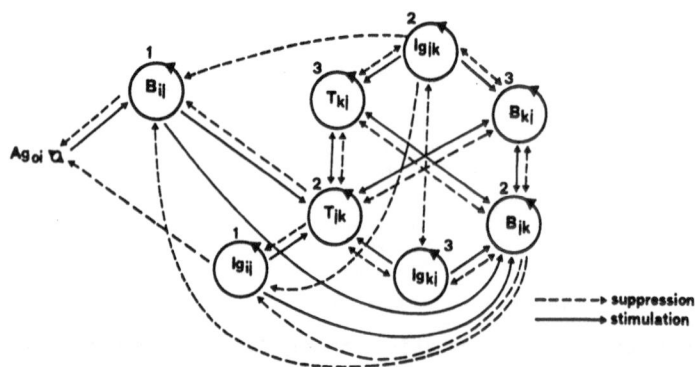

Fig. 3. Systemic network regulation hypothesis. The initial stage 1 of Ag recognition (stated as T-independent for simplicity although not excluding accessory events of higher complexity) is separated from the real regulatory "core", where two sets of components (stage 2) counteract with suppressive effects to moderate or enhance the immune response versus Ag_{oi}. The modulatory effect is obtained by two sets with intrinsic "suppressive behaviour", although not excluding the accessory participation of T helper lymphocytes. -----> suppression; ———> stimulation.

Fig. 3 reports the operative details of such network: Ag_{oi} stimulates the growth of B_{ij} clone which subsequently produces Ig_{ij} antibodies. Ig_{ij} interact with the antigen, forming Ag_{oi} Ig_{ij} complexes (stage 1). When the dose of Ag_{oi} is able to stimulate suitable expansion of B_{ij} clone, stage 2 is switched on by triggering Ab_2 set. Such events initiate the regulatory control stage.

This stage of control may allow the development of NRP or induces a state of tolerance according to the growth rates of the sets. A tolerant state (HZT or LZT) can occur when Ab_2 set suppresses efficiently Ab_1 set. Therefore, a NRP will take place if the growth rate of Ab_2 set is lower than of Ab_1 set.

It emerges that the self regulation of the immune system brings to a prevalence of a suppressive state over a stimulatory event, either during NRP or in tolerance.

The general equations which describe this network as well as its behaviour are reported in Appendix A and B.

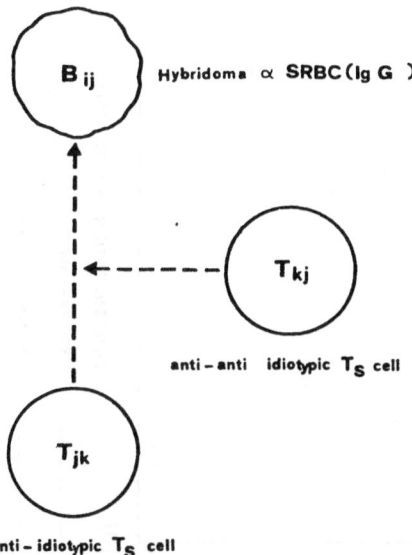

Fig.4. Outline of experimental model of idiotypic regulation. The action of T_{jk} cells on B_{ij} target is expected to be suppressive and the addition of T_{kj} on T_{jk} cells should rescue the production of anti-SRBC hybridoma antibodies.

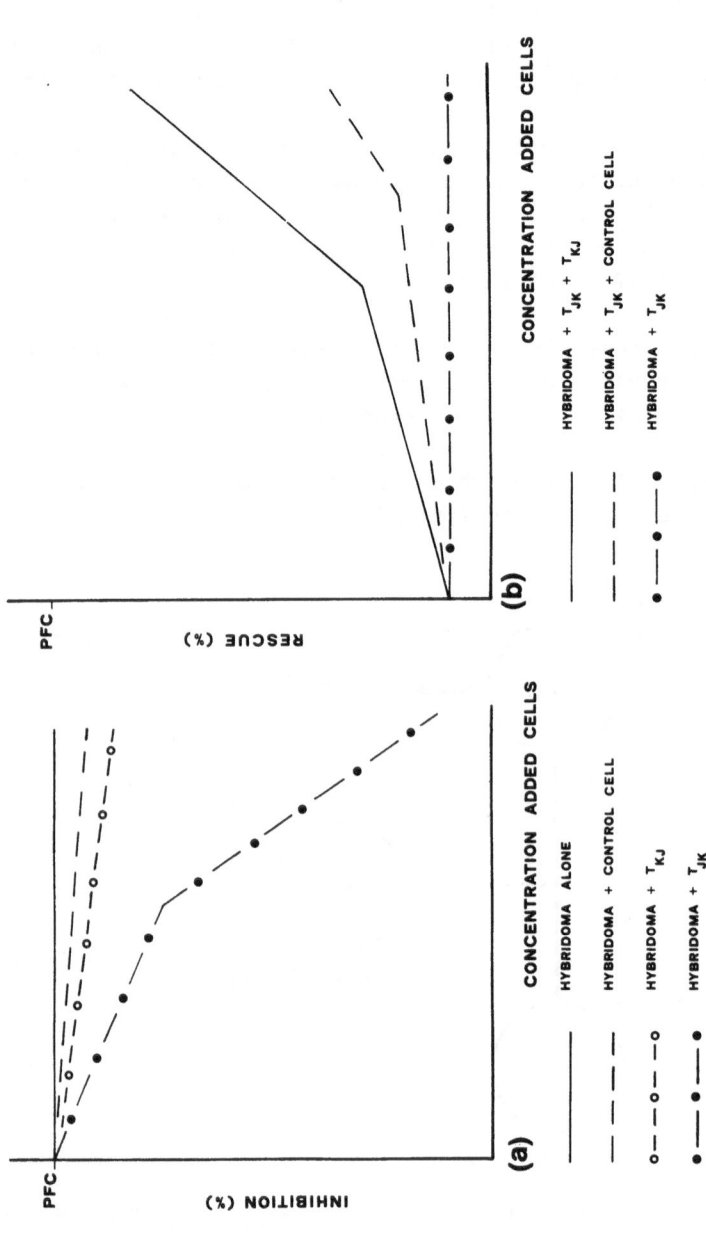

Fig. 5. Experimental evidence of suppressive idiotypic regulation (the units are arbitrary). The production of anti-SRBC IgG PFC from the hybridoma line is not affected either by control cells or T_{kj} cells, but is affected by T_{jk} alone (a). The rescue of hybridoma activity is clearly enhanced after addition of both T suppressor cells (b).

5. EMPIRICAL APPROACH TO THE SYSTEMIC
NETWORK REGULATION HYPOTHESIS

It is evident that the core of the proposed regulatory network is composed of two suppressor sets, idiotypically conjugated, which drive either normal responses or tolerant states.
This theoretical assumption gives to the network a maximum of reliability with a minimum of complexity and therefore is critical for the systemic regulation. Although some available experimental evidence may be interpreted in this sense (Gershon et al., 1981; Tilkin et al., 1981) there is no direct evidence of enhancing immune mechanism directed by a double suppressive T cell activity, and therefore, we consider of prior importance the empirical investigation of such phenomena.

We approached the problem "in vitro" as outlined in Fig. 4. The hypothetical B_{ij} cell was identified as an hybridoma cell (fusion Balb x CBA) line producing IgG anti sheep red cells (SRBC). The anti-idiotypic T suppressor cell (T_{jk}) was generated by injecting F_1 mice syngeneic spleen cells coated with IgG SRBC (Abbas et al., 1980). After seven days, the animals were sacrificed and their spleen cells passed on nylon wool columns and subsequently positively selected on plates coated with idiotype-positive IgG--α-SRBC.

The generation of the second suppressive cell, namely the anti-anti-idiotypic T suppressor cells (T_{kj}), was similarly obtained by injecting in syngeneic hosts spleen cells coated with an autologous anti-idiotypic (anti IgG-α-SRBC) antibody. Spleen cells of the recipients were then filtered through a nylon column.

After obtaining the T cell components "in vivo" the experiment was carried out "in vitro" by co-culturing hybridoma cells (B_{ij}) with anti-idiotypic T suppressor cells (T_{jk}) and addition of anti-anti-idiotypic suppressor cells (T_{kj}), with the relative controls, and measuring the amount of anti SRBC anti bodies produced by the hybrid line, by plaque forming cell technique (PFC). The results are schematically reported in Fig 5.

Antibody production by the hybridoma cell line is inhibited by an adequate number of T_{jk} suppressor cells, with a dose response effect, reaching 80% inhibition of PFC. By adding adequate numbers of T_{kj} suppressor anti-T_{jk} suppressor cells to a standard mixture of hybrid cells and T_{jk} cells in their maximal range of suppression, the number of PFC is progressively restored to about 70% of the original values. It is important to stress that, as expected, T suppressor cells of the second generation did not affect directly the hybridoma cell line and clearly needed the presence of the first T_{jk} cell to restore the activity of the hybrid cell antibody production. Alternative addition to the system of T suppressor cells generated by injecting syngeneic cells coated with an unrelated monoclonal IgG (anti-TNP) did not significantly affect the suppressive effect of the first anti-idiotype T_{jk} cells although partially interfering at maximal cell concentration. Similarly, when these cells were mixed only with the hybridoma cells, they did not show any direct effect on PFC production.

Finally, as further control for specificity, an unrelated IgG producing hybridoma cell line was also employed on which neither the first or the second suppressive T cells exerted inhibiting effects. That suppressive effects tested were of the T cell type was proved by abolition of such effects by anti Thy1 antiserum pretreatment.

6. DISCUSSION

The proposed model is a systematic interpretation of Jerne's and Richter's theories, taking into account some of the available experimental evidence. The systematic approach offers the advantage of analyzing single elementary processes without losing their systematic significance.

The model is structured to give the maximum of reliability with minimum of complexity by using the minimum number of components and interactions for autoregulating the system. The model uses a two index notation particularly useful since it allows a formalization of experimental data and their interpolation in equations necessary to define a mathematical model (see Appendix A and B).

The model focuses the existence of two different operative stages: the first concerning with the presentation of the antigen (presentation stage) the second with the regulatory control of the immune response (regulatory stage) (see Fig.3). It is important to stress that the function of the regulatory stage is not affected by the complexity of the presentation stage. The core of the regulatory stage is the interaction between two idiotypically correlated population: Ig_{jk}, T_{jk}, B_{jk} and Ig_{kj}, T_{kj}, B_{kj}

Using this minimum number of populations and interactions the behaviour of the model fits with experimental situations of NRP, LZT, HZT.

The working model is structured on the interactions of 3 sets:

Ab_1 set= Ig_{ij}, T_{ij}, B_{ij} Ab_2 set= Ig_{jk}, T_{jk}, B_{jk}

Ab_3 set= Ig_{kj}, T_{kj}, B_{kj}

These sets are linked together so that set 2 identifies set 1, set 3 identifies set 2; set 3 shows the same idiotype of set 1 but does not recognize the antigen. The model is a generalization of Wikler's data on mutual recognition of Ab_1, Ab_2, Ab_3 antibodies, and it is confirmed by our data "in vitro" on anti-idiotypic T cell mediated suppression, obtained in the hybridoma model, on which syngeneic T suppressor cells either anti-idiotypic or anti--anti-idiotypic, have shown to suppress and restore PFC capacity of the hybrid cell line. Similarly, Tilkin (1981) in an "in vivo" tumor growth system, controlled by T suppressive cells, was able to raise anti-idiotypic effectors directed against T suppressor cells which brought to enhnace anti-tumor cytotoxic activity. The reliability of the proposed systemic regulation emerges when different conditions of reactivity of the immune system are analyzed and compared. In case of NPR, Ab_1 and Ab_2 sets grow at different rates and at a certain moment the progressive growth of Ab_3 set (systemic helper), triggered by Ab_2, allow Ab_1 to emerge.

In case of the network-induced Ag dose dependent LZT and HZT, the tolerogenic doses of the antigen determine a rate of Ab_1 growth which is constantly controlled by higher level of Ab_2. Under these circumstance Ab_3 remains suppressed by Ab_2.

It is evident from the analysis of the dynamics of the regulatory processes, as well as from preliminary experimental evidences, that this network regulation is based on suppression and on suppression of its suppression (systemic helper function).

On the other hand, extensive experimental evidence is stressing the important role of helper cells and factors in the expression of immune responses. Such direct helper functions may appear to be excluded from the core of the proposed network model. However, from the theoretical point of view, one can distinguish active and passive helper function: the active helper function pertaining to peculiar cell types, while the passive helper function being a property of cells to behave like antigens, that is to stimulate a recognizing population. Under these conditions the same network component may act as helper and/or active suppressor in an systemic idiotypic recognizing process.

It emerges that in this model only active helper functions are excluded from the core of the network, while the passive helper function is very important for the systemic functioning. Obviously the existence of important active helper functions in other phases of immune system activity, such as antigen presentation, or in other auxiliary circuits related to the regulatory core of the network, is not at all excluded by the present formulation (Herzenberg et al, 1980).

7. SUMMARY

A systemic interpretation of Jerne's network hypothesis, where the elementary process is the recognition between the idiotype and an anti-idiotype, is presented. In the model structuring a maximum of reliability with a minimum of complexity and fitting with experimental evidence was allowed. The model suggests the presence of two operative stages: the first concerning with the presentation of the antigen and the second with the regulation of immune response. The core of the regulation stage operates through two sets of elements (Ig, T and B cells) idiotypically conjugated, whose net function is suppressive, but whose behaviour can be helper or suppressor according to the "systemic" phase in which they operate. An "ad hoc" experimental approach to prove the systemic network regulation hypothesis, is reported.

ACKNOWLEDGEMENTS

This work is supported in part by CNR grant 8001665961154721 of finalized project "Control of tumor growth".

APPENDIX A

1. GENERAL EQUATIONS

In order to write the equations that describe the size profiles of each population we have to sum all elementary processes, the source term and exponential decay terms (Hiernaux 1977). We obtain:

$$\frac{d\,Ag_{oi}}{dt} = Z_{oi} - e_{oi}Ag_{oi} - Ag_{oi}(d_{011i}Ig_{ij} + d_{03i}B_{ij})$$

$$\frac{d\,Ig_{ij}}{dt} = Q_{ij} - m_{ij}Ig_{ij} - Ig_{ij}(d_{11j}Ig_{jk} + d_{13j}B_{jk}) - b_{011i}Ag_{oi}Ig_{ij}$$

$$\frac{d\,B_{ij}}{dt} = Y_{ij} - f_{ij}B_{ij} - B_{ij}(d_{31j}Ig_{jk} + d_{32j}T_{jk} + d_{33j}B_{jk}) + b_{03i}Ag_{oi}B_{ij}$$

$$\frac{d\,Ig_{jk}}{dt} = Q_{jk} - m_{jk}Ig_{jk} - Ig_{jk}(d_{11k}Ig_{kj} + d_{12k}T_{kj} + d_{13k}B_{kj}) - (b_{11j}Ig_{kj} + b_{21j}T_{kj} + b_{31j}B_{kj} + b_{11j}Ig_{ij} + b_{31j}B_{ij})Ig_{jk}$$

$$\frac{d\,T_{jk}}{dt} = W_{jk} - h_{jk}T_{jk} - T_{jk}(d_{21k}Ig_{kj} + d_{22k}T_{kj} + d_{23k}B_{kj}) + (b_{12j}Ig_{kj} + b_{22j}T_{kj} + b_{32j}B_{kj} + b_{12j}Ig_{ij} + b_{32j}B_{ij})T_{jk}$$

$$\frac{d\,B_{jk}}{dt} = Y_{jk} - f_{jk}B_{jk} - B_{jk}(d_{31k}Ig_{kj} + d_{32k}T_{kj} + d_{33k}B_{kj}) + (b_{13J}Ig_{kj} + b_{23j}T_{kj} + b_{33j}B_{kj} + b_{13j}Ig_{ij} + b_{33j}B_{ij})B_{jk}$$

$$\frac{d\,Ig_{kj}}{dt} = Q_{kj} - m_{kj}Ig_{kj} - Ig_{kj}(d_{11j}Ig_{jk} + d_{12j}T_{jk} + d_{13j}B_{jk}) - (b_{11k}Ig_{jk} + b_{21k}T_{jk} + b_{13k}B_{jk})Ig_{kj}$$

$$\frac{d\,T_{kj}}{dt} = W_{kj} - h_{kj}T_{kj} - T_{kj}(d_{21j}Ig_{jk} + d_{22j}T_{jk} + d_{23j}B_{jk}) + (b_{12k}Ig_{jk} + b_{22k}T_{jk} + b_{32k}B_{jk})T_{kj}$$

$$\frac{d\,B_{kj}}{dt} = Y_{kj} - f_{kj}B_{kj} - B_{kj}(d_{31j}Ig_{jk} + d_{32j}T_{jk} + d_{33j}B_{jk}) + (b_{13k}Ig_{jk} + b_{23k}T_{jk} + b_{33k}B_{jk})B_{kj}$$

In these equations the symbol Ig_{ij} indicates the size, at instant t, of Ig population whose paratope is ' i ' and idiotype is

' j '. The same apply for the other symbols. Z, Q, W, Y, are source terms and e, m, h, f, are natural decay constants. Q, (source term for Ig) are governed by peculiar conditions: in fact they are functions of B, when they are activated at time 't-p', where 'p' is the lapse of time that B needs to differentiate. For simplicity we put Q = B so that the source term is proportional to the instantaneous value of B.

We introduce the following operators

$$
\hat{D}_i = \begin{pmatrix} d_{01i} & 0 & d_{03i} \\ 0 & 0 & 0 \\ 0 & 0 & 0 \end{pmatrix}
\qquad
\hat{D}_j = \begin{pmatrix} d_{11j} & d_{12j} & d_{13j} \\ d_{21j} & d_{22j} & d_{23j} \\ d_{31j} & d_{32j} & d_{33j} \end{pmatrix}
$$

$$
\hat{D}_k = \begin{pmatrix} d_{11k} & d_{12k} & d_{13k} \\ d_{21k} & d_{22k} & d_{23k} \\ d_{31k} & d_{32k} & d_{33k} \end{pmatrix}
\qquad
\hat{B}_i = \begin{pmatrix} -b_{01i} & 0 & b_{03i} \\ 0 & 0 & 0 \\ 0 & 0 & 0 \end{pmatrix}
$$

$$
\hat{B}_j = \begin{pmatrix} -b_{11j} & b_{12j} & b_{13j} \\ -b_{21j} & b_{22j} & b_{23j} \\ -b_{31j} & b_{32j} & b_{33j} \end{pmatrix}
\qquad
\hat{B}_k = \begin{pmatrix} -b_{11k} & b_{12k} & b_{13k} \\ -b_{21k} & b_{22k} & b_{23k} \\ -b_{31k} & b_{32k} & b_{33k} \end{pmatrix}
$$

$$
\hat{Ag} = \begin{pmatrix} Ag_{oi} & 0 & 0 \\ 0 & 0 & 0 \\ 0 & 0 & 0 \end{pmatrix}
\qquad
\hat{Ab}_1 = \begin{pmatrix} Ig_{ij} & 0 & 0 \\ 0 & 0 & 0 \\ 0 & 0 & B_{ij} \end{pmatrix}
$$

$$
\hat{Ab}_2 = \begin{pmatrix} Ig_{jk} & 0 & 0 \\ 0 & T_{jk} & 0 \\ 0 & 0 & B_{jk} \end{pmatrix}
\qquad
\hat{Ab}_3 = \begin{pmatrix} Ig_{kj} & 0 & 0 \\ 0 & T_{kj} & 0 \\ 0 & 0 & B_{kj} \end{pmatrix}
$$

$$
\hat{K}_0 = \begin{pmatrix} e_{oi} & 0 & 0 \\ 0 & 0 & 0 \\ 0 & 0 & 0 \end{pmatrix}
\qquad
\hat{K}_1 = \begin{pmatrix} m_{ij} & 0 & 0 \\ 0 & 0 & 0 \\ 0 & 0 & f_{ij} \end{pmatrix}
$$

$$\hat{K}_2 = \begin{pmatrix} m_{jk} & 0 & 0 \\ 0 & h_{jk} & 0 \\ 0 & 0 & f_{jk} \end{pmatrix} \qquad \hat{K}_3 = \begin{pmatrix} m_{kj} & 0 & 0 \\ 0 & h_{kj} & 0 \\ 0 & 0 & f_{kj} \end{pmatrix}$$

$$\hat{a}_1 = \begin{pmatrix} 0 & 0 & a_{ij} \\ 0 & 0 & 0 \\ 0 & 0 & 0 \end{pmatrix} \qquad \hat{a}_2 = \begin{pmatrix} 0 & 0 & a_{jk} \\ 0 & 0 & 0 \\ 0 & 0 & 0 \end{pmatrix}$$

$$\hat{a}_3 = \begin{pmatrix} 0 & 0 & a_{kj} \\ 0 & 0 & 0 \\ 0 & 0 & 0 \end{pmatrix}$$

(a_{ij} is the production rate of Ig_{ij} by activated B_{ij} and so on) and the vectors

$$Ag = \begin{pmatrix} Ag_{oi} \\ 0 \\ 0 \end{pmatrix} \quad Ab_1 = \begin{pmatrix} Ig_{ij} \\ 0 \\ B_{ij} \end{pmatrix} \quad Ab_2 = \begin{pmatrix} Ig_{jk} \\ T_{jk} \\ B_{jk} \end{pmatrix} \quad Ab_3 = \begin{pmatrix} Ig_{kj} \\ T_{kj} \\ B_{kj} \end{pmatrix}$$

We need also

$$S = \begin{pmatrix} Z_{oi} \\ 0 \\ \hline 0 \\ 0 \\ Y_{ij} \\ \hline 0 \\ W_{jk} \\ Y_{jk} \\ \hline 0 \\ W_{kj} \\ Y_{kj} \end{pmatrix} = \begin{pmatrix} S_0 \\ \hline S_1 \\ \hline S_2 \\ \hline S_3 \end{pmatrix}$$

as source term for the cellular populations.

We define also the operators

$$
\hat{D} = \begin{pmatrix} 0 & \hat{D}_i & 0 & 0 \\ 0 & 0 & \hat{D}_j & 0 \\ 0 & 0 & 0 & \hat{D}_k \\ 0 & 0 & \hat{D}_j & 0 \end{pmatrix} \quad
\hat{B} = \begin{pmatrix} 0 & 0 & 0 & 0 \\ \hat{B}^t_i & 0 & 0 & 0 \\ 0 & \hat{B}^t_j & 0 & \hat{B}^t_j \\ 0 & 0 & \hat{B}^t_k & 0 \end{pmatrix}
$$

$$
X = \begin{pmatrix} A_g & 0 & 0 & 0 \\ 0 & Ab_1 & 0 & 0 \\ 0 & 0 & Ab_2 & 0 \\ 0 & 0 & 0 & Ab_3 \end{pmatrix} \quad
\hat{\alpha} = \begin{pmatrix} 0 & 0 & 0 & 0 \\ 0 & \hat{\alpha}_1 & 0 & 0 \\ 0 & 0 & \hat{\alpha}_2 & 0 \\ 0 & 0 & 0 & \hat{\alpha}_3 \end{pmatrix}
$$

$$
\hat{K} = \begin{pmatrix} \hat{K}_0 & 0 & 0 & 0 \\ 0 & \hat{K}_1 & 0 & 0 \\ 0 & 0 & \hat{K}_2 & 0 \\ 0 & 0 & 0 & \hat{K}_3 \end{pmatrix}
$$

($\hat{B}_i$ means the transport of $\hat{B}_i$).

We consider the vector space V whose generic vector X is:

$$
X = \begin{pmatrix} X_1 \\ X_2 \\ X_3 \\ X_4 \\ X_5 \\ X_6 \\ X_7 \\ X_8 \\ X_9 \\ X_{10} \\ X_{11} \\ X_{12} \end{pmatrix} = \begin{pmatrix} Ag_{oi} \\ 0 \\ 0 \\ \hline Ig_{ij} \\ 0 \\ B_{ij} \\ \hline Ig_{jk} \\ T_{jk} \\ B_{jk} \\ \hline Ig_{kj} \\ T_{kj} \\ B_{kj} \end{pmatrix} = \begin{pmatrix} Ag \\ \hline Ab_1 \\ \hline Ab_2 \\ \hline Ab_3 \end{pmatrix}
$$

This vector represents the status of the system at time t. The size of each population changes with time and therefore X traces a trajectory in V.

The equations (1) assume the form (2) by using the above defined vectors and operators:

$$(2) \quad \frac{d^{Ag}}{dt} = S_0 - \hat{K}_0 \, Ag - \hat{Ag} \, \hat{D}_i \, Ag$$

$$\frac{d^{Ab_1}}{dt} = S_1 + \hat{\alpha}_1 \, Ab_1 - \hat{K}_1 Ab_1 + \hat{Ab}_1 \, \hat{B}_i^t \, Ag - \hat{Ab}_1 \, \hat{D}_j Ab_2$$

$$\frac{d^{Ab_2}}{dt} = S_2 + \hat{\alpha}_2 \, Ab_2 - \hat{K}_2 Ab_2 + \hat{Ab}_2 \, \hat{B}_k^t \, (Ab_1 + Ab_3) - \hat{Ab}_2 \, \hat{D}_k \, Ab_3$$

$$\frac{d^{Ab_3}}{dt} = S_3 + \hat{\alpha}_3 \, Ab_3 - \hat{K}_3 + Ab_3 + \hat{Ab}_3 \, \hat{B}_k^t \, Ab_2 - \hat{Ab}_3 \, \hat{D}_j \, Ab_2$$

This form better shows the interactions among the Ab-sets. ($\hat{B}^t$ means "transpost" of B operator).

Another compact form is:

$$(3a) \quad \frac{d^X}{dt} = S + \hat{\alpha} X - \hat{K}X + \hat{X}(\hat{B} - \hat{D})X$$

or, in components:

$$(3b) \quad X_1 = \Lambda_1(X) \qquad (1 = 1, \ldots, 12)$$

Were S is the source term of the cell populations and of the antigen, X is the source term for Ig, K is the decay operator (intrinsic cathabolism) B and D are respectively stimulation and suppression operators, X is the state of the system considered as "target" operator.

2. DYNAMICS OF THE SYSTEM

Since the interacting coefficients between populations "b" and "d" are unknown the dynamic analysis of the system needs the formulation of some general hypothesis:
1. the stimulation coefficients (e.g. b_{13j} et similia) are functions of the size stimulating populations. That is, the stimulation of a certain population needs an optimal concentration of the stimulating population: concentration far from the optimal rango do not give any appreciable stimulation.

2. The inferior threshold for the stimulation corresponds to the steady state concentration X between the source coefficient and the spontaneous decay of the stimulating population. That is the stimulation is "switched on" if $X_1 > X_1^*$

and is "switched off" if $X_1 \leq X_1^*$, $X_1^* = \dfrac{S_1}{k_1}$

3. The suppression is, in general, more efficient than the stimulation: at optimal concentrations the suppression rate of a clone mediated by an idiotypic mechanism (e.g. T_{jk} suppressed by T_{kj}) is in general more efficient than the growth rate due to the stimulation by the conjugated process (e.g. T_{kj} stimulated by T_{jk})

i.e. $d_{22k} T_{jk} T_{kj} > b_{22j} T_{kj} T_{jk}$

4. The suppression is regulated by the same rules as in 1 and 2.

2.1. Dynamics in Absence of Antigen Triggering.

If Ag=D the system is in steady state $\overline{X}$ and the size of interacting populations are equal to the threshold value, e.g. $\overline{X}_1 = X_1^*$.

This steady state is stable. We use the analysis of the normal mode of the linearized problem to prove this sentence (Eigen and Schuster, 1977). By introducing the variables: $X_1 = X_1 - X_1^*$

the system $\dot{X}_1 = \Lambda_1(X)$

is, in the neighbourhood of $X,\overline{o}$ linearized system: $\dot{x}=Ax$
where A is the matrix:

$$\left\| a_{lm} \right\| = \left\| \frac{\delta \Lambda_1}{\delta X_m} \right\|_{X=X^*} \qquad (l,m=1 \ldots \ldots 12)$$

One can verify that, in the hypotheses 7: 1, 2, 3, 4 the matrix A is diagonal and has the **eigenvalues** negative (see Appendix B).

The conclusion is that $X^*$is a "stable sink"

2.2. Dinamics of the System in Presence of Antigenic Triggering.

If $Ag \neq 0$, and for each clone, the sum of suppression rate is equal to the sum of the stimulatory rate, steady states X different from X, are possible. These steady states are solutions of the system of algebric equations:

3)
$$S_0 = \hat{K}_0 \, \hat{\overline{Ag}} + \overline{Ag} \, \hat{D}_i \, \overline{Ab}_1$$
$$S_1 = - \alpha_1 \overline{Ab}_1 + \hat{K}_1 \, \overline{Ab}_1 - \overline{Ab}_1 \, \hat{B}_i^t \, \overline{Ag} + \overline{Ab}_1 \, \hat{D}_j \, \overline{Ab}_2$$
$$S_2 = - \alpha_2 \overline{Ab}_2 + \hat{K}_2 \, \overline{Ab}_2 - \overline{Ab}_2 \, \hat{B}_j^t \, \overline{Ab}_1$$
$$\overline{Ab}_3 = Ab_3^*$$

In these steady states we have simultaneously

$$\overline{Ag} \neq 0 \qquad \overline{Ab}_1 > Ab_1^* \qquad \overline{Ab}_2 > Ab_2^* \qquad \overline{Ab}_3 = Ab_3^*$$

These steady states may be comparable from the biological point of view to LZT and HZT.

The critical parameters to establish LZT and HZT are:
- the source term Z_{oi} for the antigen Ag_{oi}
- the stimulatory coefficient b_{o3i} of the responsive clone B_{ij}

High and low values of Z_{oi} (and of Ag_{oi} which it its linear function) can stimulate in the same way B_{ij} by the term b_{o3i} which has the behaviour described in the figure.

Therefore, steady states such as $\overline{X}$ may be reached if Z_{oi} brings B_{ij} (and Ig_{ij}) to values which allow the leveling of stimulation and of suppression rates in the equation 2.

On the other hand, if Z_{oi} stimulates optimally B_{ij} then it is possible that the development of this clone (and of Ig_{ij}) is so fast that B_{ij} in a short time is out of the optimal range for Ab_2 stimulation, so that Ab_2 is not significantly stimulated.

In this situation, while B_{ij} produces NRP Ab_2 and Ab_3 remain near the state as in absence of antigenic signal.

At the end the immune system tends to the X*.

· APPENDIX B

$$\|a_{lm}\| = \left\| \frac{\delta \; \Lambda_1}{\delta \; X_m} \right\| \qquad \text{has the following non zero entries}$$

$$(1, \; m \; = \; 1, \; \dots\dots, \; 12)$$

$$a_{1\,1} = - e_{oi} - (d_{01i}\,^{Ig}_{ij} + d_{03i}\,^{B}_{ij})$$

$$a_{1\,4} = - d_{01i}\,^{Ag}_{oi}$$

$$a_{1\,6} = - d_{03i}\,^{Ag}_{oi}$$

$$a_{4\,1} = - b_{01i}\,^{Ig}_{ij}$$

$$a_{4\,4} = - m_{ij} - (d_{11j}\,^{Ig}_{jk} + d_{12j}\,^{T}_{jk} + d_{13j}\,^{B}_{jk}) - b_{01i}\,^{Ag}_{oi}$$

$$a_{4\,7} = - d_{11j}\,^{Ig}_{ij}$$

$$a_{4\,8} = - d_{12j}\,^{Ig}_{ij}$$

$$a_{4\,9} = - d_{13j}\,^{Ig}_{ij}$$

$$a_{6\,1} = - b_{03i}\,^{b}_{ij}$$

$$a_{6\,6} = - f_{ij} - (d_{31j}\,^{Ig}_{jk} + d_{32j}\,^{T}_{jk} + d_{33j}\,^{B}_{jk}) + b_{03i}\,^{Ag}_{oi}$$

$$a_{6\,7} = - d_{31j}\,^{B}_{ij}$$

$$a_{6\,8} = - d_{32j}\,^{B}_{ij}$$

$$a_{6\,9} = - d_{33j}\,^{Bi}_{j}$$

$$a_{7\,4} = - b_{11j}\,^{Ig}_{jk}$$

$$a_{7\,6} = - b_{31j}\,^{Ig}_{jk}$$

$$a_{7\,7} = - m_{jk} - (d_{11k}\,^{Ig}_{kj} + d_{12k}\,^{T}_{kj} + d_{13k}\,^{B}_{KJ}) - (b_{11j}\,^{Ig}_{21j}\,^{T}_{kj} + $$
$$- b_{31j}\,^{B}_{kj} + b_{11j}\,^{Ig}_{ij} + b_{31j}\,^{B}_{ij})$$

$$a_{7\ 10} = -(d_{11k} + b_{11j})Ig_{jk}$$

$$a_{7\ 11} = -(d_{12k} + b_{21j})Ig_{jk}$$

$$a_{7\ 12} = -(d_{13k} + b_{31j})Ig_{jk}$$

$$a_{8\ 4} = -b_{12j}T_{jk}$$

$$a_{8\ 6} = -b_{32j}T_{jk}$$

$$a_{8\ 8} = -h_{jk} - (d_{21k}Ig_{kj} + d_{22k}T_{kj} + d_{23k}B_{kj}) + (b_{12j}Ig_{kj} + b_{32j}B_{ij})$$

$$a_{8\ 10} = (-d_{21k} + b_{12j})\,T_{jk}$$

$$a_{8\ 11} = (-d_{22k} + b_{22j})\,T_{jk}$$

$$a_{8\ 12} = (-d_{23k} + b_{32j})\,T_{jk}$$

$$a_{9\ 4} = b_{33j}B_{jk}$$

$$a_{9\ 6} = b_{33j}B_{jk}$$

$$a_{9\ 9} = -f_{jk} - (d_{31k}Ig_{kj} + d_{32k}T_{kj} + d_{33k}B_{kj}) + (b_{13j}Ig_{kj} + b_{23j}T_{kj} + b_{33j}B_{kj} + b_{13j}Ig_{ij} + b_{33j}B_{ij})$$

$$a_{9\ 10} = (-d_{31k} + b_{13j})\,B_{jk}$$

$$a_{9\ 11} = (-d_{33k} + b_{33j})\,B_{jk}$$

$$a_{9\ 12} = (-d_{33k} + b_{33j})\,B_{jk}$$

$$a_{10\ 7} = (-d_{11j} - b_{11k})\,Ig_{kj}$$

$$a_{10\ 8} = (-d_{12j} - b_{21k})\,Ig_{kj}$$

$$a_{10\ 9} = (-d_{13j} - b_{31k})\,Ig_{kj}$$

$$a_{10\ 10} = m_{kj} - (d_{11j}Ig_{jk} + d_{12j}T_{jk} + d_{13j}B_{jk}) - (b_{11k}Ig_{jk} +$$

$$+ b_{21k}T_{jk} + b_{13k}B_{jk})$$

$$a_{11\ 7} = (- d_{21j} + b_{12k}) T_{kj}$$

$$a_{11\ 8} = (- d_{22j} + b_{22k}) T_{kj}$$

$$a_{11\ 9} = (- d_{23j} + b_{32k}) T_{kj}$$

$$a_{11\ 11} = -h_{kj} - (d_{21j}Ig_{jk} + d_{22j}T_{jk} + d_{23j}B_{jk}) + (b_{12k}Ig_{jk} + + b_{22k}T_{jk} + b_{32k}B_{jk})$$

$$a_{12\ 7} = (- d_{31j} + b_{13k}) B_{kj}$$

$$a_{12\ 8} = (- d_{32j} + b_{23k}) B_{kj}$$

$$a_{12\ 9} = (- d_{33j} + b_{33k}) B_{kj}$$

$$a_{12\ 12} = f_{kj} - (d_{31j}Ig_{jk} + d_{32j}T_{jk} + d_{33j}B_{jk}) + (b_{13k}Ig_{jk} + + b_{23k}T_{jk} + b_{33k}B_{jk})$$

In the hypotheses 6 I), II), IV), we have

$$\left\| \frac{\delta \Lambda_1}{\delta X_m} \right\|_{X=X^*} = \begin{pmatrix} - e_{oi} & & \\ 0 & & \\ 0 & & \\ -m_{ij} & & \\ 0 & & \\ -f_{ij} & & \\ 0 & -m_{jk} & 0 \\ & -h_{jk} & \\ & -f_{jk} & \\ & -m_{kj} & \\ & -h_{kj} & \\ & -f_{kj} & \end{pmatrix}$$

REFERENCES

Abbas, A.K., Burakoff, S.J., Gefter, M.L. and Greene, M.I., 1980, T lymphocyte-mediate suppression of myeloma function in vitro. III. Regulation of antibody production in hybrid myeloma cells by T lymphocytes, J. Exp. Med., 154:968.

Binz, H. and Wigzell, H., 1976, Antigen-binding, idiotypic receptors from T lymphocytes: An analysis of their biochemistry, genetics, and use as immunogens to produce specific immune tolerance, Cold Spring Harbor Symp. Quant. Biol., 41:275.

Binz, H., Frischknecht, H., Shen, F.W. and Wigzell, H., 1979, Idiotypic determinants on T cells subpopulations, J. Exp. Med., 149:910.

Bona, C. and Paul, W.E., 1979a, Cellular basic of regulation of expression of idiotype. I. T suppressor cells specific for MOPC 460 idiotype regulate the expression of cells secreting anti--TNP antibodies bearing 460 idiotype, J. Exp. Med., 149:592.

Bona, C., Hooge, R., Cazenave, P.A., Leguern, C., and Paul, W.E., 1979b, Cellular basis of regulation of expression of idiotype. II. Immunity to anti MOPC-460 idiotypes increases the level of anti-trinitrophenyl antibodies bearing 460 idiotypes, J. Exp. Med., 149:815.

Cazenave, P.A., Cavaillon, S.M. and Bona, C., 1977, Idiotypic determinats on rabbit B-and T-derived lymphocytes, Immunological Rev., 34:34.

Cosenza, H., Julius, M.H. and Augustin, A.A., 1977, Idiotypes as variable region markers: Analogies between receptors on phosphorylcoline-specific T and B lymphocytes, Immunological Rev., 34:3.

Edelman, G.M., 1976, Summary: understanding selective molecular recognition, Cold Spring Harbor Symp. Quant. Biol., 41:891.

Eichmann, K., 1975, Idiotype suppression.II. Amplification of a suppressor T cell with anti-idiotypic activity, Eur. J. Immunol., 5:511.

Eichmann, K., 1978, Expression and function of idiotypes on lymphocytes, Advances Immunol., 26:195.

Figen, M. and Schuster, P., 1979, The Hypercycle: A principle of natural self-organization, Spriger-Verlag Berlin and New York.

Gershon, R.K., Eardley, D.D., Durum, S., Green, D.R., Shen, S.W., Yamauchi, R., Cantor, H. and Murphy, D.B., 1981, Contrasuppression. A novel immunoregulatory activity, J. Exp. Med., 153:1533.

Herzenberg, L.A., Black, S.J. and Herzenberg, L.A., 1980, Regulatory circuits and antibody response, Eur. J. Immunol., 10:1.

Hiermaux, J., 1977, Some remarks on the stability of the idiotypic
    network, Immunochemistry, 14:733.

Hoffman, G.W., 1975, A theory of regulation and self-nonself discri-
    mination in an immune network, Eur. J. Immunol., 5:638.

Hoffman, G.W., 1978, Incorporation of a non specific helper factor
    into a network theory of the regulation of the immune response,
    in: "Theoretical Immunology," Bell, G.I., Perelson, A.S. and
    Pimbley, G.H., eds., M. Dekker, Basel, p. 571.

Jerne, N.K., 1974, Towards a network theory of the immune System,
    Ann. Immunol. Inst. Pasteur, 125c:373.

Morgan, A.C., Rossen, R.D., and Twomey, J.J., 1979, Naturally occur-
    ring circulating immune complexes: Normal human serum contain
    idiotype-anti-idiotype complexes dissociable by certain IgG an-
    tiglobulins, J. Immunol., 122:1672.

Pernis, B., 1978, Lymphocytes membrane immunoglobulins: An overview,
    in: "Comprehensive Immunology," Good, R.A. and Litman G.L.,
    eds., Plenum, New York, p. 357.

Richter, P.H., 1975, A network theory of Immune System, Eur. J.
    Immunol., 5:350.

Richter, P.H., 1978, The network idea and the Immune response, in:
    "Theoretical Immunology," Bell, G.I., Perelson, A.S. and Pim-
    bley, G.H., eds., M. Dekker, Basel. p. 539.

Tilkin, A.F., Schaaf-Lafontaine, N., VanAcker, A., Boccadoro, M.
    and Urbain, J., 1981, Reduced tumour growth after low-dose ir-
    radiation or immunization against blastic suppressor T cells,
    Proc. Natl. Acad. Sci., USA, 78:1809.

Urbain, J., Wikler, M., Franssen, J.D. and Collignon, 1977, Idioty-
    pic regulation of the immune system by the induction of anti-
    bodies against anti-idictypic antibodies, Proc. Nat. Acad.
    Sci., USA, 74:5126.

Wikler, M., Franssen, J.D., Collignon, C., Leo, O., Mariame, B.,
    Van De Walle, P., De Groote, D. and Urbain, J., 1979, Idioty-
    pic regulation of the immune system. Common specificities be-
    tween idiotypes and antibodies raised against anti-idiotypic
    antibodies in rabbits, J. Exp. Med., 150:184.

Woodland, R. and Cantor, H., 1978, Idiotype specific T helper
    cells, are required to induce idiotype-positive B memory
    cells to secrete antibody, Eur. J. Immunol., 8:600.

ANTIGEN SPECIFIC HELPER FACTORS:

AN OVERVIEW AFTER TEN YEARS

Marc Feldmann, Alain Fischer, Roger James,
Eric Culbert, Mike Cecka, Ian Todd, Edward Zanders,
Geoffrey Sunshine, David Katz, and Sirkka Kontiainen[*]

Imperial Cancer Research Fund, Tumour Immunology Unit
Department of Zoology, University College London
Gower Street London WC1E 6BT

[*]Department of Bacteriology and Immunology
University of Helsinki Haartmaninkatu
00290 Helsinki, 29 Finland

1. INTRODUCTION

Immunology in the late 1960's was a time of rapidly changing concepts. The functional dichotomy of T cells and B cells had been enunciated (reviewed Roitt et al., 1969, Greaves et al., 1972), the puzzle of Immune Response genes had been uncovered (Kantor et al., 1963) and receptor antibodies had been visualized on B cells but not T cells (Taylor et al., 1971). The carrier effect had been described and the phenomenon of linked recognition had suggested various molecular models (Mitchison et al., 1970) to account for the mechanism of T cell cooperation (or help). These models, represented in Fig.1, involved a 'carrier antibody' derived from the T cell recognizing carrier determinants on the antigen, whose 'haptenic' determinants interacted with B cell receptors. This could either occur with direct T-B contact, or indirectly with the 'carrier antibody' being released from the T cell. No formal test of the direct contact hypothesis was possible in 1971, and no direct test has yet been performed. However, a test to determine

whether effective help could occur without T-B contact was feasible in tissue culture, by separating T cells and B cells by a cell
impermeable membrane, which nevertheless permitted macromolecules
to pass through.

The results were unequivocal, and indicated that cell contact
was not essential. They did not rule out the possibility that cell
contact was an alternative pathway. The presence of helper
activity in the 'test tube' promised a rapid characterization of
the molecules involved but regrettably this aim has not been
fulfilled, for a variety of reasons. This communication discusses
the trials and tribulations of work in this field, and reviews
current concepts of the role of antigen specific helper factor.

2. BASIC OBSERVATION

In 1972, Feldmann and Basten (1972a) reported that in double
chamber cultures activated T cells, separated by a nucleopore
membrane of 0.1μ pore size, but not dialysis membranes, produced

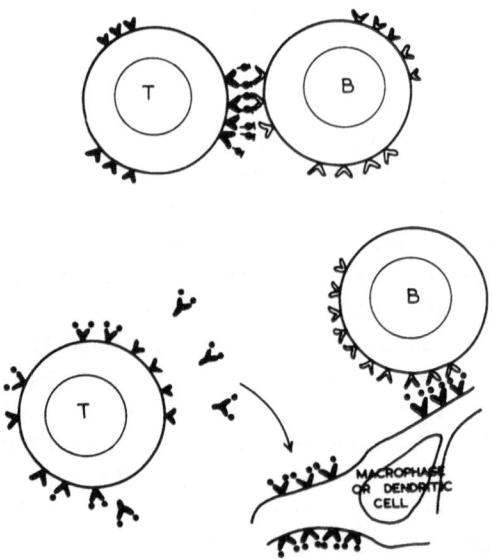

Fig. 1. Schematic models of T-B interaction, based upon the carrier
        effect. Above direct interaction of T and B cell receptors,
        below indirect interaction of T and B cell receptors. Re-
        printed from Feldmann, M., Transplant.Proc., V:43, 1973.

antigen-specific helper material to pass and induce B cell responses as efficiently as admixed T cells. This was demonstrated with red cell antigens, such as sheep red cells (SRC) and donkey red cells (DRC) or proteins, such as keyhole limpet haemocyanin (KLH) or fowl gamma globulin (FGG) using either primed or unprimed spleen cells depleted of T cells with anti-Thy-1 antiserum.
Fig. 2, reprinted from that original report, summarizes these results and also demonstrates that excess helper cells inhibited the response. These results excluded the necessity for cell contact, provided that leakage of helper cells across the membrane could be excluded. This was accomplished in a variety of ways, (Feldmann and Basten, 1972a), but most conclusively, by simplifying the protocols and using supernatants of helper cells which could be frozen and stored.

At around the same time, Schimpl and Wecker (1972) observed that mixed lymphocyte culture supernatants were able to restore the responses to SRC of nude mouse spleen cells. They termed this non antigen specific activity 'T cell replacing factor', or TRF.

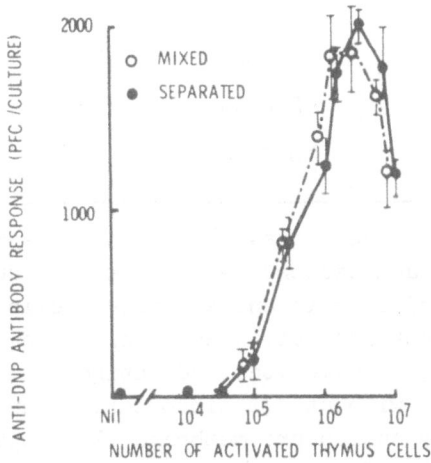

Fig. 2. Cell interactions across a cell impermeable membrane. Anti DNP response to DNP-KLH generated using KLH activated T cells and DNP Flagellon primed B cells, either cultured together (o – – o) or separated by a 1μ pore size nucleopore membrane (●——●). Note that excess T cells diminish the response. Reprinted from Feldmann, M. and Basten, A., J. Exp. Med., 136:49, 1972.

Table 1. Synergy of specific and non-specific factors.

| Culture chamber | | Antigen | Memb | Response | |
Upper	Lower			DNP	DRC
ATC$_{KLH}$	nude spleen	DNPKLH	DIALYSIS	20	120
"	"	DNPFGG	"	10	160
"	"	DNPFla	"	510	145
ATC$_{KLH}$+ nude	"	DNPKLH	"	100	860
"	"	DNPFGG	"	80	900
"	"	DNPFla	"	1640	1240
ATC$_{KLH}$+ nude	"	DNPKLH	NUCLEOPORE	890	1640
"	"	DNPFGG	"	0	880
"	"	DNPFla	"	2050	1080
ATC$_{FGG}$+ nude	"	DNPKLH	"	60	990
"	"	DNPFGG	"	950	1230
"	"	DNPFla	"	1850	1180

Double chambers were constructed in Marbrook flasks as described
elsewhere (Feldmann and Basten, 1972a) Unprimed nude spleen was
used as the source of B cells and accessory cells and cultured in
the bottom compartment and activated T cells from CBA irradiated
mice injected with CBA thymocytes and antigen cultured in the top
compartment, with or without histoincompatible nude spleen cells.
Dialysis membrane or nucleopore membrane (1) separated the two
compartments. With the former, only the thymus-independent response to DNPFlagellin was augmented, appreciably in the presence of
allogeneic interaction as well as the response to donkey red cells.
With the nucleopore membrane responses were increased with the
thymus-dependent DNP antigens provided that the appropriate specific T cells were present. Data redrawn from Feldmann and Basten,
1972 b, with permission.

We compared these activities using double chamber cultures, and it was found that their effects were quite distinct (Feldmann and Basten, 1972b). Mixed lymphocyte culture supernatants were sufficient to drive the response to erythrocyte antigens, and to the thymus-independent antigen, DNP-Flagellin, but not to thymus-dependent hapten-proteins e.g. DNP-KLH. The latter antigens required the supernatant of specific helper cells if responses were to be elicited. These results are summarized in Table 1, reproduced from Feldmann and Basten (1972b). The conclusion from this study was that, while non antigen specific factors were sufficient to restore the response of nude spleen to red cells, (and augmented the response to thymus-independent antigens), responses to hapten-proteins additionally required antigen specific factors. The two types of factor were separable on the basis of molecular size, as only the 'allogeneic factor' activity passed through dialysis membranes. Partly because 'allogeneic factor' by itself did not induce responses to hapten proteins, while it augmented already initiated responses, such as those to red cells, it was concluded that induction of B cell responses was due to antigen specific helper factor, while expansion was due to the non-specific factor (Feldmann and Basten, 1972b).

The nature of the antigen specific factor, and its target of action was investigated. Depletion of adherent cells in the B cell compartment abrogated the response to specific helper factor (HF) (Feldmann, 1972). Peritoneal exudate cells restored this response indicating that macrophage like cells were required in order to induce B cells. Absorption experiments indicated that 'macrophages' absorbed HF.

Experiments to examine the nature of the HF indicated that some antisera against Ig, μ chains or antigen abrogated the helper effect (Feldmann, 1972). These results suggested that HF was a complex of antigen and an IgM like entity. On basis of surface radioiodination of activated T cells releasing HF, it was found that material of 150,000 dalton, reactive with anti μ was obtained which bound to the surface of macrophages. It was inferred that the entity was HF (Feldmann, et al. 1973), although this could not be tested directly.

Table 2. A brief history of mouse antigen-specific helper factors.

Nomenclature	Author		Characteristics						
			Ag binding	IgV	IgC	MW	Ia	GR	Target
IgX (theoretical)	Bretscher & Cohn	1968,							
	Mitchison et al.	1970	+	+	+	NR	NR	NR	?
IgT	Feldmann & Basten	1972	+	NT	μ	?150K	NR	NT	AC
"	Taniguchi & Tada	1974	+	NT	μ	100-200K	NT	NT	?
HF	Taussig & Munro	1975	+	-	-	50K	I-A	-	B
"	Mozes	1976	+	+	-	50K	I-A	-	B
"	Howie & Feldmann	1977	+	+	Chicken	70K	I-A or I-J	-	AC (Ir+)
"	Shiozawa & Diener	1978	+	NT	NT	50K		+	+
"	Lonai et al.	1980	+	+	-				
"	Andersson & Melchers	1981	+	+	-	125K	-	+	NT

Conclusion: Heterogeneity of GR, Ia, MW, IgC and target

Similar results obtained by Kilburn and Levy, McDougal and Gordon, Rieber and Riethmuller

3. PROBLEMS VS CHARACTERISTICS OF HELPER FACTORS AND THEIR ACTIONS

3.1. Reproducibility Problem

It has been implied that specific helper factor assays are
'very difficult' and can only be performed in occasional laboratories. This was certainly not our initial experience at the
Walter and Eliza Hall Institute in Australia, but our experience
in London and of others elsewhere is that there have been spans
of time when these assays do not work. Much the same can be said
for virtually all complex in vitro immunological technology - from
growing T cell lines in TCGF to fusing myeloma cells to yield
hybridomas - the number of experimental failure are very numerous,
although never formally recorded - due to imperfections in media
and incubators, infection "in vitro" and mouse infections which
activate macrophages, release prostaglandins and carry mycoplasma
and viruses into cultures, etc. Much the same can be said for some
"in vivo" experiments, such as producing irradiation chimaeras.

The reasons for the failures are not difficult to appreciate
-HF can only be titrated if all the other parameters are functional - resting B cells (Feldmann and Basten, 1972b; Andersson and
Melchers, 1981), adequate media, sera and cofactors, culture conditions, assays etc. The same holds for other "in vitro" techno-

logy, which cannot be performed without sufficient commitment of time and resources.

Within these constraints, it is interesting to note that many independent groups have overcome these problems, and a brief summary is listed in Table 2, which also summarizes the variable characteristics of the HF reported. No less than 10 independent groups have described rodent helper factors for IgM/IgG responses, and others have reported IgE specific helper factors and primate helper factors (Table 2). Others have reported antigen specific factors involved in cell mediated responses (e.g. Kindred and Corley, 1977; Kilburn et al. 1979).

3.2. Are Helper Factors 'Secreted', or are They Shed Membrane Receptors?

The demonstration of cell free supernatants with helper activity (Fig. 2, Table 1), active "in vitro", form an 'a priori' case that help does not involve T-B contact. However it is not sufficient 'proof', as it can be argued that the same molecules present in the supernatant would trigger just as efficiently when they are still on the cell surface.

Several lines of argument have tendend to point towards an active release of helper factors. Initially, it was shown that metabolic inhibitors such as actinomycin A, an irreversible inhibitor of protein synthesis, or actinomycin D, an irreversible inhibitor of DNA dependent RNA synthesis, and hence of protein synthesis requiring new messenger RNA inhibited help (Feldmann and Basten, 1972c), whether the T cells were mixed or separated from B cells by a membrane (Feldmann and Basten, 1972 a,c). This indicated that passive membrane shedding of T cell receptors was not sufficient to yield help and that factor release was a more active process.

More recent studies while still not definite, again do not support the concept that helper factors are shed T cell receptors. A very indirect argument comes from dilution analysis: titres of helper factors can be higher than those of the helper cells from which they are derived (Howie and Feldmann, 1977; Fisher et al., 1981). This suggests a continuous secretion of factors.

It was found that human TCGF-dependent helper lines reactive to Influenza A strain viruses, yield high titres of HF, after 18 hours culture in horse serum either in the absence or presence of antigen (A/X31 virus). However, 10-100 times more HF was obtained after restimulation with E⁻ cells (B cells and monocytes) of the appropriate donor. As the T line cells are much healthier and more viable in the presence of their antigen and accessory cells, these results are most compatible with an active release of factor.

Proteolytic inhibitors such as aprotinin do not reduce the titres of factors, which may have been expected if factors are proteolytically cleaved from the cell membranes. Adult serum, as used in the cultures would also be expected to contain a number of proteolytic enzyme inhibitors. However a definitive understanding of the relationship of factor to receptor awaits further biochemical analysis, until HF can be biosynthetically labelled, and receptors biosynthetically and surface labelled.

3.3. Role of Helper Factor "in vivo"

"In vitro" analysis has the advantage that cell interactions can be identified, as can molecular messengers. However there are major difficulties in extrapolating back to "in vivo" system with their greater complexity of lymphoid architecture, cell trafficking and the like. If the concept of multiplicity of pathways is accepted, with lymphocyte triggering induced by a number of different combinations of 'signals', then it cannot be assumed that the results obtained with a single "in vitro" system, with its arbitary yet critical parameters of cell density, sera and media, reflects the entire complexity of the lymphoid function. However, it is equally unlikely that the mechanisms uncovered "in vitro" do not operate under some circumstances "in vivo".

Within these constraints of interpretation, it has been demonstrated that HF does stimulate antibody production "in vivo" (Taussig, 1974; Taussig et al., 1979). Most of these experiments have involved irradiated mice, repopulated with cells preincubated in factor "in vitro" or in the syringe, so that the relevance to the situation in intact animals is not entirely clear.

Attempts to induce responses in non-irradiated mice with HF have been relatively disappointing, as only 2-3 fold augmentation has been obtained (Woody et al., 1979). However, this may be the best possible stimulation, if other components of the immune induction pathway, which would be released by helper cells, are not also injected, such as non-specific factors involved in activating B cells (Schimpl and Wecker, 1972). It is also important to note that intravenously injected factor does not necessarily home to the appropriate site of the lymphoid tissue. It would also be subject to catabolism, and so it is unlikely that any 'single' injection would ever yield the high local concentrations of HF achieved by cells releasing factor into their immediate environment, which as it is cytophilic (Feldmann et al., 1973), would be retained locally. Multiple injections would help overcome problems of catabolism.

It is interesting to note that the effects of other entities immunologically active "in vitro", are even more uncertain "in vivo". We are not aware of any reports of T cell replacing factor (TRF) or allogenic effect factors (AEF) injected "in vivo". Antigen suppressor factors have been reported to work "in vivo", but their effects are not incredibly dramatic in the effector phase (e.g. Kapp et al., 1977; Theze et al., 1977).

3.4. MHC Restriction or Recognition

There is much evidence that in some instances T cell help of B cells is genetically restricted, while it is not in others (reviewed Sprent, 1978). The reasons for these differences are not fully resolved, but it would appear that cellular heterogeneity may explain differences. For example, Singer et al. (1981) have shown that Lyb5$^+$ cells are not restricted, whereas Lyb5$^-$ cells are.

Results with antigen specific helper factors have been as varied as those with T cells. As shown in Table 2, some HF effects are non restricted, while others are restricted. The reasons for this difference are not yet known, but could reflect a heterogeneity of the T helper cell pool. This pool is increasingly known to be highly heterogeneous: for example Schreier et al. (1981) have reported 30 egg albumin specific TCGF-dependent T cell clones, which help antibody responses in 3 clear cut patterns, i.e. some help SRC responses only, some help responses to both SRC and thymus-independent antigens while others help SRC and thymus-independent antigen as well providing egg albumin specific help in a hapten carrier system.

This degree of heterogeneity has also been fould with human TCGF-dependent T cell lines reactive to influenza virus, where some lines generate only antigen specific HF, while others generate in addition, non specific help (Fischer et al., 1981).
One individual has been of interest as cell lines were generated which helped specifically in a genetically restricted manner and other in an unrestricted manner.

The reasons for the unrestricted action of some HF (Mozes et al.,1975;Howie and Feldmann,1977) but not others (Shiozawa et al., 1977; Geha, 1979; Andersson and Melchers, 1981; Fischer et al., 1981) is not known. It is possible that these 2 types of factors should be viewed in the same way as subclasses of other groups of molecules, such as IgG. However without more information, it is possible to discriminate this from two other possibilities.
i) Lack of genetic restriction is due to mixtures of factors: non-specific activation of B cells, by factors from T cells, or by serum components, may abrogate genetic restriction. This was shown to be the case with influenza cell line H , which yielded a restricted HF of 70,000 daltons, and non-restricted helper activity in the range of 20,000 daltons (Fig. 3). The mixture acted as a non-restricted specific factor in all but the highest concentrations.
ii) Partial degradation: restricted HF may have two binding sites, one for Ia, another for antigen, whereas unrestricted HF may have only the latter. Analysis of MW data does not clarify this issue as yet, as restricted HF may have MW varying from 50,000 to 125,000 daltons (Table 2).

At the moment it is possible to discriminate between these possibilities. The situation with suppressor factors is analogous, with reports of restricted and unrestricted factors (see Kontiainen and Feldmann, 1978).

3.5. Cellular Target of Helper Factor

While the eventual functional target of HF is the B cell which is triggered to produce antibody, the immediate target is still not known with any certainty. Attempts to investigate this question have not yielded any consensus. We found in 1972 that adherent cell depleted spleen cells were not triggered by HF (Feldmann and Basten, 1972a) and that peritoneal exudate cells adsorbed sufficient HF to subsequently trigger B cells (Feldmann, 1972). On re-examining this question with HF to antigens under Ir gene control, we confirmed these observations and noted that only high responder adherent cells would trigger responder B cells (Howie and Feldmann, 1978).

Taussig and associates have suggested that HF acts directly on B cells, on the basis of absorption with bone marrow cells (Taussig et al., 1974). This cell population contains abundant accessory cells and so these results do not necessarily implicate a direct B cell target. Experiments with anti-Ig treated lymph node cells do not discriminate between either possibility, and it remains to be ascertained whether HF interacts with accessory cells, B cells, or both.

Shiozawa et al. (1977) have reported that HF acts directly on B cells provided Interleukin is present on the basis that HF triggered the response of small number (2000) of rosette forming cells which would mostly be B cells. However, these results do not determine the initial cellular target, and can be reconciled with an accessory cell target, as it is likely that one role of HF is as a signal for the release of IL-1. There is evidence to support this suggestion, as cytophilic HF-like products of T cell tumours were found to augment the IgG response of spleen cell cultures in a non-antigen-specific manner (Feldmann et al., 1975).

3.6. Role of Accessory Cells in HF Function

So far, the available data includes a role for accessory cells in HF action, although the precise type of accessory cell involved, or the nature of their role is not known at present. The limited data available merely indicates that not all accessory cells are capable of binding HF. Thus Cone et al. (1974) found that only a subpopulation of peritoneal cells bound radiolabelled T cell surface material. As there is evidence that HF requires Ir gene expressing accessory cells (Howie and Feldmann, 1978) whose function is abrogated by treatment with anti-Ia antisera (Howie, Parish and Feldmann, unpublished data), it seems likely that the relevant accessory cells bear Ia antigens.

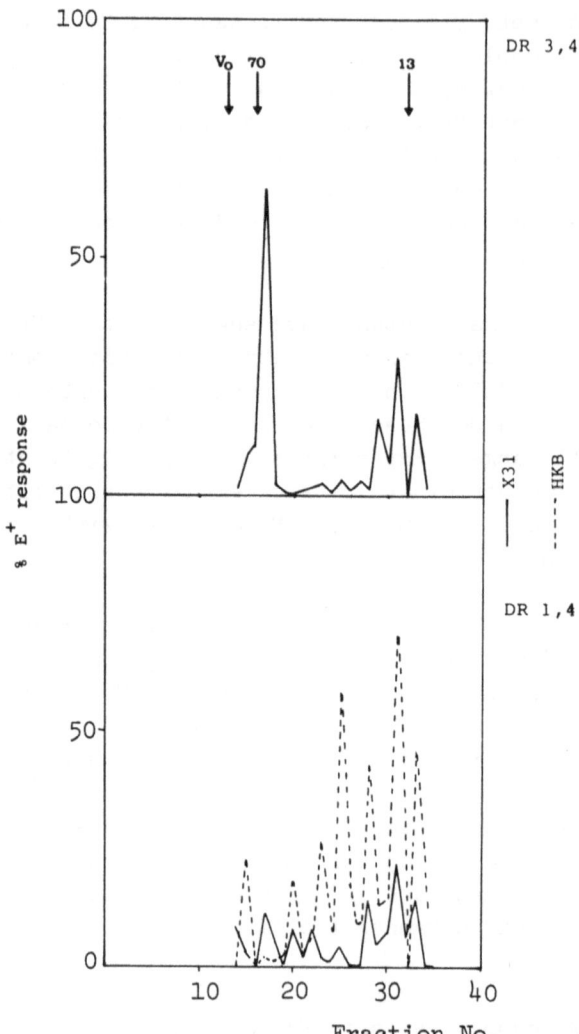

Fig. 3. Antibody response of human peripheral blood cells to Influenza virus in vitro induced by a genetically restricted
HF (——) response to A/X31 virus (---) response to HKB virus.
Top graph: Response of an HLA-D3,4 individual to or HF derived from an HLA-D3,7 helper T cell line reacting to A/X31.
The HLA-D3 specificity is shared. Peaks of activity at about
70 K daltons and around 10-20 K daltons.
Bottom graph: Response of an HLA-D1,4 individual to the
same factor from the HLA-D3,7 cell line. Peaks to both antigens are only detected at 10-20 K daltons. The 70 K dalton
HF (top graph is thus both restricted and antigen specific).

A variety of antigen trapping accessory cells have been
described in the lymphoid tissues, distinct from classical macro
phages. Dendritic follicular cells have long processes intert-
wining throughout the follicles, and marginal zone macrophages
have long processes in the marginal zone. Both these cells are
present in the B cell areas and would be involved in B cell triggering, rather than the interdigitating dendritic cells present in
the T cell areas (see Immunol. Reviews, Vol 53 on Accessory
cells). As techniques for isolating the various accessory cells
have been developed (Steinman and Cohn, 1973; Humphrey, 1981) it
should be possible to determine which accessory cell reacts with
HF. Based on the experiments of Shiozawa et al. (1977), the major
role of the accessory cells may be to generate IL-1 locally. HF
may be a trigger for the release of IL-1.

3.7. Nature of Helper Factor

Essentially all the information available was obtained by
simple procedures, e.g. immunoadsorption and column chromatogra-
phy, coupled with bioassays. To date T cell lines or hybridomas
have confirmed functional data, but have not yet permitted further
biochemical characterization.

Serological analyses, while easy to perform, are very difficult to interpret. The chief problem lies in the unknown, and
presumable very low, concentration of factor (ng or pg/ml) which
causes serological problems, as antisera usually cannot be assayed
by other techniques for such low levels of contaminants, and it is
always possible that contaminating antibodies in the sera may be
responsible for some of the reactions observed.

Serology: IgG_H .The earliest serological experiments were
mixing experiments which tested whether antisera would block
binding HF to peritoneal exudate cells, and prevent them from
subsequently immunizing cultures. These experiments indicated that
polyvalent rabbit anti-Ig, anti-μ and anti-K antisera reacted with
HF (Feldmann, 1972). These initial studies were performed with
only one anti serum of each type, and led to the notion that HF
was IgM like.

However, subsequent analysis by immunoadsorption revealed
that the reaction with anti-Ig reagents was variable: we have

found some anti-μ reagents which react with HF (e.g. Greaves et al., 1974), but others which do not. Other workers have also found this serological cross reaction, e.g. Rieber and Riethmuller (1974), Taniguchi and Tada (1974) in the rat; Zanders et al. (1980) in monkeys. However, other did not detect reactivity with the antisera they had available, e.g. Taussig and Munro (1974), Mozes et al. (1975), McDougal and Gordon (1977), Andersson and Melchers (1981).

In some experiments, chicken, but not rabbit, antisera to Ig reacted with HF, e.g. Howie and Feldmann (1977). As it is known that chicken antisera contain a high proportion of anti-carbo-hydrate antibodies, there is a possibility that all the anti-Ig reactions may due to anti-carbohydrate antibodies cross-reacting with the carbohydrate part of HF. Layton (1980) demonstrated with one chicken anti-Ig antiserum reacting with T cells, that the antibodies which stained thymus cells were all anti-carbohydrate. It is not known if all reports of chicken antisera reacting with thymus (e.g. Marchalonis et al., 1980; Hammerling, 1976) are due to anti-carbohydrate antibodies, but this remains a strong possi-bility.

Recent studies which have indicated that HF bears V_H and Idiotypic determinants (reviewed Feldmann and Kontianen, 1981) may provide another explanation for the variable reactions of HF with anti Ig antisera: the minor subpopulation of antibodies to the variable reaction in the antisera may react with the 'V_H -like' region of HF.

An alternative interpretation is that the 'constant region' of HF (see Kontiainen and Feldmann, 1979) is cross reactive with μ chain sequences, as HF and μ chains may both be products of descendents of common ancestral genes. Such a possibility is reinforced by recent experiments which demonstrated that some anti-human β_2 microglobulin antisera, and a monoclonal anti-β_2 microglobulin antibody preparation, reacted with helper factor (Lamb et al., 1981).

To summarize, the reaction of anti-μ reagents with HF, where it is detected, is currently not well understood, and could be due to anti-V_H or anti-carbohydrate antibodies, or may be detecting conserved sequences indicating a common ancestral origin of HF and chains. Studies with monoclonal anti-μ may be informative.

Serology: IgV_H . Various rabbit antisera raised against the variable region MOPC 315 by Givol and Ben-Neriah (Ben-Neriah et al., 1978) have been shown to react with T cells, notably antibodies against V_H . These also react with HF (Feldmann et al., 1979., Eshhar et al., 1980 and Andersson and Melchers, 1981).

There is a contrasting report from Taussig and associates; in the mouse, anti-F_V antibodies, which did not react with T cells by fluorescence (McConnell et al., 1975) did not absorb HF, and rabbit anti-a allotype antibodies (a variable region allotype) did not react with rabbit HF. In contrast to the latter, it was found by Krawinkel et al. (1977) that rabbit T cell receptors to nylon nets coupled with NP were reactive with anti-a-allotype antibody, an allotype marker in the F_V region.

Idiotype markers. Mozes and Haimovich (1979) detected the (T,G)-A--L idiotype marker on HF reactive to (T,G)-A--L. The phosphorylcholine (PC) idiotype marker found on myeloma T15 was found on HF_{PC} (Feldmann et al., 1979). Human HF to tetanus toxoid bears the anti-tetanus idiotype marker (Geha, 1979).

Ia antigen. Munro, Taussig and colleagues (1974) were first to demonstrate that anti Ia antisera react with HF. Since then, the basic observations have been confirmed, but their significance is still not fully appreciated. Detailed analysis, using anti I subregion antisera initially demonstrated that anti I-A antisera absorbed HF specific for the synthetic polypeptide (T,G)-A--L. Subsequently, it was noted that HF specific for another synthetic antigen, GAT, reacted with anti I-J antisera (Howie et al., 1979). By reactivity with anti I-A or anti I-J, two classes of HF were defined, with two antigens (GAT and the hapten NP) reacting with anti I-J antisera, and others - (T,G)-A--L, KLH, streptococcal antigen - with other I-A antisera. The significance of this difference remains obscure (Feldmann and Kontiainen, 1981).

Parish and McKenzie (1977) have described rabbit antisera which recognise Ia antigens present in the dialyzable portion of serum. Analyses indicate that the Ia determinants were carbohydrate in nature (reviewed Parish et al., 1981). While Parish was on sabbatical in London, he found that his antisera reacted with HF (Howie et al., 1979). However, there was not time to prove that this was due to anti-carbohydrate antibodies, as sugar inhibition experiments were not performed. But in view of the glycoprotein nature of HF, and of its relatively low MW to incorporate numerous antigenic determinants, the possibility that the Ia of factors is carbohydrate in nature, remains until proven or excluded by bio-chemical analysis.

In the past two to three years numerous monoclonal antibodies to Ia controlled antigens have been produced by various groups. Some of these have been tested on HF. The results of these studies have not been systematically reported, but at least one, 10.3.6, an anti I-A^K, reacts with HF. Others also react (Lonai et al., 1981).

The simplest interpretation of the anti Ia serology is that HF contains Ia antigenic determinants. It seems clear that HF cannot contain a whole $\beta-\alpha$ chain complex of MW 55,000, as found on B cells, as this is in the same MW range as HF, and such chains have not been identified in HF preparations. One possibility is that only a part of Ia is present, and we have recent evidence to support this, based on data with a panel of monospecific or monoclonal mouse anti human Ia antisera, of which some, but not all, were found to react with HF (Fischer et al, unpublished data).

In view of the fact that HF may also recognise Ia, in order also to have target restriction allied to Ia, it is possible that the anti Ia antisera reactions with HF have been misleading. Such antisera would be expected to contain, based on network concepts, some anti-idiotype antibodies, reacting against the combining site of the anti Ia antibodies. These may react with an anti Ia combining site of HF. This possibility could be excluded by use of anti Ia monoclonal supernatants, and not ascites. We do not know whether this issue has yet been clarified. Certainly the results have not been published by July 1981.

Miscellaneous. Other reagents have been shown to react with T cell products. Protein A derived from Staphylococcus aureus Cowan I strain was found by Cone et al. (1981) to react with a suppressor factor, and we have noted this reaction with both suppressor factors and helper factors, but not with all factors of any type (Cecka et al., unpublished). This reaction complicates biochemical analysis of factors, as the usual precipitations with antisera/antibodies and protein A cannot be performed. As protein A reacts with immunoglobulins of most species (classes vary between species), this reaction suggests that T cell factors contain sequences which resemble immunoglobulin sequences. Fig. 4 shows some of these results with a human HF.

Another puzzling serological reaction is that between anti-sera to β_2-microglobulin and helper factors. This was found by Lamb et al. (1981) with both monkey and mouse HF, and has been extended to human HF (Zanders, Lamb, Fisher, Sanderson and Feldmann, un-published data). The initial results were obtained with a panel of immunochemically purified antibodies raised against human β_2-mi-croglobulin in different species of experimental animals, with the aim of raising antibodies against different determinants on the β_2-microglobulin molecule. With these antisera, and one monoclonal mouse antibody (M8), it was found that monkey HF reacted with chicken, rat and rabbit antibody and the mouse monoclonal but not with guinea pig antibody, whereas mouse HF reacted with chicken antibody but not with rabbit antibody or the monoclonal.

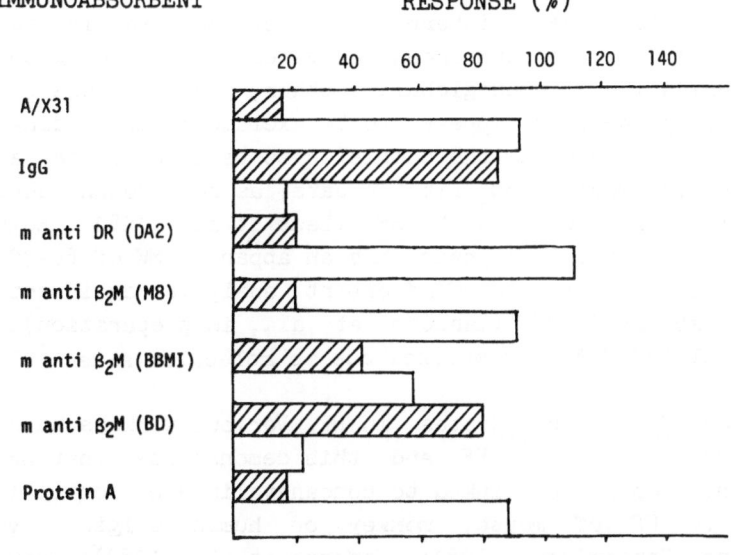

Fig. 4. Serological analysis of Human HF. Influenza A strain specific HF from a long term T cell line, F_7 was passed over Immunoadsorbent columns of antigen, or various monoclonal antibodies as indicated. Hatched bars indicate material which
flowed through i.e. not absorbed, open column the eluted material. Note that some anti-β_2M react, some do not. Protein
A reacts.

Table 3. Primate helper factors.

Report	Characteristics						
	Ag	IgV	IgC	MW	Ia	GR	Target
Geha et al., 1978–80	+	+	−	50K	DR$^+$	+	NT
Kantor & Feldmann 1979	+	NT	−	70K	Ia$^+$	−	NT
Zanders et al., 1980	+	NT		70K	Ia$^+$	−	NT
Fischer et al., 1981	+	NT	±	70K	Ia$^+$	+	NT
Heijnen et al., 1981	+	NT	NT	70K	Ia$^+$	−	NT

With human HF, we have concentrated on monoclonals and are beginning to test a panel of mouse anti human β_2-microglobulin monoclonals. Some preliminary results are shown in Fig. 4. M8 binds all HF, BBM1 shows partial binding, and BD no absorption of a human HF. The simplest interpretation of these results is that HF is derived from the same ancestral genes as β_2-microglobulin, and its derivative, immunoglobulin. Other, possibly less controversial, interpretations appear to be excluded; HLA binding non-specifically to HF, causing the complexes to be absorbed to anti-β_2-microglobulin would not fit the data, as some potent anti-β_2--microglobulin did not absorb HF (Lamb et al., 1981). Human HF fractionated by size in Sephadex has an apparent MW of 60-70,000. This was subjected to immunoadsorbent analysis: again anti-β_2M monoclonals absorbed HF (Zanders et al., in preparation). This excludes a role of HLA-β_2 complexes due to molecular size.

Evidence for carbohydrates in HF. Various workers have used lectin columnes to bind HF and this demonstrates that HF is a glycoprotein. Sepharose linked to concanavalin A or lentil lectin will bind to HF of mouse, monkey or human origin (reviewed Feldmann and Kontiainen, 1981; Zanders et al., 1980). Enzymatic treatment has also suggested that the HF is a glycprotein since neuraminidase was found to abrogate HF activity (Zanders et al., 1980). Proteolytic activity in the neuraminidase was not excluded, but is not likely as the HF preparations contain 5% serum.
There has not yet been any detailed analys is of the carbohydrate composition of HF.

Molecular weight. As shown in Table 2 and 3, MW estimates for HF have ranged widely from 50,000-200,000 daltons. As all of these are based on bioassays, and as the HF activity was unstable these results have to be interpreted cautiously. There is no information available as to the valency of HF, and it is possible that the higher MW estimates are for divalent HF, and the lower for monovalent HF. Alternatively, it is possible that the higher MW estimates involved MHC and antigen recognition sites coupled together while in the case of lower estimates these are separated. In the view of the above gaps in our information there is no definitive knowledge as to peptide chain composition.

Nature of HF - Summary. We have marshalled evidence for a two region model of factor structure (Feldmann et al., 1981), and the evidence still fits this hypothesis. The recognition site for Ia in genetically restricted factors is not understood, whether it is an immunoglobulin V region, or a totally different structure. A representation of this concept is shown in Figure 5.

For a variety of reasons we believe that the constant region has resemblances to Ig constant regions based on the immunoadsorbtion data already discussed.

7. Heterogeneity of Helper Factor

There is evidence that T cell function is highly heterogeneous,

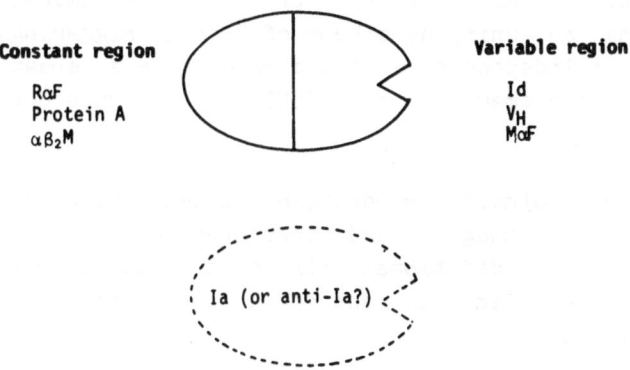

Fig. 5. A minimal model of Antigen Specific Factor. Valency not known, nor the exact nature of Ia or anti Ia.

even within the augmentation pathway. T cell clones may help in
different ways (Schreier et al., 1981) although the full extent of
this heterogeneity is not yet known. Thus it is not inconceivable
that there may be different 'subclasses' of antigen secific helper
factors to explain the different observations (see Table 1).
However there is as yet no compelling reason to invoke this. The
discrepant results (e.g. MW, genetic restriction or not, cross
reactivity with Ig) can at the moment all be explained on the
basis of partly degraded factors, or mixtures of HF and other
activating entities.

Further work with monoclonal T cells and with monoclonal
antifactor antibodies should clarify this issue. It seems likely,
however, that T cell enhancing factors which modulate responses
(i.e. alter Ig class and subclass) only in the presence of helper
cells (e.g. Tokuhisa et al., 1978) are different from HF. This
would fit in with reports of T cells modulating class/subclass
(e.g. Rosenberg and Chiller, 1979).

Many of the biological effects of HF may be mimicked by
'allogeneic effect factor', AEF, initially described by Katz and
his colleague (Armerding and Katz, 1974), but more recently
analysed by Delovitch and his colleagues (1981).The data at
present do not exclude the possibility that AEF is an antigen
specific HF, with Ia as its target.

3.9. Mechanism of HF Action

Our initial model of the action of HF (Feldmann, 1972) aimed
at providing an unifying scheme of B cell triggering, whether it
was by thymus independent antigens which have a repeating array of
determinants (Feldmann et al., 1975) or by thymus dependent antigens.

In this hypothesis, HF-antigen complexes were arranged on the
surface of macrophages, and presented a repeating array of
determinants. An addditional virtue of this concept was that it
yielded a mechanism for antigenic competition (Feldmann and
Schrader, 1974).

It is not clear where this model stands at present. There is
no doubt that B cells are readily stimulated by polymers with

repeating determinants (e.g. Feldmann et al., 1974) but evidence has accumulated to suggest that the B cells responding to thymus--independent antigens and to thymus-dependent antigens are not identical (Gorczyinski and Feldmann, 1975; Tittle and Rittenberg, (1978); Mosier et al., 1977). Thus the requirement to have a single mechanism of triggering both types of B cells is no longer essential. A visual representation of our concept of the molecules involved and their receptors is shown in Fig. 6.

There is evidence that IL-1 is of major importance in the triggering of B cells (Wood and Cameron, 1978) and a reasonable hypothesis is that HF presents antigen which induces the release of IL-1 and possible other activating signals. Further analysis with highly purified preparations of HF will be essential to clarify mechanisms of action.

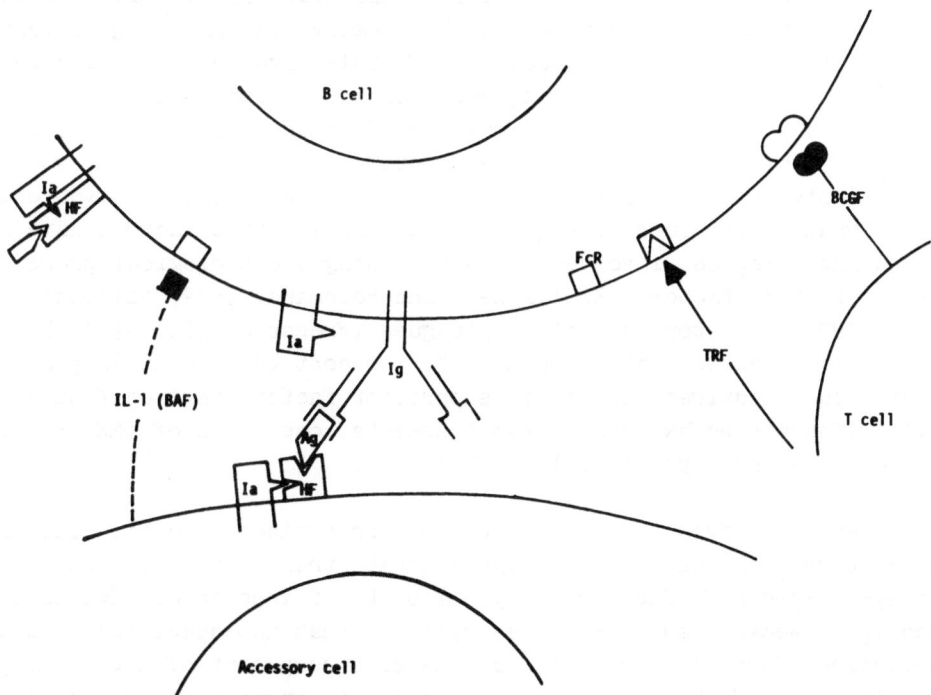

Fig. 6. A schematic representation of the molecules involved in T
        cell help, and their receptors. HF: antigen specific helper
        factor; IL-1: Interleukin - 1,B cell Activating Factor; FcR:
        Fc receptors; TRF: 'T cell replacing' factor; BCGF: B cell
        growth factor.

3.10. Experiments which do not fit in with 'HF' Concept

The virtues of the 'HF' concept is that it provides an amplifying mechanism for interlinking rare cells, and reconciles complex cell interactions with the known architecture and recirculation patterns of the lymphoid system.

Certain observations have been interpreted to argue against the relevance or importance of HF in B cell triggering.The first of these was based on the genetic restriction of T-B interaction. Katz and his colleagues (e.g. Katz et al., 1974) suggested that as HF was not known to be genetically restricted, it could not be active "in vivo". This argument is based on a single component or mechanism of help, and the limitations are apparent. The subsequent discovery of genetically restricted HF renders the proposition invalid.

More recently the possibility has been raised that B cells may present antigen, and again this observation only argues very indirectly against the concept of HF. This argument is elaborated by Mitchison in this volume, and this has already been discussed at length in this volume (comment by Feldmann, following Mitchison's article). Again these experiments, if generally valid, would only imply that HF must contain the signal for T cell activation. This would fit in perfectly with our concept that factors have a 'constant' region involved in determining the biological properties of the factor (Kontiainen and Feldmann, 1979; Feldmann et al., 1979). Cantor and his colleagues (Fresno et al., 1981) have pro- vided additional evidence to support this idea. They have found that antigen specific suppressor factors derived from a T cell line may break down to two fragments, one which of (MW 45,000 daltons) was non specifically suppressive.

Certain advocates of the role of non antigen specific factors have been reluctant to recognise that other components, such as antigen specific factors, may also be of importance. Initially Schimpl, Wecker and associates believed that non specific' T cell replacing factor', or TRF, was the sole component of T cell help (Schimpl and Wecker, 1972) on the basis of experiments, first with red cell antigens, and subsequently, with very recently primed B cells. However, it was shown that certain responses, e.g. to haptenated proteins, could not be generated "in vitro" with TRF or non specific factors alone, and that there was synergy between

antigen specific and non specific cells and factors. (Waldmann and
Munro, 1975; Waldmann et al., 1976). More recently, other workers
have shown that B cell blasts can be induced to produce Ig by
non-antigen specific and genetically unrestricted factors (Melchers et al., 1980), On that basis, it was suggested that the role
of antigen specific factors (if there was a role) must be restricted to turn the resting B cell into a blast cell (Schreier et al.,
1981). It is interesting to note that this is exactly what our
concept has been for many years (Feldmann and Basten, 1972). Our
view is that the evidence for the existence of antigen specific HF
is overwhelming, and that it cannot easily be shaken by the 'odd'
data that does not easily fit in. However, that does not imply
that we fully understand the role of HF. Rather, acceptance of the
basic observations permits us to focus more avidly on the great
gaps in our understanding of the nature, function and mode of
action of HF, and its relevance in immune regulation.

4. CONCLUSIONS : PROSPECTS

     Immunology in the 1970's has not been able to provide answers
to a number of immunological problems, despite much effort. Thus
there is still much controversy, for example the nature of the T
cell receptor(s) for antigen, the role of the thymus in the
development of the T cell repertoire, the relevance of idiotypic
networks to the regulation of immune responses, etc, as well as
about the nature and relevance of HF.

     Recent methodological advances have increased the prospect
for resolving these controversies, and it seems likely that many
of the problems, caused by the lack of available material and its
heterogeneity, may be overcome in the near future. Thus T cell
lines generated by cell fusion, viral oncogenesis, or by using
growth factors will be highly useful. Recent developments in this
field have been recently reviewed by the active proponents (see
Lymphokines, Vol 5) and it seems unnecessary to elaborate these in
detail. The existence of cloned T cells in large numbers with
helper activity, should yield answers to the problems of the
nature of T cell receptors and factors. They should also yield
sufficient material to understand the mechanisms by which these
molecules function as receptors, transducers, etc.

     Monoclonal antibodies offer another promising approach to furthering our understanding of T cell factors. We have begun to develop a panel of such reagents, and our initial efforts are documented elsewhere (Feldmann et al., 1981; James et al., in preparation).

Possibly by the time of the next conference on this topic much more insight into T cell immune regulation will have been gained by the use of newer techniques. A practical guide to the depth of understanding which has been reached, is the efficiency with which the information can be applied. There are many clear cut examples of disordered immune regulation in the autoimmune diseases of man and experimental animals. These are profound tests of our understanding of immune regulation, and we expect that it will take some time before their immunological abnormalities can be logically controlled by applying a profound understanding of immune regulation.

ACKNOWLEDGEMENTS

This work was supported by the Imperial Cancer Research Fund, MRC, Wellcome Trust, Arthritis Foundation, and National Institutes of Health, Grants A1-15636, 15653 and 13145.

REFERENCES

Andersson, J., and Melchers, F., 1981, T cell-dependent activation of resting B cells: requirement for both non-specific Ia-restricted soluble factors, Proc. Natl. Acad. Sci., 78:2497.

Andersson, J., Schreier, M.H., and Melchers, F., 1980, T cell dependent B cell stimulation is H2 restricted and antigen-dependent only at the resting B cell level, Proc. Natl. Acad. Sci., U.S.A., 77:1612.

Armerding, D., and Katz, D.H., 1974, Activation of T and B lymphocyte "in vitro". II. Biological and biochemical properties of an allogeneic effect factor (AEF) active in triggered specific B lymphocyte, J. Exp. Med., 140:19.

Ben-Neriah, Y., Wilmart, C., Lonai, P. and Givol, D., 1978, Preparation and characterisation of anti-framework antibodies to the heavy chain variable-region (VH) of mouse immunoglobulins, Eur. J. Immunol., 8:797.

Cone, R.E., Feldmann, M., Marchalonis, J.J., and Nossal, G.J.V.,

1974, Adherence of T cell receptor Ig to the macrophages surface, Immunology, 26:49.

Cone, R.E., Murray, J., Rosenstein, R.W.Ptak, W., Iverson, G.M.,
and Gersham, R.K., The use of heteroantisera to T cell antigen
binding proteins as probes for T cell receptors, in: "Immunoglobulin idiotypes and their suppression", C. Janeway, E. sercarz, H. Wigzell, L.C.F. Fox, Eds. Academic Press, in press.

Delovitch, T.L., 1980, Ia antigens: signals for lymphocyte communication, Compendium in Immunology, 3:5.

Eshhar, Z., Apte, R.N., Lowy, I., Ben-Neriah, Y., Givol, D. and
Mozes, E., 1980, T cell hybridoma bearing heavy chain variable
region determinants producing (T, G)-A--L specific helper factor, Nature, (London), 286:270.

Feldmann, M., 1972, Cell interaction in the immune response "in
vitro". V. Specific collaboration with complexes of antigen
and thymus derived cell immunoglobulin, J. Exp. Med., 136:737.

Feldmann, M., and Basten, A., 1972a, Cell interaction in the immune
response "in vitro". III. Specific co-operation across a cell
impermeable membrane, J. Exp. Med., 136:49.

Feldmann, M. and Basten, A., 1972b, Cell interaction in the immune
response "in vitro". IV. Comparison of the effects of antigen
specific and allogeneic thymus-derived cell factors, J. Exp.
Med., 136:722.

Feldmann, M. and Basten, S., 1972c, Cell interaction in the immune
response "in vitro". I. Metabolic activities of T cells in a
collaborative antibody response, Eur. J. Immunol., 2:213.

Feldmann, M., Boylston, A., and Hogg, N.M., 1975, Immunological
effects of IgT synthesized by theta positive cell lines,
Eur. J. Immunol., 5:429.

Feldmann, M., Cone, R.E. and Marchalonis, J.J., 1973, Cell interaction in the immune response "in vitro". IV. Mediation by T cell
surface IgM, Cell. Immunol., 9:1.

Feldmann, M., Howard, J.G., and Desaymard, C., 1975, Role of antigen
structure in the discrimination between tolerance and immunity
by B cells, Transplant. Rev., 23:78.

Feldmann, M. and Kontiainen, S., 1981, The role of antigen specific
factors in the immune response, Lymphokines, 2:87.

Feldmann, M. and Schrader, J.W., 1974, Mechanism of antigenic com-
petion. II. Induction by specific T cell products, Cell. Immunol., 14:235.

Fischer, A., Zanders, E.D., Beverly, P.C.L., and Feldmann, M., 1981,
Human long term helper lines, Lymphokines, Vol. 5, in press.

Fischer, A., Beverley, P.C.L. and Feldmann, M., 1981, Long term human T helper lines producing specific helper factor reactive to influenza virus, Nature, 294:166.

Fresno, M., McVay-Boudreau, L., Nabel,G., and Cantor, H., 1981b, Antigen-specific T lymphocyte clones. II. Purification and biological characterization of an antigen-specific suppressive protein synthesized by cloned T cells, J. Exp. Med., 153:1260.

Fresno M., Nabel, G., McVay-Boudreau, L., Furthermayer, H. and Cantor, H., 1981a, Antigen-specific T lymphocyte clones. I. Characterization of a T lymphocyte clone expressing antigen-specific suppressive activity, J. Exp. Med., 153:1246.

Geha, R., 1979, Regulation of human B cell activation, Immunol. Rev., 45:275.

Gorzynski, R., and Feldmann, M., 1975, B cell heterogeneity-difference in the size of B lymphocytes responding to T dependent and T independent antigens, Cell. Immunol., 15:88.

Greaves, M., Janussy, G., Feldmann, M. and Doenhoff, M., 1974, Polyclonal mitogens and the nature of B lymphocyte activation mechanisms, in "The immune system: genes, receptors, signals", E. Sercarz and C. Fox, Eds. Academic Press., N.Y., p. 271.

Greaves, M.F., Owen, J.J.T., and Raff, M.C., 1973, T and B lymphocytes: origins properties and roles in immune response, in: "T and B Lymphocytes", Eds. Elsevier-Excerpta Medica, North Holland, Amsterdam.

Hammerling, U., Pickel, H.G., Mack, C. and Masters, D., 1976, Immunochemical study of an immunoglobulin-like molecule of murine thymocytes, Immunochemistry, 15:533.

Howie, S., and Feldmann, M., 1978, Immune response (Ir) gene expressed at macrophage B-lymphocyte interactions, Nature, (London), 273:664.

Howie, S., Parish, C.R., David, C.S., McKenzie, I.F.C., Maurer, P.H. and Feldmann, M., 1979, Serological analysis of antigen specific helper factors specific for (T,G)-A--L and GAT, Eur. J. Immunol., 9:501.

Humphrey, J.H. and Grennon, D., 1981, Different macrophage populations distinguished by means of fluorescent polysaccharides. Recognition and properties of marginal-zone macrophages, Eur. J. Immunol., 11:221.

Kantor, F.S., Ojeda, A., and Benacerraf, B.,1963, Studies on artificial antigens. I. Antigenicity of DNP-Polylysine and DNP copolymer of lysine and glutamic acid in guinea pigs, J. Exp. Med., 117:55.

Kapp, J.A., Pierce, C.W., de la Croiz, F., and Benacerraf, B., 1977, Immunosuppressive factor(s) extracted from lymphoid cells of

non responder mice primed with L-glutamic acid [60] -L-alanine
[30]-L-tyrosine [10] (GAT). I. Activity and antigenic specificity,
J. Exp. Med., 145:828.

Kilburn, D.G., Talbot, F.O., Teh, H.S. and Levy, J.G., 1979, A specific helper factor which enhances the cytotoxic response to
a syngeneic tumour, Nature, 277:474.

Kindred, B. and Corley, R.B., 1977, A T cell-replacing factor specific for histocompatibility antigens in mice, Nature, (London), 268:531.

Kontiainen, S. and Feldmann, M., 1978, Suppressor cell induction
"in vitro". IV. Target of antigen specific suppressor factor
and its genetic relationship, J. Exp. Med., 147:110.

Kontiainen, S. and Feldmann, M., 1979, Structural characteristics
of antigen-specific suppressor factors: definition of 'costant'
region and 'variable' region determinants, Thymus, 1:39.

Krawinkel, U., Cramer, M., Imanishi-Kari, T.R.S., Rajewsky, K., and
Makela, O., 1977, Isolated hapten-binding receptors of sensi-
tised lymphocytes. I. Receptors from nylon wool-enriched mouse
T lymphocytes lack serological markers of immunoglobulin con-
stant domains but express heavy chain variable portions, Eur.
J. Immunol., 7:566.

Lamb, J.R., Zanders, E.D., Sanderson, A.R., Ward, P.J., Feldmann,
M., KontiainenS., Lehner, J. and Woody, J.N., 1981, Antigen specific helper factor reacts with antibodies to human β_2 microglobulin, J. Immunol., 127:231.

Layton, J.E., 1980, Anti-carbohydrate activity of T cell-reactive
chicken anti-mouse immunoglobulin antibodies, J. Immunol.,
125:1993.

Marchalonis, J.J., Warr, G.W., Santucci, L.A., Szenberg, A., von
Fallenberg, R. and Burckhart, J.J., 1980, The immunoglobulin-
-like T cell receptor. IV. Quantitative cellular assay and
partial characterization of a heavy chain cross-reactive with
the Fd fragment of serum μ chain, Mol. Immunol., 17,985.

McConnell, I., Lachmann, P.J., and Givol, D., 1975, Variable region
(Fv) determinants on mouse lymphocytes, Immunol., 30:841.

McDougal, J.S. and Gordon, D.S., 1977, Generation of T helper cells
"in vitro". I. Cellular and antigen requirements, J. Exp. Med.,
145:676.

Melchers, F., Andersson, J., Lernhardt, W., and Schreier, M.H., 1980,
H-2 unrestricted polyclonal maturation without replication of
small B cells induced by antigen-activated T cell help factors,
Eur. J. Immunol., 10:679.

Mitchison, N.A., Rajewsky, K. and Taylor, R.B., 1970, Co-operation of antigenic determinants and of cells in the induction of antibodies, in: "Stertz, J., Prague Symposium on Developmental aspects of antibody formation and structure", Ed. Publishing House of the Czechoslovakia Academy of Sciences, Prague, 2:547.

Mosier, D.E., Mond, J.J. and Goldings, E.A., 1977, The ontogeny of thymic independent antibody responses "in vitro" in normal mice and mice with an X-linked B cell defect, J. Immunol., 119:1874.

Mozes, E. and Haimovich, J., 1979, Antigen-specific T cell helper factor cross reacts idiotypically with antibodies of the same specificity, Nature, (London), 278:56.

Mozes, E., Isaac, R. and Taussig, M.J., 1975, Antigen-specific T cell factors in the genetic control of the immune response to poly (Tyr GPhe)-poly D,LAla-poly Lys. Evidence or T and B cell defects in SJL mice, J. Exp. Med., 141:703.

Parish, C. and McKenzie, I.F., 1977, Direct visualization of T lymphocytes bearing Ia antigens controlled by the I-J subregion, J. Exp. Med., 146:332.

Parish, C.R., O'Neill, H.C., and Higgins, T.J., 1981, Glycosyltransferases and T cell recognition, Immunology Today, 2:98.

Rieber, E.P. and Riethmuller, G., 1974, Surface immunoglobulin on thymus cells. I. Increased immunogenicity of heterologous anti--Ig bound to thymus cells, Immunitaetsforsch. Exp. Klin. Immunol., 147:262.

Roitt, I.M., Greaves, M.F., Torrigiani, G., Brostoff, J. and Playfair, J.H.L., 1969, The cellular basis of immunological responses, Lancet, 2:367.

Rosenberg, Y.J. and Chiller, J.M., 1979, Ability of antigen-specific helper cells to effect a class-restricted increase in total Ig-secreting cells in spleens after immunization with the antigen, J. Exp. Med., 150:517.

Schimpl, A. and Wecker, E., 1972, Replacement of T cell function by a T cell product, Nature New Biol., (London), 237:15.

Schreier, M.H., Tees, R. and Nordin, A.A., 1981, Establishment and characterisation of helper T cell clones: Their functional heterogeneity and effect on the B cell responses to particulate, soluble and T-independent antigens, Lymphokines, Vol 5, in press.

Schiozawa, C., Singh, B., Rubinstein, S., and Diener, E., 1977, Molecular control of B cell triggering by antigen-specific T cell-derived helper factor, J. Immunol., 118:2199.

Schiozawa, C., Longenecker, M.B. and Diener, E., 1980, "In vitro" cooperation of antigen-specific T cell derived helper factor, B cells, and adherent cells or their secretory product in a

primary IgM response to chicken MHC antigens, J. Immunol.,
125:68.

Singer, A., Cowing, C., Hathock, K.S., Dickler, H.B. and Hodes, R.J.,
1981, Role of the major histocompatibility complex in T cell
activation of B cell subpopulation. Lyb-5 B cell subpopulations differ in their requirement for major histocompatibility
complex-restricted T cell recognition, J. Exp. Med., 154:501.

Sprent, J., 1978, Role of H-2 gene products in the function of T
helper cells from normal and chimeric mice "in vivo", Immunol.
Rev., 42:108.

Steinmann, R.M. and Cohn, Z.A., 1973, Identification of a novel cell
type in peripheral lymphoid organs of mice, J. Exp. Med.,
137:1142.

Taniguchi, M. and Tada, R., 1974, Regulation of homocytotropic antibody formation in the rat. X. Ig T-like molecule for the induction of homocytotropic antibody response, J. Immunol., 113:1757.

Taussig, M.J., 1974, T cell factor which can replace T cells "in
vivo", Nature, (London), 248:234.

Taussig, M.J., 1981, Studies on an antigen-specific suppressor factor produced by a T-hybrid line, Lymphokines, Vol 5 in press.

Taussig, M.J., Mozes, E. and Isac, R., 1974, Antigen-specific thymus
cell factors in the genetic control of the immune response to
poly-(tyrosyl,glutamyl)-poly-DL-alanyl-poly-lysyl, J. Exp.
Med., 140:301.

Taussig, M.J. and Munro, A.J., 1974, Specific co-operative T cell
factor: removal by anti-H-2 but not by anti-Ig sera, Nature,
(London), 251:63.

Taylor, R.B., Duffus, W.P.H., Raff, M.C. and de Petris, S., 1971,
Re-distribution and pinocytosis of lymphocytes surface immuno-
globulin molecules induced by anti-immunoglobulin antibody,
Nature New Biol., 233:225.

Theze, J., Waterbaugh, C., Dorf, M.E. and Benacerraf, B., 1977, Immunosuppressive factor(s) for L-glutamic acid[50]-L-thyroxine[50]
(GT). II. Presence of I-J determinants on the GT suppressive
factor, J. Exp. Med., 146:287.

Tittle, T.V. and Rittenberg, M.B., 1978, Expression of IgG memory
response "in vitro" to thymus-dependent and thymus-independent
antigens, Cell. Immunol., 35:180.

Tokuhisa, T., Taniguchi, M., Okumura, K. and Tada, T., 1978, An antigen-specific I-region gene product that augments the antibody
response, J. Immunol., 120:414.

Wood, D.D. and Cameron, P.M., 1978, The relationship between bacterial endotoxin and human B cell activating factor, J.

Immunol., 121:53.

Woody, J., Howie, S. and Feldmann, M., 1979, Induction of antibody responses "in vivo" by antigen specific helper factor, Immunobiology, 156:13.

Zanders, E.D., Lamb, J.R., Kontiainen, S. and Lehner, T., 1980, Partial characterisation of murine and monkey helper factor to a streptococcal antigen, Immunol., 41:587.

FINE SPECIFICITY OF H-2-RESTRICTED,

LYSOZYME SPECIFIC SUPPRESSOR T CELL FACTOR

Luciano Adorini*, Carlo Pini**, Camillo Mancini*
Gino Doria* and Paola Ricciardi-Castagnoli***

*CNEN-Euratom Immunogenetics Group, Laboratory of
Radiopathology, C.N.S. Casaccia, 00060 Roma, Italy
**Laboratory of Cell Biology and Immunology
Istituto Superiore di Sanità, 00100, Roma, Italy
***CNR Center of Cytopharmacology, Department of
Pharmacology, University of Milano, 20129 Milano
Italy

1. INTRODUCTION

Antigen-specific T cells play a major role in the complex network of cellular interactions which regulate the immune response. These cellular interactions are mediated by soluble factors which may represent antigen-specific T cell recognition structures. T cell factors induced by different antigens have several features in common: they are antigen-specific, bear I-region encoded and idiotypic determinants, lack immunoglobulin constant region determinants and their molecular weight is usually in the range of 50,000 - 70,000 daltons. However, the structural definition and the precise immunoregulatory function of the antigen--specific T cell receptor is still unclear largely because, until recently, antigen-specific, functional T cell clones were not available. Substantial progresses towards the biochemical and functional characterization of antigen-specific T cell products cannot be achieved by studies of conventional T cell populations because of the low frequency of antigen-specific T cells, the short life span of lymphocytes and the heterogeneity of T cell subsets. Three different techniques have now been developed to obtain antigen-specific T cell clones: somatic cell hybridization between T lymphocytes and T cell lymphomas, continuous growth of T cells in interleukin 2-containing media, and virus-induced transformation of T cells.

The radiation leukemia virus (RadLV)-induced T cell transformation technique, originally developed by Kaplan and coworkers (Finn et al, 1979), represents a very useful approach to the production of antigen-specific, functional T cell clones and overcomes some of the problems encountered with the T cell hybridoma and IL-2-dependent long term culture technologies.

In this paper, we will briefly review some characteristics of hen egg-white lysozyme (HEL)-specific suppressor T cells as well as the establishment of HEL-specific suppressor T cell lines by RadLV-induced transformation of specifically enriched suppressor T cells. In addition, we will describe an H-2 restricted suppressive factor, obtained from a transformed cell line, specific for a restricted portion of the HEL molecule.

2. CHARACTERISTICS OF HEL SPECIFIC SUPPRESSOR T CELLS

HEL-specific suppressor T cells are easily induced in genetically non responder C57BL/10 (H-2^b) mice after intraperitoneal injection of HEL-CFA (Adorini et al., 1979a).
These suppressor T cells demonstrate an exquisite fine specificity because they are unable to suppress helper T cells induced by the closely related ring-necked pheasant egg-white lysozyme (REL). HEL and REL differ at 10 out of 129 amino acid residues and comparative analysis of lysozyme sequences and antibody responses indicate that a determinant including phenylalanine at position 3 is critical for the induction of suppressor T cells in genetically non responder mice (Sercarz et al., 1978). By using defined peptides obtained from HEL the specificity of these suppressor T cells has been shown to be restricted to an epitope present on the N-terminal, C-terminal (N-C, aminoacid residues 1-17: cys 6 - cys 127: 120-129) peptide of HEL. Although N-C priming induces help in B10.A mice, injection of N-C in the congenic B10 strain raises suppressor T cells which, when confronted with native HEL, are able to counteract the helper activity induced by determinants present in other regions of the molecule (Adorini et al., 1979b;

Yowell   et al.,   1979). Experiments with HEL-derived peptides
composed   of amino acids 1-17 and 1-12 are also consistent with the
presence   of the suppressive determinant within the N region of the
HEL   molecule   (Adorini and Harvey, unpublished observations). One
cell   in   the   HEL-specific suppressive pathway bears idiotypic
determinants   since   suppression   is   abrogated   by   treatment   of
suppressor   cells with anti-idiotype and complement (Harvey et al.,
1979; Adorini et al., 1980).

Therefore,   HEL-specific   suppressor   T   cells,   submitted to a
stringent genetic,   epitopic   and   idiotypic   control, represent a
very   interesting   and   versatile   system to analyze functional and
structural   characteristics   of antigen-specific T cell factors and
T cell receptors.

3. ESTABLISHMENT OF HEL-SPECIFIC SUPPRESSOR T CELL LINES

Intraperitoneal HEL-CFA priming in mice of H-2^b haplotype,
genetically non responder to HEL (Hill and Sercarz, 1975) induces
suppressor   T   cells   which   are   antigen-specific and I-J positive
(Adorini   et   al.,   1979a).   The   procedure   we   have   followed   to
establish HEL-specific T cell lines from this cell population has
recently   been   described   (Ricciardi-Castagnoli et al., 1981; Adorini   et   al.,   1981).   Briefly,   suppressor T cells from HEL-primed
C57BL/6   (H-2^b)   mice   have been enriched by a sequential positive
selection   on   anti-mouse Ig and HEL-coated plates. This enriched
suppressor   T   cell   population   (80% I-J$^+$) has been infected "in
vitro"   with RadLV/Nu$_1$ virus harvested from culture supernatants of
the BALB/nu$_1$ cell line (Ricciardi-Castagnoli et al., 1978), and
the   infected   cells   subsequently   injected into sublethally irradiated   syngeneic   recipients.   Within   4-6 months, 30% of the
injected mice developed large thymomas which were analyzed for T
cell   markers   by   immunofluorescence. Among the six thymomas tested
one   showed   the   expected   surface   markers for suppressor T cells
(Thy 1,2$^+$, Lyt 2$^+$, I-J$^+$, sIg$^-$) and cell-free extracts obtained
from this lymphoma showed HEL-specific suppressive activity in a T
cell-dependent lymph node proliferative assay. A cell line (LH8)
was   then   established   "in   vitro"   from this thymoma. Culture
supernatants   from   the   LH8   cell   line   demonstrated HEL-specific
suppressive activity of antigen-specific T cell proliferation and
of "in vitro" anti-HEL antibody response (Adorini et al., 1981).

Table 1. HEL-Specific suppressive activity of LH8 culture superna-
         tant.

Factor	Priming	Developed anti-HEL PFC/10^6 PT-LN cells	Priming	Developed anti-TNP PFC/10^6 PT-LN cells
-	HEL-CFA	4166 (1.33)	TNP-KLH-CFA	1460 (1.37)
LH8	HEL-CFA	1433 (1.65)	TNP-KLH-CFA	1798 (1.37)
RL 12	HEL-CFA	3950 (1.35)		

BDF1 mice (5 mice/group) were injected i.p. with 100 ug HEL or TNP-
KLH in CFA and the developed PFC response measured 8 days later in
the parathymic lymph node (PT-LN) cells. Culture supernatant from
LH8 or RL 12 cell lines (1 ml/mouse) was injected i.v. at the same
time of antigen priming and one day later. Values refer to geometric mean PFC and numbers in parentheses represent a factor by
which the mean should be multiplied or divided to give one standard error.

4. FINE ANTIGENIC SPECIFICITY OF HEL-SPECIFIC SUPPRESSOR T CELL FACTOR

The HEL-specific suppressor T cell factor produced by the LH8
cell line is not only able to specifically suppress T cell
proliferation and antibody responses, when added to "in vitro"
cultures, but it can also suppress the anti-HEL PFC responses when
injected in vivo. The next two sections will summarize the results
of experiments in which the suppressive factor activity has been
assessed "in vivo".

The antigenic specificity of HRL-specific suppressor T cell
factor is demonstrated in Table 1. In BDF$_1$ mice, responder to HEL,
injection of LH8 culture supernatant induces a considerable
suppression of the primary anti-HEL PFC response whereas injection
of culture supernatants from a control RadLV-producing lymphoblastoid cell line is ineffective. Moreover, LH8 culture supernatants injection does not suppress the antibody response to an
unrelated antigen confirming the HEL specificity of this suppressive factor.

Table 2. HEL-specific suppressive factor does not suppress the response induced by a closely related lysozyme.

LH8 Factor	Priming	Developed PFC/10^6 anti-HEL	PT-LN cells anti-REL	Suppression (%)	Cross-reac. at the PFC level[a] (%)
−	HEL-CFA	<u>21056</u> (1.09)	14286 (1.17)		68
+	HEL-CFA	<u>5052</u> (1.26)	4656 (1.38)	77	92
−	REL-CFA	18346 (1.08)	<u>21815</u> (1.09)		84
+	REL-CFA	12487 (1.13)	<u>18781</u> (1.13)	14	66

BDF1 mice (6 mice/group) were injected i.p. with 100 ug HEL or REL in CFA and the developed PFC response measured 8 days later in the parathymic lymph node (PT-LN) cells. Culture supernatant from LH8 cell line (1 ml/mouse) was injected i.v. at the same time of antigen priming and one day later. PFC values are expressed as geometric mean and number in parentheses represent a factor by which the mean should be multiplied or divided to give one standard error. [a]HEL-REL cross-reactivity at the PFC level has been estimated taking as 100 % the response to homologous lysozyme.

As mentioned earlier HEL-specific suppressor T cells display an exquisite fine specificity for an antigenic epitope present in the N-terminal region of the HEL molecule. This conclusion stems from two observations: the N-C (a.a. 1-17: cys 6 - cys 127: 120-129) but not the L_{II} (a.a. 13-205) peptide is able to induce suppressor T cells in non responder mice, and HEL-induced suppressor T cells are unable to suppress helper T cells induced by L_{II} or by lysozymes, as REL, lacking the suppressive determinant (Adorini et al., 1979a; Adorini et al., 1979b).

Therefore it was of interest to ascertain whether or not the HEL-specific suppressor T cell factor was able to suppress the antibody response induced by REL. Data in Table 2 demonstrate that the anti-REL response induced by REL-CFA priming is not significantly suppressed by injection of LH8 culture supernatant, indicating that this factor is able to discriminate between helper T cells induced by two closely related lysozymes. Conversely, the HEL-REL cross-reactivity at the antibody level is very high, sug-

Table 3. Fine specificity of LH8 suppressive factor.

Factor	Priming	Challenge	Developed anti-HEL PFC/10^6 PT-LN cells	% suppression
−	HEL-CFA	HEL	5141 (1.13)	
+	N-C-CFA	HEL	1017 (1.79)	80
−	N-C-CFA	HEL	2221 (1.37)	
+	N-C-CFA	HEL	776 (1.45)	65
−	L_{II}-CFA	HEL	1804 (1.35)	
+	L_{II}-CFA	HEL	1598 (1.22)	11
−	−	HEL	161 (1.45)	

BDF1 mice (6 mice/group) were injected i.p. with 100 ug HEL or 20 ug N-C or 70 ug L_{II} in CFA and challenged 28 days later with 100 ug soluble HEL. Developed anti-HEL PFC were measured 6 days after challenge in the parathymic lymph node cells. Culture supernatant from LH8 cells line (1 ml/mouse) was injected i.v. at the same time of antigen priming and one day later. Values refer to geometric mean PFC and number in parentheses represent a factor by which the mean should be multiplied or divided to give one standard error.

gesting that suppressor T cells and B cell products exhibit a different specificity repertoire. Furthermore, lack of crossreactivity of the suppressive factor in presence of high B cell cross--reactivity indicates that helper T cells and not B cells are probably the target of suppression.

The fine antigenic specificity of HEL-specific suppressor T cell factors is confirmed by peptide priming experiments. Results in Table 3 demonstrated that N-C-induced helper cells are suppressed by factor injection, whereas L -induced helper cells are not. Therefore, the suppressive factor displays a very precise fine specificity restricted to an antigenic epitope present in the N-terminal, C-terminal region of the HEL-molecule. It is also interesting to note that data in Table 3 refer to suppression of the secondary "in vivo" anti-HEL antibody response which was tested 36 days after LH8 supernatant injection. This result indicates that suppressive factor injection induces a very stable and

Table 4. H-2 restriction of LH8 suppressive factor activity.

Exp. no.	Mice	Developed anti-HEL PFC/10^6 PT/LN cells	% Suppression
1	BDF1	10995 (1.16)	
	BDF1	2547 (1.25)	77
	DBA/2	7834 (1.54)	
	DBA/2	9593 (1.51)	0
2	BDF1	22944 (1.23)	
	BDF1	8926 (1.20)	61
	B01.D2	14572 (1.16)	
	B10.D2	18183 (1.19)	0

Six mice/group were injected i.p. with 100 ug HEL in CFA and the developed anti-HEL PFC response measured 8 days later in the parathymic lymph node (PT-LN) cells. Culture supernatant from LH8 cell line (1ml/mouse) was injected i.v. at the same day of antigen priming and one day later. Value refer to geometric mean PFC and number in parentheses represent a factor by which the mean should be multiplied or divided to give one standard error.

long-lasting epitope-specific suppression.

5. H-2 RESTRICTION OF HEL-SPECIFIC SUPPRESSOR T CELL FACTOR ACTIVITY

The HEL-specific suppressor T cell factor produced by the LH8 cell line, which was established from suppressor T cells obtained by genetically non responder B6 (H-2^b) mice, has been routinely tested on semisyngeneic BDF$_1$(H-$2^{b/d}$)mice (responders to HEL). This suppressive activity is restricted by genes located within the H-2 complex since the anti-HEL antibody response in DBA/2 and B10.D2 mice is not suppressed by factor injection (Table 4). Experiments are in progress to precisely map the H-2 region(s) that controls an effective interation between the suppressive factor and its target. The presence of H-2 restriction also indicates that suppression is not the resultant of peripheral removal or masking of antigenic determinants by the injected suppressive factor.

Recent experiments (data not shown) demonstrate that the entire suppressive activity of the LH8 culture supernatant is specifically bound and can be eluted from an HEL cross-reactive idiotype (IdX) immunoadsorbent column. Therefore this suppressor T cell factor bears anti-idiotypic determinants which are able to recognize a cross-reactive idiotype present on the majority of anti-HEL antibodies.

6. CONCLUSIONS

The precise relationship between antigen-specific T cell-derived factors and T cell receptors is not yet defined but it is very likely that antigen-specific factors represent, at least in part, specific cell surface recognition structures.

Results from several antigenic systems indicate that the suppressor T cell pathway involves at least two different types of suppressor T cell factors termed TsF1 and TsF2 (Germain and Benacerraf, 1980). TsF1 binds to antigen and anti-idiotype immuno-adsorbents, acts across the H-2 barrier, does not exert directly suppressive activity but induces TsF2 producing cells.
TsF2 does not bind to antigen-coated columns but bears anti-idiotypic determinants, is H-2 restricted and exerts suppressive activity also when the response is fully established.
The HEL-specific suppressor T cell factor we have described shares most properties with TsF2 type factors: it bears anti-idiotypic determinants and it is H-2 restricted but it does not suppress, when injected shortly before the assay, an ongoing anti-HEL antibody response.

The molecular organization of antigen-specific T cell receptors is still undefined. According to Taniguchi et al., (1980) the T cell receptor could be composed of two chains, one carrying V_H-like gene products which determine antigenic and idiotypic specificity and the other including I-region encoded determinants which mediate effector functions. Alternatively, the antigen--specific T cell receptor could be constitued by a single polypeptide composed of two distinct regions, one that binds antigen and the other that mediate effector function (Fresno et al., 1980). The inability to decide for single chain vs two chains receptor models clearly exemplifies our imprecise knowledge of T cell recognition structures. However, the availability of cloned, antigen-specific, functional T cell lines should provide soon a clearer picture of the antigen-specific T cell receptor. In addition, virus-transformed T cell lines represent a very promising material to analize the arrangements of genes encoding for the different elements of the T cell receptor. A correct molecular biology approach may eventually prove to be the most straight forward way to obtain clear-cut and definitive information not only on the molecular organization but also on the biological function of antigen-specific T cell receptors.

ACKNOWLEDGEMENTS

Work supported by Istituto Pasteur-Fondazione Cenci Bolognetti.

REFERENCES

Adorini, L., Miller, A., and Sercarz, E.E., 1979a, The fine specificity of regulatory T cells. I. Hen egg-white lysozyme-induced suppressor T cells in a genetically non responder mouse strain do not recognize a closely related immunogenic lysozyme, J. Immunol., 122:871.

Adorini, L., Harvey, M., Miller, A., and Sercarz, E.E., 1979b, The fine specificity of regulatory T cells. II. Suppressor and helper T cells are induced by different regions of hen egg--white lysozyme (HEL) in a gentically non responder mouse strain, J. Exp. Med., 150:293.

Adorini, L., Harvey, M.A., Rozyka-Jackson, D., Miller, A., and Sercarz, E.E., 1980, Differential major histocompatibility complex-related activation of idiotypic suppressor T cells. Suppressor T cells cross-reactive to two distantly related lysozyme are not induced by one of them, J. Exp. Med., 152:521.

Adorini, L., Doria, G. and Ricciardi-Castagnoli, P., 1981, Biochemical and functional analysis of antigen-specific products obtained from virus-transformed, lysozyme-specific suppressor T cell lines, Lymphokines, in press.

Finn, O.J., Boniver, J., and Kaplan, H.S., 1979, Induction, establishment "in vitro", and characterization of functional, antigen-specific, carrier-primed murine T cell lymphomas, Proc. Natl. cad. Sci., USA, 76:4033.

Fresno, M., McVay-Boudreau, L., Furthmayer, H., and Cantor, H., 1981, Antigen-specific T lymphocyte clones. II. Purification and biological characterization of an antigen-specific suppressive protein synthesized by cloned T cells, J. Exp. Med., 153:1260.

Germain, R.N., and Benacerraf, B., 1980, Helper and suppressor T cell factors, Springer Semin. Immunopathol., 3:93.

Harvey, M.A., Adorini, L., Miller, A., and Sercarz, E.E., 1979, Lysozyme induced T suppressor cells and antibodies bear a predominant idiotype, Nature, 281:594.

Hill, S.W., and Sercarz, E.E., 1975, Fine specificity of the H-2 linked immune response gene for the gallinaceous lysozyme, Eur. J. Immunol., 5:317.

Ricciardi-Castagnoli, P., Lieberman, M., Finn, O., and Kaplan, H.S., 1978, T-cell lymphoma induction by radiation leukemia virus in athymic nude mice, J. Exp. Med., 148:1292.

Ricciardi-Castagnoli, P., Doria, G., and Adorini, L., 1981, Production of antigen-specific suppressive T cell factor by radiation leukemia virus-transformed suppressor T cells, Proc. Natl. Acad. Sci., USA, in press.

Sercarz, E.E., Yowell, R.L., Turkin, D., Miller, A., Araneo, B.A., and Adorini, L., 1978, Different functional specificity repertoire for suppressor and helper T cells, Immunological Rev., 39:108.

Taniguchi, M., Takei, I., and Tada, T., 1980, Functional and molecular organization of an antigen-specific suppressor factor from a T-cell hybridoma, Nature, 283:227.

Yowell, R.L., Araneo, B.A., Miller, A., and Sercarz, E.E., 1979, Amputation of a suppressor determinant on lysozyme reveals underlying T-cell reactivity to other determinants, Nature, 279:70.

MARROW REGULATING FACTORS (MRF) AND RADIATION CHIMERAS :

A MODEL FOR BONE MARROW-DIRECTED IMMUNITY

Walter Pierpaoli and Georges J.M. Maestroni*

Institute for Integrative Biomedical Research
Lohwisstrasse 50,8123 Ebmatingen, Switzerland

1. THE BONE MARROW MICROENVIRONMENT

The bone marrow microenvironment still constitutes a completely unexplored continent in spite of the fact that, in adult organisms, the bone marrow is the principal hemopoietic organ and that lympho-hemopoiesis represents the vital and ultimate result of a finely modulated course of proliferative and differentiative events. The bone marrow is populated by a huge variety of cells of very different embryologic origin (bone, nerve, endothelial, reticular, hemopoietic) which live in close contact and show very different stages of maturation. Signals of disparate origin and character (neural, hormonal, chemical mediators, blood pressure variations, temperature, oxygen tension, ionic changes, pH, a.o.) are all detected, elaborated and transmitted in the bone marrow. We know practically nothing of the complexity, significance and functions of this ancient organ, except that it delivers mature cells to the lymphatic tissues and to the blood and that some of these cells (B cells) are relevant for synthesis of antibodies (Kelemen et al., 1979; Wolf, 1979; Lichtman, 1981).

We have proposed recently a broader, prioritary function of

*New address: Istituto Cantonale di Patologia - Laboratorio di Patologia Cellulare - 6604, Locarno-Solduno, Switzerland.

the bone marrow for regulation of immune or, as we like to call
them, identity-defense functions (Pierpaoli, 1981; Pierpaoli and
Maestroni, in press). This concept is based on the experimental
observation that immune identity resides in the bone marrow itself
and that transplantation of allogeneic, incompatible bone marrow
(BMT) across the H-2 barrier is a possibility, provided the
integrity of the marrow transferred is maintained and the unmanipulated marrow is infused in the irradiated host together with
some basic microenvironmental components, the so-called marrow
regulating factors (MRF). Thus, we view BMT as a complex hemato-
logical problem which can be solved if a more profound knowledge
of bone marrow physiology is aquired (Pierpaoli, 1981; Pierpaoli
and Maestroni, in press).

2. BONE MARROW TRANSPLANTATION AS A MODEL FOR THE STUDY OF BONE MARROW PHYSIOLOGY AND OF ITS FUNCTION IN IMMUNITY

Transplantation of organs, tissues, and cells from histoincompatible donors has recently been given new impetus and fresh
prospects by the development of more comprehensive modes of
immunosuppression of the recipient such as fractionated total
lymphoid irradiation (Slavin et al., 1977). For the most part,
however, transplantation of bone marrow between genetically dissi-
milar individuals is presently restricted to the best possible
match; in practical terms, this generally limits the choice to
sibling or parental marrow. This continues to be based on traditional immunological concepts and essentially empirical approaches
(Storb et al., 1977). The fact is that marrow transplantation is
presently utilized solely to correct aplastic anemia and immunodeficiencies, i.e. replacement of host marrow to restore function;
for this purpose, histocompatibility of donor and recipient is the
"sine qua non". Its use for immunotherapy requires a quite different orientation. If BMT is to go beyond mere restoration of
hematopietic function, a more ambitious goal, for example, would
be to achieve by such passive transfer, host adoption of additional, new donor attributes such as "resistance-defense" for the
tumor-bearing, non-resistant host. Accordingly it is allogeneic
BMT that constitutes the principal remaining prospect in tumor
immunology, as an unique means of achieving tumor therapy (Blume
et al.,1980; Newburger et al., 1981).

Hemopoietic reconstitution and immune reactivity of allogeneic bone marrow chimeras has received considerable study (Mae-

stroni et al., submitted for publication). Our methodology diver-
ges radically from prior work in as much as fully allogeneic and
clinically Graft-versus-Host Disease (GvHD)-free chimeras have
heretofore been limited to special situations in which the recipients of allogeneic marrow had either been raised and maintained
under germ-free conditions,or the cellular composition of the bone
marrow to be transplanted has been manipulated so as to remove cytotoxic T cells. Furthermore, only recently reports of fully allogeneic, conventionally bred radiation chimeras surviving longer
than six months after irradiation and marrow transplantation have
been published (Norin et al., 1981; Krown et al., 1981).

From our studies on BMT there has evolved a system which
makes for induction of enduring engraftment of fully allogeneic,
H-2 incompatible marrow in mice and the establishment of GvHD-
free hemopoietic chimeras which survive at least as long as synge-
neically reconstituted mice. This system is based on the concept
that the problem of BMT is more hematologic than immunogenetic in
character and that maintenance of the integrity of cellular
composition of donor marrow (including T cells) and its microenvironmental components is a "sine qua non" for harmonious
engraftment of allogeneic marrow, eradication of resistance in
recipients and avoidance of graft versus host disease.

3. A NOVEL MODEL FOR ALLOGENEIC BONE MARROW TRANSPLANTATION

In the course of recent investigations on the pharmacologic
control of the immune response we progressively recognized the
presence of a potent regulator of lympho-hemopoiesis, in the bone
marrow microenvironment. While studying the effect of a new
combination of neuroactive drugs on the immune response (Pierpaoli and Maestroni, 1977; Pierpaoli 1978) we found this mixture
to be highly immunosuppressive. One of the experimental models
utilized was allogeneic BMT in mice.

An interesting feature of the methodology was that the
combination of drugs was able to induce antigen-specific and long
lasting immune unresponsiveness (Pierpaoli and Maestroni, 1978;
Maestroni and Pierpaoli, 1981). We thought of applying this
property to allogeneic BMT, in the attempt to induce in the
recipient mice a specific "tolerance" towards donor antigens by
treating them with donor bone marrow cells and the drugs before

Table 1. Marrow regulating factors (MRF) promote engraftment of allogeneic, H-2 incompatible bone marrow and permanent chimerism in lethally irradiated mice.

Group	No. of mice	TBI 950 rad	Post-conditioning	Survival (%) (3 months)	Chimerism (%)
A	22		-	0	-
B	43		$15-20 \times 10^6$ BM cells, iv + 2-5 mg MRF/mouse	31 (72%)	31 (72%)
C	44		$15-20 \times 10^6$ BM cells, iv	4 (9%)	4 (9%)
D	10		$15-20 \times 10^6$ BM cells, iv +3 mg Kidney extract	0	-

Donors of bone marrow (BM) were adult, DBA/2 ($H-2^d$). Recipients were adult, C5B1/6 ($H-2^b$) mice. The BM was suspended in medium TC 199, the cells were dissociated, filtered and adjusted to the wished volume and concentration. Supernatant was eliminated by centrifugation and the cells resuspended in medium with or without MRF. The BM was injected over 24 hours after TBI (between 25 and 29 hours). Chimerism was evaluated in all the surviving mice by skin grafting, hemoglobin electrophoretic pattern and analysis of chimerism spleen cells for susceptibility to cytolysis by specific anti-H-2 antisera. All the surviving mice were perfectly healthy and showed no clinical symptoms of GVHD. They lived over 2 years and maintained their chimerism. The results shown above derive from five similar or identical experiments. The mice of group D died with a symptomatology similar to that of group B (GVHD). MRF is the lyophilized material obtained by ultrafiltration on Amicon Dialfo membranes (MW 100.000) of supernatant of rabbit bone marrow cell suspensions in TC 199 medium. MRF is endotoxin-free (< 1 ng/mg MRF).

total body irradiation (TBI) and BMT. Surprisingly, it turned out that the simple inoculation of viable bone marrow cells alone before lethal irradiation was sufficient to allow a significative number (40%) of the bone-marrow-transplanted semiallogeneic recipient mice to be reconstituted and to become healthy, GvHD-free, bone marrow chimeras (Pierpaoli and Maestroni, 1980). This effect was demonstrated to be organ-specific but not species-specific. Therefore, we excluded pre-TBI, allogeneic stimulation as the possible mechanism inducing allochimerism. We started thinking of humoral factors released by bone marrow cells and able to induce a particular "receptive" state in the treated mice. In fact, successive experiments showed the presence of active factors in supernatants of suspensions of bone marrow cells (Maestroni and Pierpaoli, 1980; Pierpaoli and Maestroni, 1980). Practically, it was found that the tissue culture medium used for collecting and dissociating the bone marrow contained agents capable of influencing the outcome of allogeneic and/or xenogeneic BMT (Maestroni and Pierpaoli, 1980; Pierpaoli, and Maestroni, 1980). We proceeded further to the analysis of these findings and finally we were able to identify a crude fraction of bone marrow supernatants which was active in allogeneic BMT. We called this fraction marrow regulating factors (MRF) (Pierpaoli, et al., 1981). MRF is defined as the material retained on a Diaflo XM 100 membrane, when supernatants of suspensions of bone marrow cells are ultrafiltrated.

The peculiar property of MRF is to induce permanent and complete allogeneic chimerism in lethally irradiated and bone marrow transplanted mice (Pierpaoli et al., 1981) (Table 1). MRF has to be inoculated i.v. into the recipient mice 24 hr after TBI, together with donor BM cells. The resulting bone marrow chimeras are perfectly healthy, GvHD-free and long-lived (over 2 years). The animals survive in an unprotected environment. This suggests that reconstitution with allogeneic bone marrow could be a suitable model for adoptive immunotherapy in man (Maestroni et al., submitted for publication).

The MRF effect is non-species-specific, in fact the majority of the studies have been and are presently done utilizing rabbit MRF in mice. However, the effect seems to be organ-specific; ultrafiltrates of supernatant of cells suspensions from other organs are ineffective in inducing chimerism (manuscript in preparation, Table 1).

In summary:

1) MRF is a physiological component of the bone marrow microenvironment.

2) MRF together with unmanipulated bone marrow cells induces a state of complete allogeneic chimerism when inoculated into lethally irradiated mice.

3) The allogeneic BM chimeras thus obtained show a donor-type, identity-defence, immune system, are long-lived and GvHD-free (Maestroni et al., submitted for publication).

4) The nature of the tolerance underlying this allogeneic chimerism is unknown. Recent experiments failed to point out either suppressor or clonal deletion mechanisms (Maestroni et al., submitted for publication).

4. CONCLUSIONS

It seems reasonable to assume that the bone marrow microenvironment contains potent regulators of hemopoiesis and that these factors are also active in the physiological control of other important functions (Pierpaoli, 1981; Pierpaoli and Maestroni, in press). As a crude fraction, MRF is still a mixture of many and completely unknown substances with presumably different physiological functions. Thus, MRF can be viewed as a primitive prototype of a new family of unknown physiological regulators of hemopoiesis and immunity (Pierpaoli, 1981; Pierpaoli and Maestroni, in press).

There are reasons for believing that the bone marrow possesses powerful autonomic and active homoeostatic qualities whose functioning is likely based on a complex network of cellular and humoral interactions, as well as on anatomical requirements peculiar to the bone marrow itself (Pierpaoli, 1981).
This intricate "tolerogenic" machinery could well play an important role in controlling the ontogenetic maturation of self-recognition and the physiological regulation of the immuno-hemopoietic system. That such active mechanisms operate continuously under physiological conditions for monitoring potentially harmful autoimmune phenomena and for modulating immune or identity-defence against potential snares of homeostasis (pathogenic microrganisms, tumor cells, etc.) is not excluded. The present experimental findings on induction of allogeneic chimerism by use of unmanipulated bone marrow and MRF are viewed as suggesting that the bone

marrow can also be considered an autonomic organ with powerful autoregulatory capabilities. In this respect it could function as a repository of the "immunologic intelligence" of the host. In such a context, allogeneic BMT would represent the basic means for passive transfer of a "new" identity-defence system and for a meaningful acquisition of fresh resistance to ongoing threats of the environment, be they intercurrent infections, tumors, auto-immune or immunodeficiency diseases (Pierpaoli, 1981; Pierpaoli and Maestroni, in press; Maestroni et al., submitted for publication.

REFERENCES

Blume, K.G., Beatler, E., Bross, K.J., 1980, Bone marrow ablation and allogeneic marrow transplantation in acute leukemia, N. Engl. J. Med., 302:1041.

Kelemen, E., Calvo, W., and Fliedner, T.M., 1979, "Atlas of human hemopoietic development," Springer-Verlag, Berlin.

Krown, S.E., Coico, R., Scheid, M.P., Fernandes, G., and Good, R.A., 1981, Immune function in fully allogeneic mouse bone marrow chimeras, Clin. Immunol. Immunopathol., 19:268.

Lichtman, M.A., 1981, The untrastructure of the hemopoietic environment of the marrow: A review, Exp. Hematol., 9:391.

Maestroni, G.J.M., and Pierpaoli, W., 1980, Factor(s) elaborated by bone marrow that promote persistent engraftment of xenogeneic and semiallogeneic marrow, J. Clin. & Lab. Immunol., 4:189.

Maestroni, G.J.M., and Pierpaoli, W., 1981, Pharmacological control of the hormonally mediated immune response, in: "Psychoneuro-immunology," R. Ader, ed., Academic Press, New York.

Maestroni, G.J.M., Pierpaoli, W., and Zinkernagel, R.M., Immunoreactivity of long-lived H-2 incompatible irradiation chimeras, submitted for publication.

Newburger, P.E., Latt, S.A., Pesando, G.M., Gustashaw, K., Powers, M., Chaganti, R.S.K., and O'Reilly, R.J., 1981, Leukemia relapse in donor cells after allogeneic bone-marrow transplantation, N. Engl. J. Med., 304:712 .

Norin, A.J., Emeson, E.E., and Veith, F.J., 1981, Long-term survival of murine allogeneic bone marrow chimeras: effect of anti-lymphocyte serum and bone marrow dose, J. Immunol., 126:428.

Pierpaoli, W., 1981, Integrated phylogenetic and ontogenetic evolution of neuroendocrine and identity-defence, immune functions, in: "Psychoneuroimmunology," R. Ader, ed., Academic Press,

New York.

Pierpaoli, W., and Maestroni, G.J.M., 1977, Pharmacological control of the immune response by blockade of the early hormonal changes following antigen injection, Cell. Immunol., 31:355.

Pierpaoli, W., and Maestroni, G.J.M., 1978, Pharmacological control of the hormonally modulate immune response. II. Blockade of antibody production by a combination of drugs acting on neuroendocrine functions. Its prevention by gonadotropins and corticotrophin, Immunology, 34:419.

Pierpaoli, W., and Maestroni, G.J.M., 1978, Pharmacologic control of the hormonally modulated immune response. III. Prolongation of allogeneic skin graft rejection and prevention of runt disease by a combination of drugs acting on neuroendocrine functions, J. Immunol., 120:1600.

Pierpaoli, W., and Maestroni, G.J.M., 1980, The facilitation of enduring engraftment of homologous bone marrow and avoidance disease in mice, Cell. Immunol., 52:62.

Pierpaoli, W., and Maestroni, G.J.M., 1980, Induction of enduring allogeneic bone marrow chimerism in rabbits via soluble marrow-derived components, Immunol. Let., 1: 244.

Pierpaoli, W., and Maestroni, G.J.M., Enduring allogeneic and xenogeneic hemopoietic engraftment via marrow-derived regulating factors (MRF), in: "Organ Transplantation, Present State, Future Goals," S. Slavin, ed., Elsevier-North-Holland Biomedical Press B.V., Amsterdam, in press.

Pierpaoli, W., Maestroni, G.J.M., and Sache, E., 1981, Enduring allogeneic marrow engraftment via non-specific bone marrow derived regulating factors (MRF), Cell. Immunol., 57:219.

Slavin, S., Strober, S., Fuks, Z., and Kaplan, H., 1977, Induction of specific tissue transplantation tolerance using fractionated total lymphoid irradiation in adult mice: long-term survival of allogeneic bone marrow and skin grafts, J. Exp. Med., 146:34.

Storb, R., Weiden, P.L., Prentice, R., Buckner, C.D., Clift, R.A., Einstein, A.B., Fefer, A., Johnson F.L., Lerner, K.G., Neiman, P.E., Sanders, J.E., and Thomas, E.E., 1977, Aplastic anemia (AA) treated by allogeneic marrow transplantation: the Seattle experience, Transplant. Proc., 9:181.

Wolf, N.S., 1979, The haemopoietic microenvironment, Clin. Haematol. 8:469.

ROLE OF THYMOSIN AND THE NEUROENDOCRINE SYSTEM

IN THE REGULATION OF IMMUNITY

Nicholas R. Hall and Allan L. Goldstein

Dept. of Biochemistry, The George Washington
University, School of Medicine and Health Sciences
Washington D.C., 20037, U.S.A.

1. INTRODUCTION

A central role for the thymus in host defense has been documented by studies correlating either surgical or genetic absence of this gland with immunodeficiency. Consequently, thymic immunity has become synonymous with cellular immunity, a component of host defense that interfaces with both phagocytic and immuno- globulin producing cells.

This role is due in part to soluble factors produced by thymic epithelial cells: soluble factors with hormonal-like action that are exerted throughout the stages of lymphoid differen- tiation. But, in addition to its influence upon immunity, it is apparent that the thymus gland is also inter-associated with endocrine physiology; a reciprocal association that is frequently ignored in the thymic literature. It is ironic that this omission has occurred since some of the earliest literature concerned with thymic extracts describes their effects upon non-immunologic phe- nomena. These range from delayed metamorphosis in tadpoles to re- tarded reproductive function in rodents (Andersen, 1932).
However, due to increasing evidence that a variety of hormones are able to, either directly or indirectly, influence the course of immunogenesis, such interactions may not necessarily represent "non-immunologic" phenomena after all. Instead, they may represent

141

evidence of multiple afferent links between the endocrine thymus and the cellular components of immunity.

In this paper, we will review the evidence of multiple regu-latory influences upon immunity with emphasis upon those systems that are interconnected with the endocrine thymus.

2. THYMIC FACTORS: BIOCHEMICAL PROPERTIES

A number of investigators have found that the impaired state of immunity that follows neonatal thymectomy can be restored by either syngeneic or allogenic thymic grafts (Davies, 1969; East and Parrott, 1964; Dalmasso et al., 1963; Leuchars et al., 1965). That soluble factors produced by thymic epithelial cells are in part responsible for this restorative effect is suggested by a number of studies in which either epithelial cells or thymus tissue contained in cell impermeable chambers were found to be effective (Bigger et al., 1973; Hays, 1967; Miller, 1966). Until recently, the chemical and biological characteristics of these factors were difficult to discern. Crude and impure extracts were frequently utilized and in paradigms that seldom controlled for the effects of stress and/or circadian release of hormones. Since the early part of this century, when some of the thymic extract experiments were initially conducted, our understanding of the chemical and biological nature of thymic preparations has expanded considerably. Those that appear to be biochemically distinct in-clude the thymosins (Goldstein et al., 1981), thymic humoral fac-tor (THF) (Trainin et al., 1975), facteur thymique serique (FTS) (Bach et al., 1977) and thymopoietin (G. Goldstein and Lau, 1980).

Thymosin was first isolated from calf thymus in 1965 (Gold-stein et al., 1966). A purer, although still heterogeneous ex-tract, was subsequently prepared and termed thymosin fraction 5 (Hooper et al., 1975). This fraction is thought to consist of 40 to 50 component peptides of which 20 have been purified to homogeneity or near homogeneity. It has been reported to include trace amounts of FTS (Dardenne et al., 1980) and thymopoietin (Gershwin et al., 1979), although the levels of FTS are about the same as those found in similar preparations of calf spleen, liver or kidney. Based upon the isoelectric focusing pattern of fraction 5, three distinct regions of polypeptides have been described (Goldstein et al., 1977). Those with isoelectric points below 5.0

lie within the alfa region; those between 5.0 and 7.0 are in the beta region; and those above 7.0 are within the gamma region. The subscript numbers α_1, β_1, β_2 eccetera are used to identify the polypeptides from each region in the order that they are isolated. The molecular weights of these peptides range from 1,000 to 15,000; however, only three have been fully characterized and sequenced. These are thymosin α_1 (Goldstein et al., 1977; Low et al. 1979; Low and Goldstein, 1979); thymosin β_4 (Low et al., 1980); and polypeptide β_1 (Low et al., 1979; Low and Goldstein, 1979). Since β_1 is not a thymic hormone, it is given the prefix "polypeptide" rather that "thymosin" (Low et al., 1979). In addition, thymosin α_7 possesses immunomodulating activity and will be included in a discussion of the biological role of thymosin peptides.

The complete amino acid sequence of thymosin α_1 and β_4 are shown in Fig. 1. Polypeptide β_1 has been found to be homologous with ubiquitin (Goldstein et al., 1978) and the N-terminal 74 aminoacids of A-24, a non-histone chromosomal protein (Hunt and Dayhoff, 1977). It has also been shown to be homologous with AFP, and ATP dependent coupling factor involved in proteolysis (Wilkinson et al., 1980).

3. BIOLOGICAL PROPERTIES

Despite the dissimilarity in chemical properties, all of the thymic factors described to date, share in common the ability to influence one or more assays of immunologic activity. In some instances, the mechanism appears to involve activation of cyclic nucleotides, while in others the peptides appear to act indirectly by stimulating other endocrine systems.

3.1. Direct Influence of Thymosin on Immunologic Measures

Immunoregulatory effects of both partially purified and purified thymosin preparations have been demonstrated in a variety of animal models (Goldstein et al., 1978; White and Goldstein, 1974; Low and Goldstein, 1978; Goldstein et al.,1981). For example, in thymectomized animals, thymosin treatment has been shown to restore: 1) graft vs. host reactivity, 2) the development of suppressor T-cells, and 3) to correct the cell cycle of lymphocytes from aging thymectomized rats (Law et al., 1968; Asherson et al., 1976; Dabrowski and Goldstein, 1976).

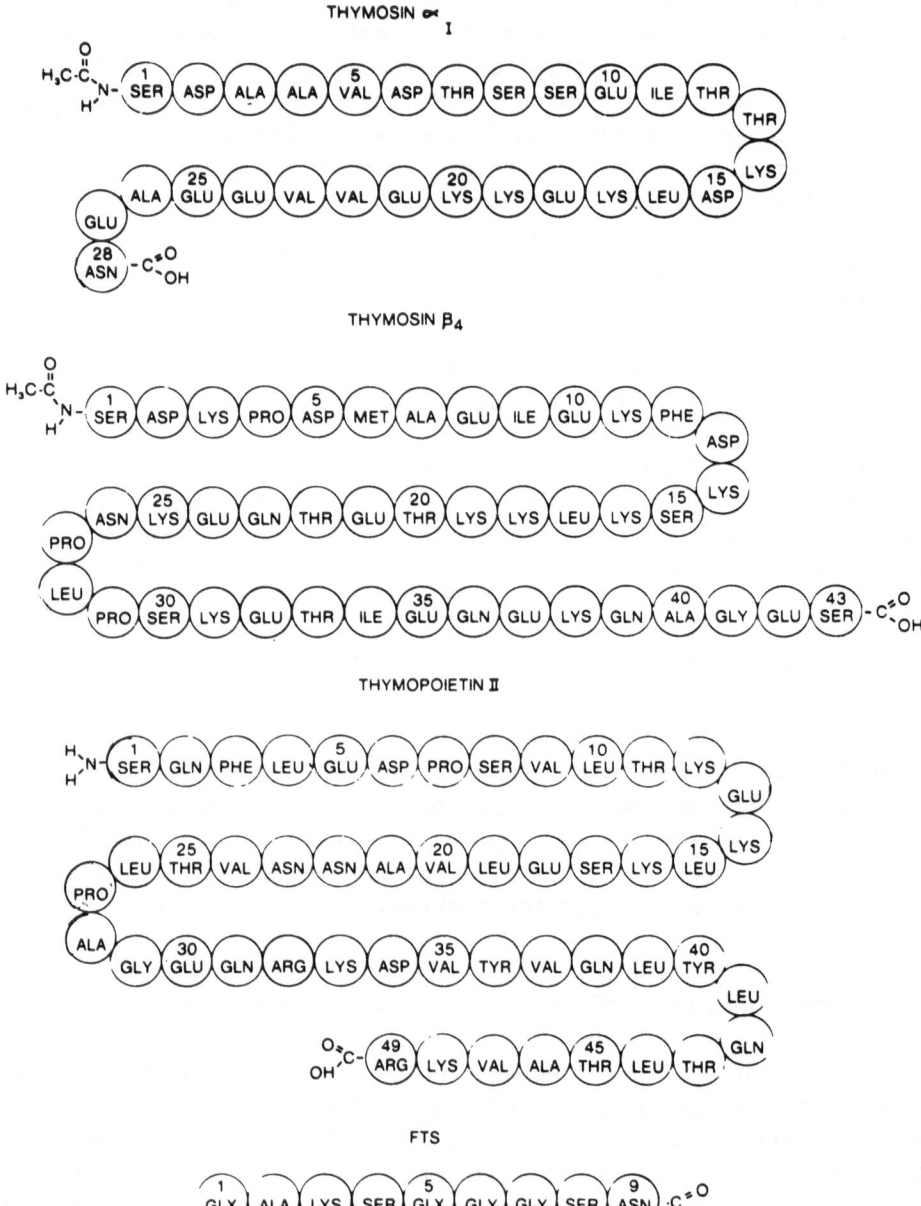

Fig. 1. Amino acid sequence of purified thymic factors.

In aged animals, thymosin treatment has been found to increase:
1) hemagglutinin responses against sheep red blood cells, 2) anti-
-hapten responses to TNP, and 3) delayed hypersensitivity responses to oxazolone (Stausser et al., 1971; D'Agostaro et al., 1980;
Bruley-Rosset, 1979). Using the autoimmune NZB mouse model, thymosin administration has been found to reconstitute suppressor and
other T-cell functions and to temporarily induce remissions in the
autoimmune disease that these animals develop (Gershwin et al.,
1974; Talal et al., 1975; Dauphinee et al., 1974). In addition to
its role in maintaining immunologic balance, thymosin peptides
have been found like other thymic factors, to influence the normal
differentiation of lymphoid cells.

Thymosin peptides have been found to be effective in inducing
the differentiation of specific subsets of T-lymphocytes, such as
killer, helper and suppressor cells (Goldstein et al., 1978, 1981;
Marshall et al., 1980) and in the induction of certain T-cell
markers such TdT, Thy-1 and Lyt (Ahmed et al., 1978, 1979; Scheid
et al., 1973; Pazmino et al., 1978; Hu et al., 1979; Goldschneider
et al., 1980). For example, thymosin fraction 5 and thymosin polypeptides β_3 and β_4 have been found to induce TdT activity "in

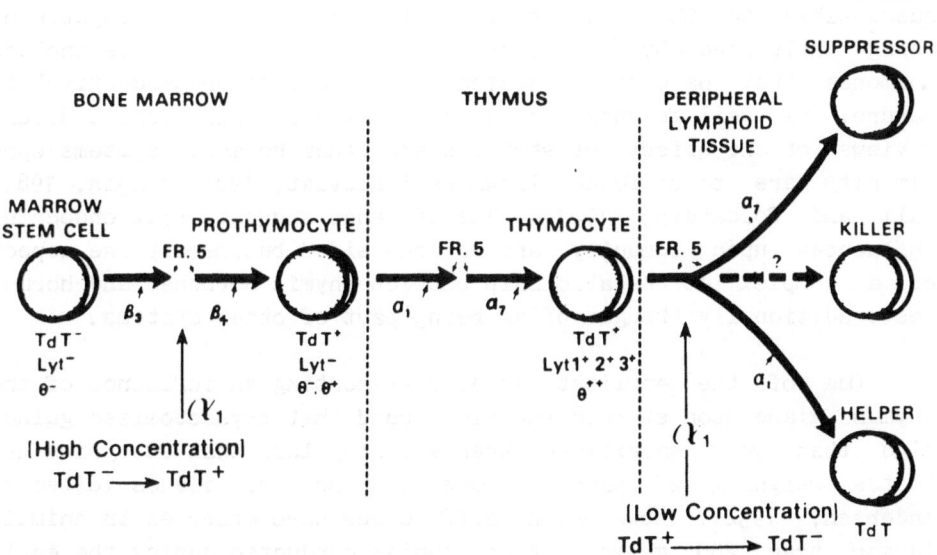

Fig. 2. Proposed role of thymosin peptides in T-cell maturation.

vitro" and "in vivo" in precursor cells from both normal and nude
mice (Pazmino et al., 1978; Hu et al., 1979). It has further been
shown that when thymosin fraction 5 or the purified thymosin β_3
polypeptide are given "in vivo", they significantly accelerate the
recovery of cell numbers and TdT positive cells in the thymus of
steroid-treated immunosuppressed mice. In contrast, thymosin α_1 a
potent inducer of helper T-cells (Goldstein et al., 1977; Ahmed et
al., 1979) decreases TdT positive thymocytes when used at low
concentrations (Wetzel et al., 1980; Hu et al., 1980) but induces
TdT positive cells when used at high concentrations (Goldschneider
et al., 1980).

These data suggest that the individual thymosin polypeptides
may exert their immunomodulatory influences at different stages of
thymocyte differentiation. Based upon the existing evidence,
thymosin β_3 and thymosin β_4 appear to act both prior to and at the
prothymocyte stage. Thymosin α_1 appears to act at both early and
late states of thymocyte maturation. A working hypothesis that
accounts for the reported data is illustrated in Fig. 2.

3.2. Indirect Influences of Thymic Factors upon Immunologic Measures

Many of the immunologic events that have been shown to be
susceptible to the actions of thymic factors are also capable of
being influenced by a variety of hormonal systems. These include
hormones that have been classically regarded as "reproductive" in
nature, as well as those released during stressful events. Recent
reviews of the effects of steroids and other hormonal systems upon
immunity are to be found elsewhere (Ahlqvist, 1981; Monjan, 1981;
Hall and Goldstein, 1981). The evidence suggests that endocrine
influences upon immunity are not one sided but merely one aspect
of a complex interrelationship between thymic hormones and hormones traditionally thought of as being part of other systems.

One of the earliest studies reporting an influence of the
thymus gland upon steroid function found that thymectomized guinea
pigs that were sacrificed when weighing less than 200 grams had
testes weighing 27 percent more than control tissues (cited by
Andersen, 1932). However, no differences were observed in animals
larger than 200 grams. Other studies conducted during the early
part of this century were not always consistent in their findings.

In a critical review of this subject, Andersen (1932) concluded
that the effects of thymectomy upon reproductive function were
most likely the result of trauma rather than of a specific action
of the thymus.

In more recent years, however, it appears that the detection
of thymic influences upon reproductive function may require
additional assays than simply the weighing of gonadal tissue.
Martin (1964) reported the effects of thymectomy upon the growth
of secondary reproductive structures in rats and found that the
removal of this gland resulted in significantly heavier ventral
prostate glands and seminal vesicles. In subsequent studies, it
was found that thymectomy can alter the enzymatic activity of
accessory reproductive structures in pubertal rats (Martin 1964;
Miller and Martin, 1969) and to influence the effects of gonadotropins upon the prostate gland (Rosoff and Martin,1971). In the
latter study, it was found that FSH enhanced the stimulatory
effects of thymectomy upon ventral and lateral prostate gland
weights. Only the lateral prostate weight of thymectomized rats
was enhanced by LH administration. The authors suggested that the
differences in lateral vs ventral prostate weight following LH
administration might have been due to the differential responsiveness of these tissues to certain hormones.

There is also evidence of a modulatory influence of the
thymus upon the female reproductive system. Athymic female mice
have been found to have several deficiencies involving the
reproductive system. The first ovulation is delayed, the ovarian
tissue is diminished in size and lacks large follicles, and the
animals display an abnormal estrus cycle (Besedovsky and Sorkin,
1974; Lintern-Moore and Pantelouris, 1975).

These changes are thought to be due to deficient levels of
pituitary serum gonadotropins with subsequent reduction of some
steroids (Rebar et al., 1981). Similar changes have been reported
in female mice that were thymectomized as neonates (Nishizuka and
Sakakura, 1971), although it has been found that treatment of
neonatally thymectomized animals with gonadotropin hormone prevents some of the histological changes associated with the ovaries
(Lintern-Moore and Pantelouris, 1976; Michael et al., 1981).

In a related study, Weinstein (1978) measured levels of gonadotropin hormones in serum and pituitary tissue from congeanitally

thymic female mice. There were no significant difference in either the gonadotropin hormone levels in pituitary and serum or of gonadotropin releasing hormone in the hypothalamus, but differences were observed in the animals hormonal feedback system. Following ovariectomy, serum LH levels in normal mice were almost 10 times higher that in non-ovariectomized animals, however, no increase was observed in the ovariectomized nude mice. Although not as great as in the control animals, serum levels of LH did increase by almost 6 fold when the athymic mice were injected with gonadotropin releasing hormone. Consequently, it was concluded that the aberrant cycling and lack of normal feedback following thymectomy were indicative of a disfunction involving the central nervous system (Weinstein, 1978). Since athymic mice implanted with thymic tissue at birth exhibited a normal elevation of LH following ovariectomy, a relationship between the thymus gland and normal functioning of neuroendocrine control systems is evident.

3.3. Effects of Thymic Extracts Upon Steroids

     Interest in thymic hormone research has intensified during the past two decades. As more sophisticated methods have been applied to evaluate the chemical and biological properties of thymic extracts, it has become apparent that they are comprised of a variety of hormonal-like polypeptides.

     Crude thymic extracts have been used in a number of studies investigating thymic influences upon the reproductive system. While inconclusive, there are claims in the literature that cryptorchidism can be cured by the injection of thymus extract (Andersen, 1932). There is also evidence of synergism between thymic extracts and ovarian hormones, although apparently not specific to the thymus gland since muscle extracts were found to be effective as well (Andersen, 1932). In 1971, Comsa reported that gonadal degeneration occurred in thymectomized guinea pigs, but that this degeneration could be prevented by the administration of a thymic extract. Deschaux et al. (1979) have extended this observation by comparing the effects of two thymic extracts upon a variety of endocrine systems. Extracts were prepared by the method of Bernardi and Comsa (1965) or by the method of Goldstein et al. (1972). Rats were thymectomized within 24 hours of birth and subsequently treated with either homeostatic thymic hormone or thymosin. Animals were sacrificed at various ages and serum levels of testosterone, corticosterone, LH and ACTH were measured. Both thymic extracts were found to restore the decreased body, adrenal and testes weight that followed thymectomy. Plasma corticosterone was decreased through 60 days in neonatally rats, while ACTH showed biphasic changes. This peptide hormone was lower than control values at 15, 30, and 45 days, higher at 60 days and normal by 90 days. These hormonal changes were not observed in thymectomized animals treated with either of the thymic extracts. Muscle extract was used as a control substance and was without effect. A similar, though opposite, biphasic pattern was exbibited by testosterone and LH. Elevations were observed at 30 days, a significant decrease at 60 days and no difference at 90 days. Administration of thymic extracts was found to reduce the extent of these changes.

The mechanism(s) by which these changes occurred appeared to be different for each hormone system. An influence at the level of the pituitary gland was suggested for the reproductive hormone changes since the thymic extracts failed to prevent them when given to thymectomized-hypophysectomized rats. However, the exracts prevented the glucocorticoid changes regardless of whether the pituitary was present. It is also possible that the thymic extracts were having an influence at the level of the central nervous system with respect to the LH and testosterone changes. Such a mechanism is consistent with Weinsteins (1978) conclusion that the thymus acts at the level of the CNS to influence LH cyclicity and feedback control in the female mouse. This conclusion is further supported by recent observation that thymosin fraction 5 can stimulate LRF and LH release when superinfused into hypothalamic tissue "in vitro" (Rebar et al., submitted).

3.4. Effects of Purified Thymosin Polypeptides upon Neuroendocrine Systems

The "in vivo" effects of the intracerebral administration of purified thymosin peptides upon endocrine and immunologic measures in adult mice and rats is currently under investigation in our laboratory. These studies utilize a paradigm in which thymic peptides are injected into the 3rd or lateral ventricle of unanesthetized animals. Preliminary studies have revealed that this procedure results in minimal stress to the animals as determined by measuring serum corticosterone levels and causes no

abnormal behavioral consequences following the injection of either
purified thymosin peptides or the more heterogeneous preparation,
thymosin fraction 5.

Antibody titers to SRBC have been found to be significantly
depressed in female mice that received thymosin fraction 5 or
thymosin α_7 when compared with saline injected control animals
(Hall et al., 1981). In contrast, female mice that received
intracerebral thymosin α_1 had slightly elevated antibody titers.
No significant differences were observed in the mixed lymphocyte
response or spleen cell response to LPS. However, spleen cell
responsiveness to PHA and Con-A were significantly depressed in
animals that received thymosin fraction 5 (Hall et al., 1981). The
possibility that some of these immunologic changes might have been
due to an altered neuroendocrine axis was suggested by the
observation that the pituitary glands and ovaries were enlarged in
the thymosin fraction 5 treated animals, but not in those that
received thymosin α_1 or thymosin α_7. Similar observations were
recorded in pilot studies using a similar procedure in adult male
rats. Thymosin fraction 5 injected into the third ventricle
resulted in a variety of changes of immunological measures, as
well as an increase in the testis-body weight ratio. These changes
were not observed in rats that received systemic injections of the
same dose of thymosin fraction 5, suggesting a role for thymosin
at the level of the CNS-pituitary axis.

While the precise mechanism of action remains to be elucidated, these findings are consistent with the previously discussed data suggesting a role for the thymus gland in modulating
gonadotropin hormone levels. If the thymic peptides are indeed
playing a physiological role in modulating various neuroendocrine
systems, their presence within the CNS should be demonstrable.
Preliminary results from our laboratory, as well as from other
laboratories, indicate that they are. Belokrylov et al., (1979)
have reported the presence of low molecular weight polypeptides
(mol. wt. < 10,000) in extracts of bovine cerebral cortex and of
white matter and evaluated their effect upon hemoagglutination
titers. Injection of extracts from the cerebral cortex, but not
from white matter was found to significantly elevate antibody
titers to SRBC. This extract has subsequently been called cortexin
and has been found to have cross-reactivity with rabbit antisera
prepared against thymosin. Since the antibodies were made against
heterogenous thymic extracts, it is possible that they contained

ubiquitin cross-reactivity. Because ubiquitin is synthetized in rat brain and human pituitary gland (Seidah et al., 1978; Scherrer et al., 1978), this peptide might have accounted for not only the cross-reactivity of the antibody against thymus extracts, but also the biological activity of the brain extract. Ubiquitin has been reported to induce the differentiation of T and B lymphocytes (G. Goldstein et al., 1975) which might have accounted for the increased antibody titers which resulted from injection of the brain extracts into mice. A low molecular weight peptide with thymocyte stimulating properties has also been extracted from anterior pituitary gland (Saxena and Talwar, 1977). This peptide has been found to cause a significant elevation in ^{3}H-TdR uptake in thymocytes.

Using a RIA, developed to measure the purified peptide thymosin α_1, we have conducted a preliminary analysis of gross brain regions in order to assess whether this particular peptide is present in discrete brain regions. Brains of adult male guinea pigs were perfused with physiological saline to remove those peptides circulating in the serum. This was done since pilot studies revealed that brain levels of thymosin α_1-like activity were elevated by up to 70% in some brain regions from non perfused tissue. Tissue was then dissected grossly into discrete regions and extracted using the procedure of Straus et al. (1977). Thymosin α_1 cross-reactivity was found to be highest in the diencephalon and lowest in the cortex. Mesencephalon and brainstem contained intermediate levels. These relative differences have also been found in discrete regions of rat brain tissue with highest levels of α_1 cross-reactivity in the hypothalamus and pituitary and lowest levels in the cortex and spinal cord (Hall et al., 1981). In all brain regions assayed, one major peak of immunoreactivity was present which had a molecular weight similar to that of thymosin α_1. It was not possible to assess the precise subcortical localization of thymosin α_1 cross-reactivity using grossly dissected tissue, however, related studies suggest that much of this cross reactivity may have been due to thymosin α_1-like material in the CSF and/or circumventricular organs.

A comparison of sagittal, horizontal and coronal sections through the brains of animals injected intraperitoneally with ^{125}I thymosin α_1 has revealed greatest radioactivity to be associated with several of the circumventricular organs, especially the median eminence, organum vasculosum of the lamina terminalis

(OVLT) and area postrema. Thus, the influences exerted by thymosin
hormones upon neuroendocrine measures probably occurs in these
specialized regions. It is also of interest that thymosin α_1 has
been detected in human CSF by RIA (McClure et al. unpublished
observation). Therefore, in addition to gaining access to circumventricular organs via the blood stream, thymic hormones might
also have access to neuroendocrine centers by transport through
tanycytes as illustrated in Fig. 3.

4. DISCUSSION

    Numerous reports of hormonal interactions with immunologic
parameters can be found in the literature. But many investigations
have been conducted using either pharmacologic doses of the
hormone under study, or analogs not normally found in the animal

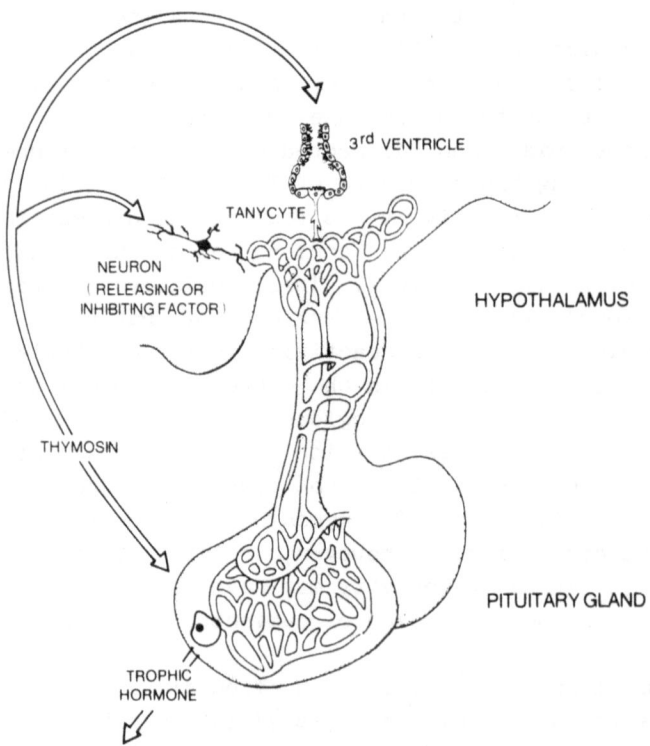

Fig. 3. Proposed sites of action of thymosin peptides in regula-
    ting neuroendocrine function.

model being utilized, i.e., the testing of hydrocortisone in rodents. Therefore, while statistically significant changes are thought provoking, of paramount importance is the physiological significance of neuroendocrine effects upon immunity.

An intriguing hypothesis that might explain the biological significance of glucocorticoid inhibition of immune functioning has been discussed by Besedovsky and Sorkin (1977). These authors have demonstrated that at the time of maximum antibody production, there occurs an increase in serum corticosterone levels. It was suggested that this increase in a potentially inhibitory hormone plays an important role in immunospecificity. This hypothesis is supported by following evidence.

Non-antigen stimulated thymocytes residing in the thymic cortex are more susceptible to the inhibitory effects of steroids than are sensitized T-cells. Consequently, the elevated steroid would more likely inhibit these lymphocytes with either low or no affinity for the antigen. This could provide a modulatory influence preventing the proliferation of cells that might otherwise be activated by soluble factors produced by either leukocytes or thymic epithelial cells. It was noted that such a model is not inconsistent with lateral or afferent inhibition of neurons in order to reduce non-specific sensory signals.

It was predicted by Besedovsky and Sorkin (1977) that if corticosteroids are playing a regulatory role, then the injection of a second immunogen at the time of elevated corticosteroid levels should result in a lower titer of antibody to that second immunogen. The predicted inhibition was observed. When SRBC were injected into rats that had previously been immunized with TNP-horse red blood cells, there was a marked depression of the PFC response to the SRNC. Corticosteroids were implicated when it was found that this depression did not occur in rats that had been adrenalectomized prior to the first sensitization.

Thus, the corticosteroids could be regarded as fine tuning the immune response by suppressing the clonal expansion of cells that lack high affinity for the inducing immunogen. As suggested by the authors, such a mechanism might also serve to reduce the probability of autoimmune disease, a concept that is supported by a number of clinical studies (Craddock, 1978).

It has also been proposed that the thymus gland may interact with the glucocorticoid axis by acting as an antistressor (Martin, 1976). This hypothesis is consistent with evidence that thymic extracts are able to prevent the rise in ACTH and corticosterone that normally follows thymectomy (Deschaux et al., 1979).

A modulatory role for the thymus upon glucocorticoid effects is further supported by the observation that thymosin administration to steroid treated mice either increased the Con-A response of spleen cells, if it were low, or decreased the response, if it were elevated (Thurman et al., 1977). There is additional evidence that thymic factors may interfere with the binding of corticosteroids and in this way perhaps suppress their activity. Bach et al. (1975) reported that FTS was able to cause a 60-70% inhibition of steroid binding when thymocyte cytosol preparations were incubated in the presence of the purified serum factor.

A possible physiological role for gonadotropins during the immune response is suggested by the demonstration that within 1 to 2 hours following the injection of allogeneic cells, there occurs a rapid increase in serum LH levels (Pierpaoli and Maestroni, 1977).

It was suggested by these authors that the rise in LH might have been due to release of lymphokines from immunoreactive lymphocytes. While previously discussed studies suggest a role for thymic hormones acting at the level of the brain or pituitary in bringing about gonadotropin release, the possibility that lymphokines may also play a role cannot be discounted, especially since lymphokine-containing supernatants from Con-A stimulated lymphocytes have been found to cause a 3 fold increase in serum corticosteroid levels within 1 to 2 hours after injection into animals (Besedovsky et al., 1981) and humans (Dumonde et al., 1981).

While none of the above hypotheses have been fully substantiated, there is sufficient evidence to suggest that the endocrine thymus is regulated in much the same way as are other endocrine tissues. A summary of the major evidence in support of this hypothesis is summarized in Table 1.

Consequently, it is proposed that the endocrine thymus is part of a neuroendocrine axis that is capable of influencing its own functioning via hormones produced by thymic epithelial cells. A diagrammatic representation of how this axis might function is illustrated in Figure 4. In addition, there is also evidence that during ontogeny, the thymus gland may play an integral role in the programming of neuroendocrine mechanisms, especially those related

Table 1. Summary of major evidence in support of a neuroendocrine-
        thymus axis.

Surgical and pharmacologic manipulation of neuroendocrine regions can influence thymic dependent immunity	(See review by Hall and Goldstein, 1981)
Some hormones under CNS control are effected by neonatal thymectomy or by genetic absence of the thymus	(Pierpaoli and Sorkin, 1972; Pierpaoli et al., 1976)
Thymic hormone administration can normalize changes in certain CNS controlled hormones following thymectomy	(Deschaux et al., 1979)
Injection of thymosin peptides directly into the brain can result in both endocrine and immunologic changes	(Hall et al., 1081)
Thymosin α_1 has been localized in hypothalamic tissue by the use of RIA	See text
Systemically injected radiolabelled thymosin α_1 can be localized in circumventricular organs	See text
During the course of immunity, electrical, morphological and neurochemical changes can be detected in the CNS	(See review by Hall and Goldstein, 1981; Hall, 1981)

to reproductive physiology (Pierpaoli et al., 1970, 1976; Pierpaoli and Sorkin, 1972, 1972b; Pierpaoli and Besedovsky, 1975).

While there is considerable evidence in support of this model, an additional possibility which accounts for nearly all of the evidence cited has to be considered. Thymic hormones and lymphokines may simply act upon phagocytic cells in the brain that are involved with defense against neurologic disease. These might include supraependymal cells, which have many of the characteristics of macrophages (Bleier and Albrecht, 1980) and certain glial cells which can be stimulated by supernatants from Con-A stimulated lymphocytes (Fontana et al., 1980). It has also been shown that immunosuppression can be correlated with suppression of trauma-induced proliferation of glial cells (Billingsley et al., 1981).

   Macrophages have been found to synthesize and secrete prostaglandins (Stradecker and Unanue, 1979). If such release were to
occur from lymphokine or thymic peptide activated macrophages in
the brain, it might account for some of the hormonal changes that
have been correlated with host defense. PGE has been shown to
cause the release of corticotropin releasing factor (CRF) and lu-
teinizing hormone releasing factor (LRF) in brain tissue (Harms et

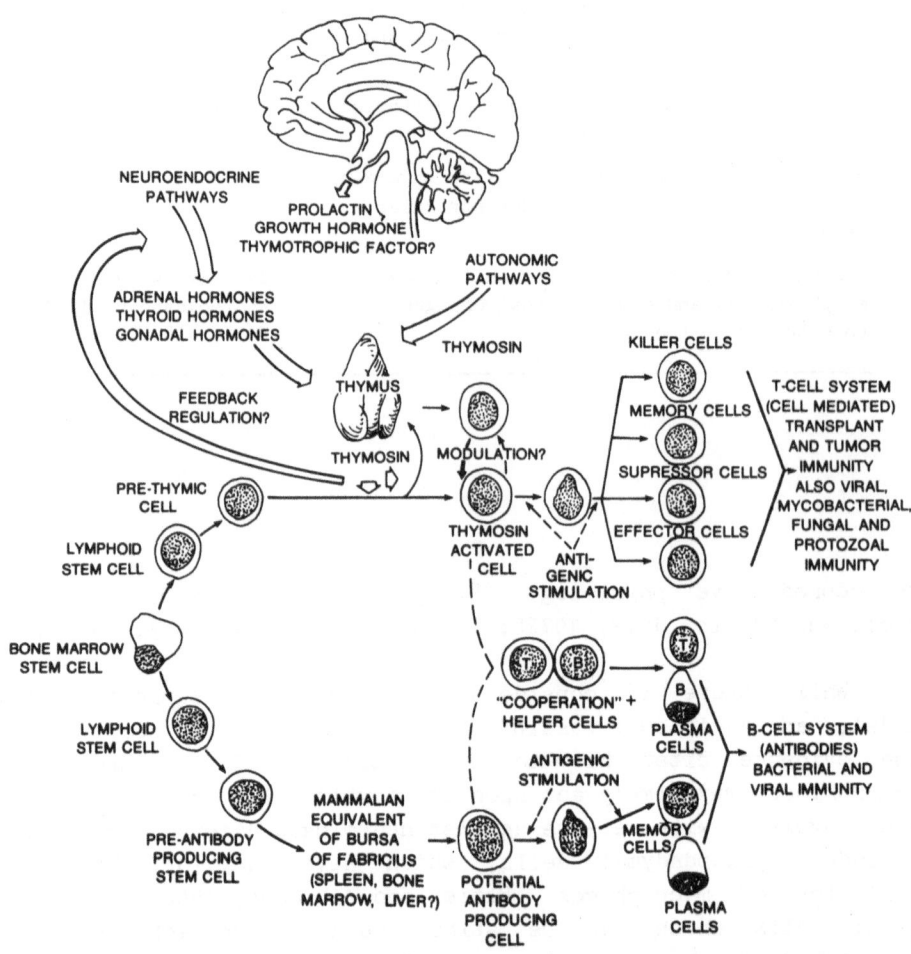

Fig. 4. Interrelationship of the endocrine thymus with the central
       nervous system.

al., 1973; Hedge, 1976) and mimic some of the biological effects
of LRF when injected into the brain (Hall et al., 1975; Hall and
Luttge, 1977). This latter hypothesis does not necessarily con-
tradict the model proposed in Figure 4. To the contrary, it
suggests a mechanism by which some of the observed hormonal changes might be brought about during the course of the immune
response.

ACKNOWLEDGEMENTS

The present work was supported in part by grants from the
National Cancer Institute (CA 2494), the National Institute on
Aging (AG 01531) and Hoffman-LaRoche, Inc., Nutley,N.J.

REFERENCES

Ahlqvist, J., 1981, Outline of endocrine influences on immune pro-
        cesses, in: "Psychoneuroimmunology", R. Ader, ed., Academic
        Press New York.
Ahmed, A., Smith, A.H., Wong, D.M., Thurman, G.B., Goldstein, A.L.
        and Sell, K.W., 1978, In vitro induction of Lyt surface markers
        on precursor cells incubated with thymosin polypeptides, Cancer
        Treat. Rep., 62:1739.
Ahmed, A., Wong, D.M., Thurman, G.B., Low, T.L.K., Goldstein, A.L.,
        Sharkis, S.J., and Goldschneider, I., 1979, T-lymphocyte matura-
        tion: Cell surface markers and immune function induced by T-
        -lymphocyte cell free products and thymosin polypeptides, Ann.
        N.Y. Acad. Sci., 332:81.
Andersen, D.H., 1932, The relationship between the thymus and repro-
        duction, Physiol. Rev., 12:1.
Asherson, G.B., Sembala, M., Nayhew, B. and Goldstein, A.L., 1976,
        Adult thymectomy: prevention of the appearance of suppressor T
        cells which depress contact sensitivity to picryl chloride and
        reversal of adult thymectomy effect by thymus extract, Eur. J.
        Immunol., 6:699.
Bach, J.F., Duval, D., Dardenne, M., Solomon, J.C., Tursz, T. and
        Fournier, C., 1975, The effects of steroids on T cells,
        Transplant. Proc., 7: 25.
Bach, J.F., Dardenne, M., Pleau, J.M. and Rosa,J., 1977, Biochemical
        characterization of serum thymic factor, Nature, 266:55.

Belokrylov, G.A., Morozov, V.G. and Khavinson, K.H.,1979, Effect of
    substances of polypeptide nature isolated from the cerebral
    cortex on the immune response in mice, Bull. Exp. Biol. Med.,
    86:1631.
Bernardi G. and Comsa, J., 1965, Purification chromatographique
    d'une preparation de thymus donée d'activité hormonale, Expe-
    rientia, 21:416.
Besedovsky, H.O. and Sorkin, E., 1974, Thymus involvement in female
    sexual maturation, Nature, 249:356.
Besedovsky, H.O. and Sorkin, E., 1977, Network of immune-neuroendo-
    crine interactions, Clin. Exp. Immunol., 27:1.
Besedovsky, H.O., Del Rey, A. and Sorkin E., 1981, Lymphokine-con-
    taining supernatants from Con-A-stimulated cells increase cor-
    ticosterone blood levels, J. Immunol., 126:385.
Biggar, W.D., Park, B.H. and Good, R.A., 1973, Immunologic recon-
    stitution, Ann. Rev. Med., 24:135.
Billingsley, M.L., Hall, N.R. and Mandel, H.G., 1981, Immunosuppres-
    sion blocks trauma induced neuroglial DNA synthesis in the rat,
    Fed. Proc., 40:526.
Bleier R., and Algrecht, R., 1980, Supraependymal macrophages of
    third ventricle of hamster: Morphological, functional and hi-
    stochemical characterization in "situ" and in culture, J. Comp.
    Neurol., 192:489.
Bruley-Rosset, M., Florentin, I., Kiger, N., Schulz, J., Davigny, M.
    and Mathé, G., 1979, in: "The immune system, functions and the-
    rapy of dysfunction," H. Faraitre, ed., Academic Press, New York.
Comsa, J., 1971, Thymic hormones, Hormones, 2:226.
Craddock, D.G., 1978, Corticosteriod-induced lymphopenia, immunosup-
    pression and body defense, Ann. Int. Med., 88:564.
Dabrowski, M.P., and Goldstein, A.L., 1976, Thymosin induced changes
    in cell cycle of lymphocytes, from aging neonatally thymectomi-
    zed rats, Immunol. Commun., 5:695.
D'Agostaro, G., Frasca, D., Garavini, M. and Doria, G., 1980, Immu-
    norestoration of old mice by injection of thymus extract;
    enhancement of T-cell, T-cell cooperation in the in vitro anti-
    body response, Cell. Immunol., 53:207.
Dalmasso, A.P., Martinez, C., Sjodin, K., and Good, A., 1963. Stu-
    dies on the role of the thymus in immunology. Reconstitution
    of immunologic capacity in mice thymectomized at birth, J.
    Exp. Med., 118:1089.
Dauphinée, M.J., Talal, N., Goldstein, A L. and White, A., 1974,
    Thymosin corrects the abnormal DNA synthetic response of NZB
    mouse thymocytes, Proc. Natl. Acad. Sci., 71:2637.

Davies, A.J.S., 1969, The thymus and the cellular basis of immuni-
    ty, Transplant. Rev., 1:43.
Deschaux, P., Massengo, and Fontanges, R., 1979, Endocrine interac-
    tion of the thymus with the hypophysis, adrenals and testes:
    effects of two thymic extracts, Thymus, 1:95.
Dumonde, D.C., Pulley, M.S., Hamblin, A.S Singh, A.K., Southcott, B.
    M., O'Connell, D., Paradinas, F.J., Robinson, M.R.G., Rigby,
    C.C., Hollander, F. den, Schurs, A., Verheul, H. and Vliet, E.
    van, Short term and long term administration of lymphoblastoid
    cell line lymphokine (LVL-LK) to patients with advanced cancer,
    in: "Lymphokines and Thymic Hormones: Their Potential Utili-
    zation in Cancer Therapeutics," A.L. Goldstein and M.A.
    Chirigos, eds., Raven Press, in press.
East, J. and Parrott, D.M.V., 1964, Prevention of wasting in mice
    thymectomized at birth and their subsequent rejection of allo-
    geneic leukemic cells, J. Natl. Cancer Inst., 33:673.
Fontana, A., Grieder, A., Arrenbrecht, S.T. and Grob, P., 1980, "In
    vitro" stimulation of glia cells by a lymphocyte-produced fac-
    tor, J. Neurological Sci., 46:55.
Gershwin, M.E., Ahmed, A., Steinberg, A.D., Thurman, G.B. and Gold-
    stein, A.L., 1974, Correction of T-cell function by thymosin
    in New Zealand mice, J. Immunol., 113:1068.
Gershwin, M.E., Kruise, W. and Goldstein G., 1979, The effect of
    thymopoietin 32=36 and ubiquitin on spontaneous immunopathology
    of New Zealand mice, J. Rheumatol., 6:610.
Goldschneider, I., Ahmed, A., Bollum, F.J. and Goldstein, A.L.,1981,
    Induction of terminal deoxynucleotidyl transferase and Lyt an-
    tigens with thymosin: Identification of multiple subsets of
    prothymocytes in mouse bone marrow and spleen, Proc. Natl.
    Acad. Sci., 78:2469.
Goldstein, A.L., Slater, F.D. and White, A., 1966, Preparation, as-
    say and partial purification of a thymic lymphocytopoietic
    factor (Thymosin), Proc. Natl. Acad. Sci., 56:1010.
Goldstein, A.L., Guha, A., Zatz, M.M. and White, A., 1972, Purifi-
    cation and biological activity of thymosin, a hormone of the
    thymus gland, Proc. Natl. Acad. Sci., 69:1800.
Goldstein, G., Scheid, M., Hammerling, U., Boyse, E.A., Schlesin-
    ger, D.H. and Nial, H.D., 1975, Isolation of a polypeptide that
    has lymphocyte-differentiating properties and is probably re-
    presented universally in living cells, Proc. Natl. Acad. Sci.,
    72:11.
Goldstein, A.L., Low, T.L.K., McAdoo, M., McClure, J., Thurman, G.
    B., Rossio, J.L., Lai, C-y, Chang, D., Wang, S-S., Harvey, C.,

Ramel, A.H., and Meienhofer, J., 1977, Thymosin α_1: Isolation
    and sequence analysis of an immunologically active thymic poly-
    peptide, Proc. Natl. Acad. Sci., 74:725.

Goldstein, A.L., Thurman, G.B., Low, T.L.K., Rossio, J.L. and Tri-
    vers, G.E., 1978, Hormonal influences on the reticuloendothe-
    lial system. Current status of the role of thymosin in the re-
    gulation and modulation of immunity, J. Reticuloend. Soc.,
    23:252.

Goldstein, A.L., Low, T.L.K., Thurman, G.B., Zatz, M.M., Hall, N.R.
    Chen, C-P., Hu, S-K., Naylor, P.B. and McClure, J.E., 1981, Cur-
    rent status of thymosin and other hormones of the thymus gland,
    Recent Progress in Hormone Res., in press.

Goldstein, G., Lau, C.Y., 1980, Immunoregulation by thymopoietin.,
    J. Supramol. Struct., 14:397.

Hall, N.r., 1980, Neural control of immunogenesis, in: Molecular
    and behavioral neuroendocrinology. C.B., Nemeroff and A.J. Dunn,
    eds., Spectrum, N.Y., in press.

Hall, N.R. and Goldstein, A.L., 1981, Endocrine regulation of host
    immunity: the role of steroids and thymosins, in: "Immunogeni-
    city," F. Borek, ed., Elsevier Press, Holland, in press.

Hall, N.R. and Luttge, W.G., 1977, Diencephalic sites responsive to
    prostaglandin E_2: facilitation of sexual receptivity in estro-
    gen primed, ovariectomized rats, Brain Res. Bull., 2:203.

Hall, N.R., Luttge, W.G. and Berry, R.B., 1975, Intracerebral pro-
    staglandin E_2: Effects upon sexual behavior, open-field acti-
    vity and body temperature in ovariectomized female rats, Pro-
    staglandins, 10:177.

Hall, N.R., Palaszynski, E.W., Moody, T.W. and Goldstein, A.L.,
    1981, Evidence for a CNS-thymus axis involving thymosin pepti-
    des, Soc. for Neuroscience, abstract.

Harms, P.G., Ojeda, S.R., and McCann, S.M., 1973, Prostaglandin in-
    volvement in hypothalamic control of gonadotropin and prolac-
    tin release, Science, 181:760.

Hays, E.F., 1967, The effects of allografts on thymic epithelial re-
    ticular cells on the tissues of neonatally thymectomized mice,
    Blood, 29:29.

Hedge, G.A., 1976, Hypothalamic and pituitary effects of prostaglan-
    dins on ACTH secretion, Prostaglandins, 11:293.

Hooper, J.A., McDaniel, M.C., Thurman, G.B., Cohen, G.H., Schulof,
    R.S., and Goldstein, A.L., 1975, Purification and properties of
    bovine thymosin, Ann. N.Y. Acad. Sci., 249:125.

Hu, S-K., Low, T.L.K., and Goldstein, A.L, 1979, "in vivo" induction
    of terminal deoxynucleotidyl transferase (TdT) by thymosin in

hydrocortisone acetate (HCA) treated mice, Proc. Fed. Am. Soc. Exp. Biol., 38:4501, abstract,

Hu, S-K., Thurman, G.B., Low, T.L.K., McClure, J., and Goldstein, A. L., 1980, Multifaced role of purified thymosin peptides in differentiation and function of T cells, New Trends Immunol. Cancer Ther., in press.

Hunt, L.T., and Dayhoff, M.D., 1977, Amino-terminal sequence identity of ubiquitin and the non histonic component of nuclear protein A24, Biochem. Biophys. Res. Commun., 74:650.

Law, L.W., Goldstein, A.L. and White, A., 1968, Influence of thymosin on immunological competence of lymphoid cells from thymectomized mice, Nature, 219:1391.

Leuchars, E., Cross, A.M., and Dukov, P., 1965, The restoration of immunologic function by thymus grafting in thymectomized irradiated mice, Transplantation, 3:28.

Lintern-Moore, S., and Pantelouris, E.M., 1975, Ovarian development in athymic nude mice. The size and composition of the follicle population, Mech. Age. Dev., 4:385.

Lintern-Moore, S., and Pantelouris, E.M., 1976, Ovarian development in athymic nude mice. III. The effect of PMSG and oestradiol upon the size and composition of the ovarian follicle population, Mech. Age. Dev., 5:33.

Low, T.L.K., Thurman, G.B., McAdoo, M., McClure, J.E., Rossio, J.L., Naylor, P.H., and Goldstein, A.L., 1979, The chemistry and biology of thymosin, J. Biol. Chem., 254:981.

Low, T.L.K. and Goldstein, A.L., 1979, The chemistry and biology of thymosin, J. Biol. Chem., 254:987.

Low, T.L.K., Hu, S-K., and Goldstein, A.L., 1981, Complete amino acid sequence of bovine thymosin B_4: A thymic hormone that induces a terminal deoxynucleotidyl transferase activity in thymocyte populations, Proc. Natl. Acad. Sci., 78:1166.

Martin, C.R., 1964, Influence of thymectomy on growth of secondary reproductive structures in rats, Am. J. Physiol., 206:193.

Martin, C.R., 1976, Textbook of Endocrine Physiology, Williams and Wilkins, Baltimore, p. 390.

Michael, S.D., Taguchi, O. and Nishijuka, Y., 1981, Changes in hypophyseal hormones associated with accelerated aging and tumorigenesis of the ovaries in neonatally thymectomized mice, Endocrinology, 108:2375.

Miller, J.F.A.P., 1966, The thymus in relation to the development of immunological capacity, in: "Experimental and clinical studies," G.E.W. Wolstenholme and R. Porter, eds., Ciba Found. Symp., Churchill, London, p. 153.

Miller, L., and Martin, C.R., 1969, Further investigation of thymic
     influence on reproductive structure maturation, Proc. Fed. Amer.
     Soc. Exp. Biol., 28:774, abstract.
Monjan, A.A., 1981, Stress and immunologic competence; studies in
     animals, in: "Psychoneuroimmunology," R. Ader, ed., in press.
Nishizuka, Y. and Sakakura, T., 1971, Ovarian dysgenesis induced
     by neonatal thymectomy in the mouse, Endocrinology, 89:886.
Pasmino, N.H., Ihle, J.N. and Goldstein, A.L., 1978, Induction "in
     vivo" and "in vitro" of terminal deoxynucleotidyl transferase by
     thymosin in bone marrow cells from athymic mice, J. Exp. Med.,
     147:708.
Pierpaoli, W., and Besedovsky, H.O., 1975, Role of the thymus in pro-
     gramming of neuroendocrine functions, Clin. Exp. Immunol.,
     20:323.
Pierpaoli, W., and Maestroni, G.J.M., 1977, Pharmacological control
     of the immune response by blockade of the early hormonal chan-
     ges following antigen injection, Cell. Immunol., 31:355.
Pierpaoli, W., and Sorkin, E., 1972a, Hormones, thymus, and lympho-
     cyte functions, Experientia, 28:1385.
Pierpaoli, W., and Sorkin, E., 1972b, Alterations of adrenal cortex
     and thyroid in mice with congenital absence of the thymus,
     Nature, New Biol., 238:282.
Pierpaoli, W., Fabris, N., and Sorkin, E., 1970, Developmental hor-
     mones and immunological maturation, in: "Hormones and the im-
     mune response," G.E.W. Wolstenholme and J. Knight, eds., Ciba
     Found. Study Group No. 36, Churchill, London, p. 126.
Pierpaoli, W., Kopp, H.G., and Bianchi, E., 1976, Interdependence of
     thymic and neuroendocrine functions in ontogeny, Clin. Exp.
     Immunol., 24:501.
Rosoff, B., and Martin, C.R., 1971, The influence of thymectomy and
     sham operation on prostate gland responses of hooded rats to
     gonadotrophins, Gen. Comp. Endocr., 16:484.
Saxena, R.K., and Talwar, G.P., 1977, An anterior pituitary factor
     stimulates thymidine incorporation in isolated thymocytes,
     Nature, 268:57.
Scheid, M.P., Hoffman, M.K., Komuro, K.,Hammerling, H., Boyse,
     E.A., Cohen, G.H., Hooper, J.A., Schulof, R.S., and Goldstein
     A.L., 1973, Differentiation of T cells induced by preparations
     from thymus and by nonthymic agents, J. Exp. Med., 138:1027.
Scherrer, H., Seidah, N.G., Benjannet, S., Crine, P., Lis, M., and
     Chretien, M.,1978, Biosynthesis of a ubiquitin-related pepti-
     de in rat brain and in human and mouse pituitary tumors, Bio-
     chem. Biophys. Res. Commun., 84:874.

Seidah, N.G., Crine, P., Benjannet, S., Scherrer, H., and Chretien, M., 1978, Isolation and partial characterization of a biosynthetic N-terminal metionyl peptide of bovine pars intermedia: Relationship to ubiquitin, Biochem. Biophys. Res. Commun., 80:600.

Stadecker, M.J., and Unanue, E.R., 1979, Macrophage secretion of micromolecules, Ann. N.Y. Acad. Sci., 332:550.

Straus, E., Muller, J.E., Choi, H-S., Paronetto, F., and Yalow, R.S., 1977, Immunohistochemical localization in rabbit brain of a peptide resembling the COOH-terminal octapeptide of cholecystokinin, Proc. Natl. Acad. Sci., 74:3033.

Strausser, H.R., Bober, L.A., Bisci, R.A. Schillcock, J.A., and Goldstein, A.L., 1971, Stimulation of the hemagglutinin response of aged mice by cell-free lymphoid tissue fractions and bacteria endotoxin, Exp. Gerontol., 6:373.

Talal, N., Dauphinée, M., Philarisetty, R., and Goldblum, R., 1975, Effect of thymosin on thymocyte proliferation and autoimmunity in NZB mice, Ann. N.Y. Acad. Sci., 249:438.

Thurman, G.B., Rossio, J.L., and Goldstein, A.L., 1977, Antibody-forming cells with specificity for syngeneic and allogeneic (Thymocyte) tissue antigens following lipopolysaccharide mitogenic stimulation, Transplant. Proc., 9:1201.

Trainin, N., Small, M., Ziport, D., Umiel, T., Kook, A.I. and Rotter, V., 1975, in: "The Biological activity of thymic hormones," D.W. VanBekkum, ed., Kooyker Scientific. Pub., Amsterdam, p.261.

Weinstein, Y., 1978, Impairment of the hypothalamo-pituitary-ovarian axis of the athymic nude mouse, Mech. Age. Dev., 8:63.

Wetzel, R., Heyneker, H.L., Goeddel, D.V., Jhurani, P., Shapiro, J., Crea, R., Low, T.L.K., McClure, J.E., and Goldstein, A.L, 1980, Production of biologically active N^{α} desacetylthymosin α_1 in Escherichia coli through expression of a chemically synthesized gene, Biochemistry, 19:6096.

Wilkinson, K.D., Uran, M.K., and Haos, A.L., 1980, Ubiquitin is the ATP-dependent proteolysis Factor I of rabbit reticulocytes, J. Biol. Chem., 255:7529.

THYMIC FACTORS IN EXPERIMENTAL DISEASES

E. Garaci*, F. Bistoni**, C. Favalli *, P. Marconi**,
V. Del Gobbo *, C. Rinaldi* and B.M. Jaffe***

Institutes of Microbiology, University of Rome*
and University of Perugia**, and from the Department
of Surgery S.U.N.Y., Brooklyn, New York***, U.S.A.

1. INTRODUCTION

As a series of methods were available for determination of
serum thymic hormone-like activity (Bach and Dardenne, 1973;
Astaldi et al., 1976; Lewis et al., 1981), studies were carried
out by several researchers in order to determine modifications of
thymic activity in different clinical and experimental conditions.
This area of investigation has been considered of primary interest
in the recent years for the following reasons:
a) understanding the pathogenesis of several diseases;
b) possibility of substitute therapy with thymic hormones;
c) contribution to a better knowledge of the pathophysiology of
   the thymus.

During the last years in our laboratory we have obtained data
concerning: (a) serum thymic factor (STF) determinations according
to the method of Bach and Dardenne (1973), in a number of clinical
and experimental models; (b) the possible use of thymic factors at
experimental level in the control of some infectious diseases and
(c) the interaction of thymic factors with prostaglandins which
may add some contribution to understand the mechanism of thymic
hormones activity. This chapter will review synthetically and
discuss our work also in the light of the data published in the
literature.

2. CHANGES OF SERUM LEVELS OF THYMIC FACTOR IN EXPERIMENTAL
   MODELS AND IN CLINICAL DISEASES

In a previous study on the ultrastructure of thymus in mice treated with anti-lymphocyte serum (Djaczenko and Garaci, 1976) we prospected the possible correlation between morphology of thymic epithelial cells and their function. In view of the importance attributed to these cells as a source of biologically active thymic factors (Bach et al., 1975), this problem was investigated by us in more detail with the preparation of a rabbit anti-serum specific for thymic epithelial cells of mice (Garaci et al., 1978), using a test for the determination of serum thymic activity. This had been performed when a suitable method was available i.e. the application of the rapid azathioprine (AZ) sensitive spleen cell rosette assay developed by Bach and Dardenne (1973).

In these studies, determinations of serum thymic factor (STF) were carried out in mice, at different times after treatment with antiserum against thymic epithelial cells, in parallel with observations on thymus ultrastructural changes. The data obtained showed evidence of a strict relationship between morphological state of thymic epithelial cells and STF levels. The results of these studies not only added support to the concept of the STF production by thymic epithelial cells but showed that the deter-

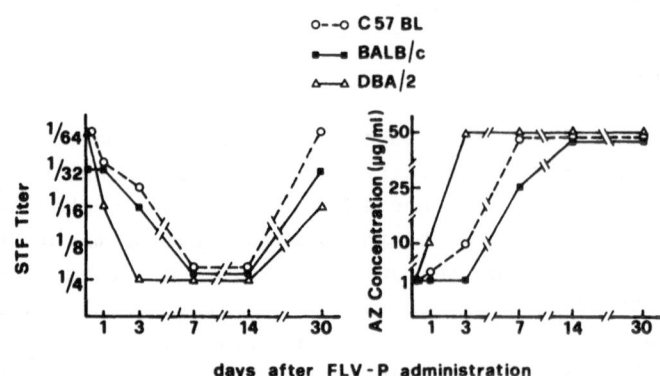

Fig. 1. Time-course study of STF levels and azathioprine sensitivity of spleen rosette-forming-cells in C57BL/6, BALB/c and DBA/2 mice inoculated with the polycythemic strain of Friend Leukemia virus.

mination of STF was a very good and sensitive indicator of the
functional activity of epithelial cells. In fact also when the
alterations of epithelial cells were not particularly evident, a
significant and constant decrease of STF was observed.

A similar approach was followed studying mice infected with
Friend Leukaemia Virus (FLV). In a previous report we observed a
fall of STF titres in some strains of susceptible mice (Garaci et
al., 1981a) infected with FLV. Therefore we decided to investigate
the problem in more detail. Several strains of mice with different
susceptibility to Friend Leukemia were infected with a polycythemic (Fig.1) or with an anemic strain (Fig.2) of FLV. The polycythemic strain comprises a competent leukemia-inducing virus and
a defective spleen focus-forming virus, while the anemic strain
lacks the focus-forming component but includes a competent leukemia virus, since it induces an erythro-leukemia, indistinguishable
from that caused by the polycythemic strain. STF determinations
were performed in parallel with a detailed ultrastructural study
of the thymus.

These investigations allowed to draw the following conclusions: early and prolonged decrease of STF appears in mice
infected with both strains of FLV. These STF changes, which seem
to be virus-dose related, are associated with early localisation
and replication of virus in thymic epithelial cells. The FLV

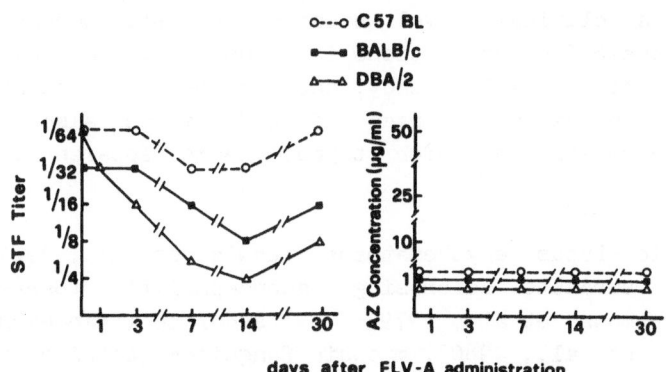

Fig. 2. Time-course study of STF levels and azathioprine sensitivi-
ty of spleen rosette-forming-cells in C57BL/6, BALB/c and
DBA/2 mice inoculated with the anemic strain of Friend
Leukemia virus.

Table 1. Serum thymic factor titer in controls and in asthmatic and in vitiligo patients (age 2-13 years).

STF Titer	1/4	1/4	1/8	1/16	1/32	1/64
Controls	-	-	-	7	10	12
Asthmatic patients	1	7	10	7	1	-
Vitiligo patients	14	7	8	-	-	-

component responsible for STF decrease seems to be the leukaemogenic virus, while the spleen focus-forming virus appears to be involved in early disappearance of theta antigen from spleen cells.

At the moment we don't know if the STF changes could have some influence on the early fate of FLV-transformed cells, but in some way these are probably involved in modifications occurring in suppressor cells populations during the course of Friend Leukaemia (Garaci et al., 1981b).

If now we concentrate our attention from these experimental models to a clinical level we can observe the increasing importance of the STF determinations in a number of human diseases. In fact, with increasing frequency, data are being accumulated in the literature, indicating changes of STF titres also in several different diseases in which thymus seemed apparently not to be involved.

Systemic Lupus erythematosus (Lewis et al., 1981; Bach et al., 1975) subacute sclerosing panencephalitis (Garaci et al., 1981b; Wijermons et al., 1979) Down syndrome (Franceschi et al., 1981; Duse et al., 1980), mycosis fungoides (Safai et al., 1979) represent examples of diseases in which serum thymic activity has been found consistently altered.

In our studies we have found a constant and significant decrease of thymic activity in Asthma (Garaci et al., 1978) and

Table 2. Mortality of several strains of mice challenged i.v.
         with graded inocula of Candida Albicans (CA) organisms.

Number of CA cells $(\times 10^6)$	Median survival time of mice strains (days)			
	CD2F1	C3H/Hej	BALB/c	C57BL/6
0,12	18	13	61	22
0,25	12	9	13	18
0,50	7	7	8	13
1	4	4	6	11
2	4	3	4	8
4	2	2	2	4

Vitiligo (Table 1). In the former case, this finding confirmed by
Fabris (Fabris, 1980) may probably have some importance in the
pathogenesis of the disease. Actually it could be postulated a
correlation between decreased STF activity and the increased
stimulation of the reaginic system via its effects on T suppressor
lymphocytes. Some recent data obtained with the use of thymic
factors by Hobbs et al. (1980) and by Shohat et al. (1980) in
athopic patients strongly support this hypothesis. Concerning the
vitiligo disease, studies are now in progress to elucidate the
possible significance of STF variations in the pathogenesis of the
disease. Interestingly, the findings of autoimmune manifestations
which occur in this disease may have some connection with thymic
disturbances.

From all the data concerning this particular area, the following general conclusions could be made: in all the experimental
models tested, STF determination reflects precisely the state and
the degree of integrity of the thymus and particularly of the
epithelial cells which are thought to be the source of thymic
factors. This fact does not obviously rule out the possibility
that a disturbance in the factors that regulate the release
and/or synthesis of STF might occur also in presence of an
integrity state of the thymus; this both in experimental models or
in the clinics. In any case we can reasonably extend our experimental findings to the clinical situation, affirming, in general,
that any damage of the thymic epithelial cells involves signifi-

cant decrease of STF levels. To this regard much attention has to
be given to viral diseases. Epithelial cells of thymus may in fact
be a privileged early site of virus replication.

Further studies are necessary to a better understanding of
the consequences of lowered STF levels in the peripheral efficiency of the immune system. However, tests on STF variations
should be extended to all diseases in which an immune disturbance
is suspected. Moreover, STF determinations should be considered a
mandatory step before beginning any therapy with thymic preparations.

3. AN APPROACH TO TREATMENT OF INFECTIOUS DISEASES
   WITH THYMIC PREPARATIONS

Mice infected with Candida albicans and treated with several

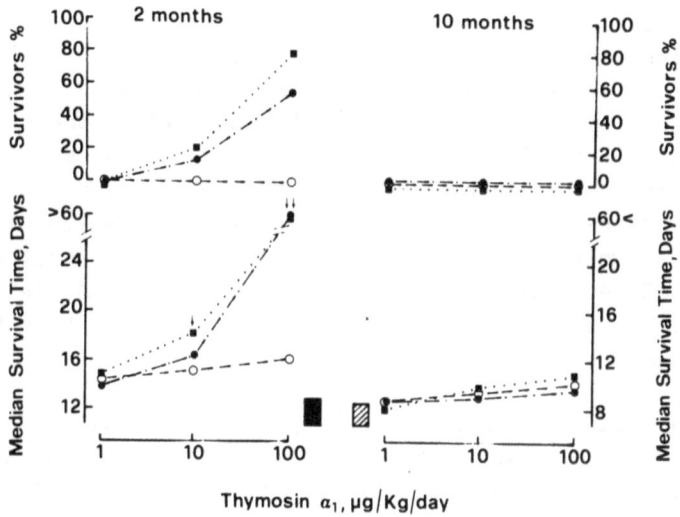

Thymosin α_1, μg/Kg/day

Fig. 3. Increased anti-infection resistance induced by thymosin α_1
administered to young or old CD2F1 mice challenge with
$2,5 \times 10^5$ CA cells iv. ■ young untreated controls; ▨
old untreated controls; ●—● thymosin α_1 on day −10 −8
−6 −4 −2; ■·····■ thymosin α_1 on day +1 +2 +3 +4 +5; O−−O
thymosin α_1 on day −10 −8 −6 −4 −2 +1 +2 +3 +4 +5. $P < 0.01$
comparing the survival times of control mice with those of
thymosin α_1 treated mice.

thymic preparations were chosen as experimental model. This model may represent a classical example of infection with opportunistic pathogens, generally occurring in hosts with impaired immunological functions. It has been established that appropriate i.v. inocula of Candida albicans cells in mice are able to kill 100% of animals.

Table 2 illustrates the median survival time (MST) of several strains of mice infected intravenously with graded doses of Candida albicans (CA) organisms. The doses of CA cells used to test the effectiveness of thymic preparations ranged from 0,5 x 10^6 to 2 x 10^6. Different doses of thymosin α_1 (Goldstein et al., 1977), given in different periods of time, are compared in (BALB/C x DBA/2) F_1 CD2F_1 mice infected with 2,5 x 10^5 CA cells (Fig.3). When thymosin α_1 is given after CA infection no effect on mice survival can be observed. When the factor is inoculated before

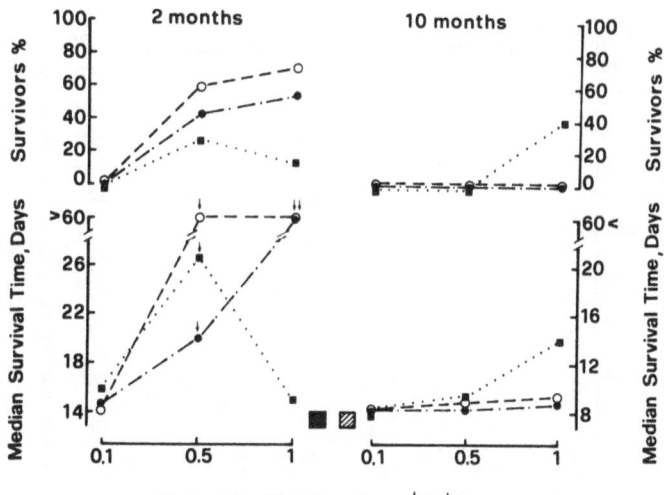

Fig. 4. Increased anti-infectious resistance induced by thymosin fraction 5 administered sc to young or old CD2F1 mice challenged with 2,5 x 10^5 CA cells iv. ■ young untreated controls; ▨ old untreated controls; ●—·—● thymosin fraction 5 on day -10 -8 -6 -5 -2; O—— O thymosin fraction 5 on day +1 +2 +3 +4 +5; ■·····■ thymosin fraction 5 on day -10 -:8 -6 -4 -2 +1 +2 +3 +4 +5. P 0.01 comparing the survival times of control mice with those of thymosin fraction 5 treated mice.

CA challenge, high doses of thymosin α_1 are able to protect mice indefinitely or to increase significantly the MST. Interestingly no protective effects or increased survival was observed when thymosin α_1 was given to old mice. Two other additional thymic preparations were tested in CA infected mice: thymosin fraction 5 (Hoffman La Roche) (Fig.4) and TP-1 (Serono) (Fig. 5). These thymic products were generally more active than thymosin α_1. This has been confirmed also in these experiments since TP-1 and Fraction 5 are effective in old mice. Moreover, both preparations show a wide range of concentrations in which they induce protective effects against CA infection.

In conclusion the results obtained clearly show that various thymic preparations are of value in controlling CA infections. This represents a promising and expanding area of application of thymic factors, presumably extensible to infections other than those provoked by CA. The mechanism of the protection induced by

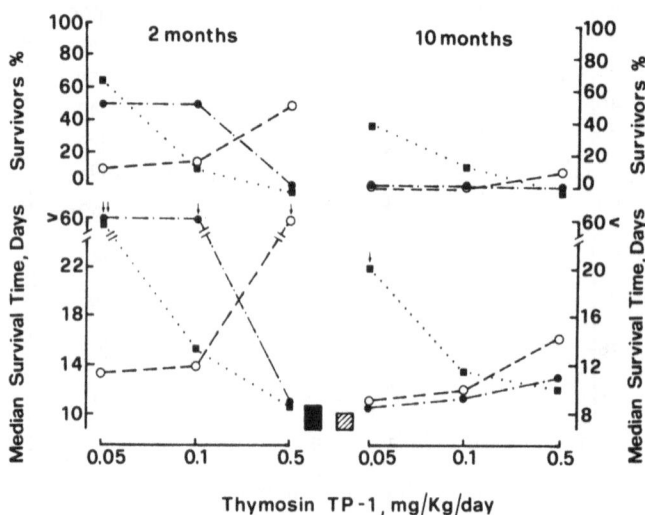

Fig. 5. Increased anti-infection resistance induced by thymosin TP-1 administered sc to young or old CD2F1 mice challenged with 2,5 x 10^5 CA cells iv. ■ young untreated controls; ▨ old untreated controls; ●–··–● thymosin TP-1 on day –10 –8 –6 –4 –2; O–––O thymosin TP-1 on day +1 +2 +3 +4 +5; ■······■ thymosin TP-1 on day –10 –8 –6 –4 –2 +1 +2 +3 +4 +5. P < 0.01 comparing the survival times of control mice with those of thymosin TP-1 treated mice.

Table 3. Effect of di-M-PGE$_2$ and of thymosin fraction 5 on the induction of Azathioprine sensitivity in spleen cells from thymectomized.

Time[b]	1 h	12 h	24 h	48 h	96 h
Di-M-PGE$_2$ (1 μg)[a]	1.5	6	48	100	100
Di-M-PGE$_2$ (10 μg)	1.5	1.5	6	12	100
Thymosin 5 (100 μg)	75	6	1.5	1.5	48
Control Tx mice	100	100	100	100	100

[a] Concentration (μg/ml of culture).
[b] Time in hours after administration of synthetic analog of PGE$_2$ and Thymosin fraction 5.

thymic preparations is not presently known. Studies are now in progress in order to clarify this problem.

4. INTERACTION OF PROSTAGLANDINS WITH THYMIC HORMONES

Several thymic preparations are able to induce the appearance of theta antigen in normal bone marrow cells and in spleen cells derived from adult thymectomized (ATx) mice "in vitro" and "in vivo". Bach and Bach (1974) have reported that cyclic AMP and products which increase the endogenous level of this nucleotide in lymphocytes, like some types of prostaglandins, mimic "in vitro" the effects of thymic hormone. All these agents are capable of converting lymphocytes from theta negative to theta positive rosette forming cells (RFC). In our experiments the administration to ATx mice of 16,16 dimethylprostaglandin E$_2$-methyl-ester (di-M-PGE$_2$), a long-acting synthetic analog of prostaglandin E$_2$, induced the appearance of theta antigen, in a fashion similar to that detectable with thymic hormone (Garaci et al., 1981c). Using the AZ rosette inhibition test, a concentration of di-M-PGE$_2$ as little as 1 μg is able to induce the appearance of theta antigen (Table 3), while Thymosin fraction 5 appears to be less effective in inducing the same effect. Interestingly indomethacin, a prostaglandin synthetase inhibitor, was able to prevent the

expression of theta antigen induced by administration of exogenous
thymosin in ATx mice (Garaci et al., 1981c). Indomethacin given in
normal mice for 7 days was also able to inhibit the effects of
endogenous thymic activity with respect to the expression of theta
antigen. Furthermore, indomethacin inhibits the effect of di-M-PGE
in inducing theta antigen, probably because a part of this effect
is mediated by endogenous prostaglandin biosynthesis stimulated by
di-M-PGE$_2$.

Interestingly (Fig. 6) the administration of di-M-PGE$_2$ was
also able to induce the appearance of consistent thymic activity
in the serum, detectable with the rosette inhibition test of Bach
(Bach and Dardenne, 1973).

The results strongly support the concept that prostaglandins
could be mediators of thymic hormones at least with regards to
some effects. In fact, thymic hormone may, at least in part, work
by inducing increase of endogenous prostaglandin biosynthesis at
the level of lymphocytes. This could be in turn responsible of
theta antigen expression probably by a change of intralymphocyte
concentration of cyclic AMP.

In fact prostaglandins play an important immunoregulatory
role (Jaffe et al., this volume) and could promote lymphocyte
maturation and differentiation. Our recent results of immuno-
restoration in tumor bearing mice treated with di-M-PGE$_2$ support

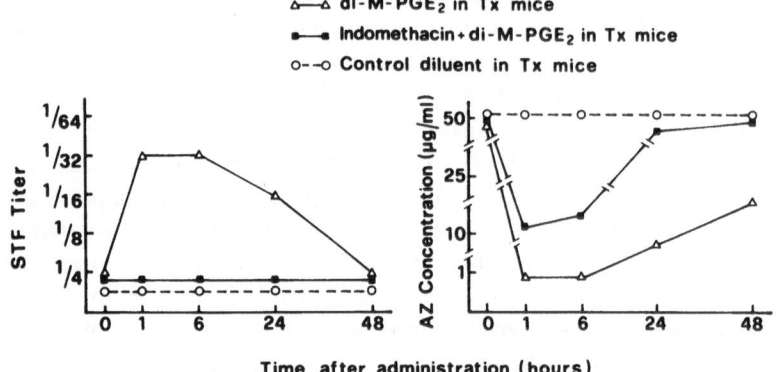

Fig. 6. Effect of di-M-PGE$_2$ in the appearance of serum thymic-like-
-activity and in the induction of theta antigen evaluated
by the Azathioprine inhibition test.

this hypothesis (Favalli et al., 1980). Further studies are under investigation to better understand the detailed mechanism of action of thymic hormones and to test this hypothesis.

REFERENCES

Astaldi, A., Astaldi, G.C.B., Schellekens, P.Th.A., and Eijsvoogel, V.P., 1976, Thymic factor in human sera demonstrable by a cyclic AMP assay, Nature, 260:713.

Bach, J.F., Dardenne, M., Pleau, J.M., and Bach, M.A., 1975, Isolation, biochemical characteristics and biological activity of a circulating thymic hormone in the mouse and in the human, Ann. N.Y. Acad. Sci., 249:186.

Bach, J.F., and Dardenne, M., 1973, Studies products. II. Demonstration and characterization of a circulating thymic hormone, Immunology, 25:353.

Bach, M.A., and Bach, J.F., 1974, in: "Prostaglandin Synthetase Inhibitors," H.J., Robinson, and J.R., Vane, eds., Raven Press, New York, p. 241.

Djaczenko, W., and Garaci, E., 1976, Dark reticular epithelial cells of the thymus as the primary target of heterologous anti--lymphocyte serum, Clin. Immunol. Immunopath., 6:213.

Duse, M., Brugo, M.A., Martini, A., Tassi, C., Ferrario, C., and Ugazio, A.G., 1980, Immunodeficiency in Down's syndrome low levels of serum thymic factor in trisomic children, Thymus, 2:127.

Fabris, N., 1980, Serum Thymic Factor determination in different human pathologies, Int. J. Immunopharm., 2:157, Abstract.

Favalli, C., Garaci, E., Etheredge, F., Santoro, M.G., and Jaffe, B.M., 1980, Influence of PGE on the immune response in melanoma-bearing mice, J. Immunol.,125:897.

Franceschi, C., Licastro, F., Chiricolo, M., Bonetti, F., Zannotti, M., Fabris, N., Mocchegiani, E., Fantini, M.P., Paolucci, P., and Masi, M., 1981, Deficiency of autologous mixed lymphocyte reactions and serum thymic factor level in Down's syndrome, J. Immunol., 12:1261.

Garaci, E., Del Gobbo, V., Santucci, L., Rossi, G.B., and Rinaldi--Garaci, C., 1981a, Changes of serum thymic factor levels in Friend Leukaemia Virus-infected mice, Leukaemia Research,3:67.

Garaci, E., Migliorati, G., Jezzi, T., Bartocci, A., Gioia, L., Rinaldi-Garaci, C., and Bonmassar, E., 1981b, Impairment of "in vitro" generation cytotoxic or T suppressor lymphocytes by

Friend Leukaemia Virus infection in mice, <u>Int. J. Cancer,</u> 28:367.

Garaci, E., Rinaldi-Garaci, C., Del Gobbo, V., Favalli, C., Santoro, M.G., and Jaffe, B.M, 1981c, A synthetic analog of Prostaglandin E is able to induce "in vivo" theta antigen on spleen cells of adult thymectomized mice, <u>Cell. Immunol.,</u> 62:8.

Garaci, E., Ronchetti, R., Del Gobbo, V., Tramutoli, G., Rinaldi--Garaci, C., and Imperato, C., 1978, Decreased serum thymic factor activity in asthmatic children, <u>J. All. Clin. Immunol.,</u> 62:357.

Garaci, E., Pecci, G., Rinaldi-Garaci, C., Del Gobbo, V., and Tonietti, G., 1978, Ultrastructural and functional changes of the mouse thymus following treatment with an antiserum specific for thymic epithelial cells, <u>Clin. Immunol. Immunopath.,</u> 11:157.

Goldstein, A.L., Low, T.L.K., Adoo, M., Clure, J. Mc., Thurman, G.B., Rossio, G., Lay, C.Y., Chang, D., Wang-Su-Sun, Harwey, C., Ramel A.H., and Meienhofer, J., 1977, Thymosin α_1:isolation and sequence analysis of an immunologically active thymic polypeptide, <u>Proc. Natl. Acad. Sci.,</u> USA, 74:725.

Hobbs, J.R., Byron, N.A., Campbell, M.A., Copeman, P.W.M., Gibbs, M., Lane, A.M., Perez, A., and Staughton, R.C.D., 1980, Thymosin-inducible lymphocytes in athopy, <u>in</u>: "Thymus, Thymic hormones and T lymphocytes," Aiuti, F. and Wigzell, H., eds., Acad. Press, p. 143.

Lewis, V.M., Twomey, J.J., Steinberg, A.D., and Goldstein, G., 1981, Serum thymic hormone activity in systemic lupus erythematosus, <u>Clin. Immunol. Immunopath.,</u> 18:61.

Safai, B., Dardenne, M., Incefy, G.S., Bach, J.F., and Good, R.A., 1979, Circulating thymic factor, facteur thymique serique (FTS) in Mycosis Fungoides and Sezary syndrome, <u>Clin. Immunol. Immunopath.,</u> 13:402.

Shohat, B., Metzker, A., and Trainin, N., 1980, Cell mediated immunity and the "in vitro" effect of thymic humoral factor (THF) on blood lymphocytes of children with athopic dermatitis, <u>Clin. Immunol. Immunopath.,</u> 15:646.

Wijermons, P., Astaldi, A., Astaldi, G.C.B., Kapsenberg, J.G., Groenewood, M., Roos, M., Lucas, C., and Schellekens, P.A., 1979, Serum thymic factor in subacute sclerosing panencephalitis patients, <u>Clin. Immunol. Immunopathol.,</u> 12:105.

LYMPHOKINES AND THE LYMPHOENDOTHELIAL SYSTEM :

AN ILLUSTRATION OF IMMUNOREGULATORY INTEGRATION

D.C. Dumonde, Anne S. Hamblin, Eva Kasp-Grochowska,
Melanie S. Pulley and R.A. Wolstencroft

Department of Immunology, St Thomas's Hospital and
Medical School, London SE1 7EH, United Kingdom

1. LYMPHOKINES AS IMMUNOREGULATORY MEDIATORS

1.1. Background

The possibility that non-antibody products of lymphocyte activation might be involved in the expression and regulation of lymphocyte function arose indirectly from consideration of the role of lymphocytes and macrophages in experimental delayed hypersensitivity (Dumonde, 1967; Dumonde et al., 1968). Analysis of experimental cell-mediated immune phenomena had pointed to the role of cellular interactions between a few specifically sensitized lymphocytes and the majority of other host cells participating in these responses (see Turk, 1967). These features were consistent with the concept that special 'mediators' of cellular immunity could well facilitate such interactions; and that this would bring the cellular immune system into line with other biological systems in which differentiated cell products (for example endocrine and neurotransmitter substances) were known to mediate complex physiological events.

In 1969 the generic term "lymphokine" was coined in order to communicate the broader concept that non-antibody protein products of lymphocyte activation may themselves activate and regulate cellular systems involved in lymphocyte-mediated immunological and

Table 1.   Accomplishments in lymphokine research in the 1970's*.

---

1. Increasing number of biological activities relevant to induction,
   regulation and expression of the immunological response.

2. Lymphokine (LK) activities demonstrated in a wide variety of
   species (rodents; birds; fish; reptiles; primates; Man).

3. Lymphokines 'appropriately' produced by both T and B lymphocytes.

4. 'Alternative' pathways of LK production (mitogen-induced; virus-
   induced; from lymphoid cell lines) viewed as relevant to the
   immuno-pathology of 'inappropriate' lymphocyte activation.

5. Biochemical characterization partially achieved but limited by
   'trace' representation and heterogeneity of (anionic) proteins/
   /glycoproteins and by reproducibility of bioassays.

6. Lymphokines clearly unrelated to immunoglobulins but some
   'factors' contain MHC products and/or exhibit antigen-dependence
   in expression of activity.

7. Semantic links began to develop between investigators studying
   different animal species (eg mouse; guinea pig) and those
   studying human disease.

8. Biological activities carefully described on most mesenchymal
   cell types involved in inflammation and defence.

9. "In vitro" metabolic and behavioural responses of cell populations
   to lymphokine preparations thought to be compatible with selected
   lymphokine actions via cell-surface receptors and mediated via
   cytoskeletal enzyme systems.

10. Work on the control of lymphokine production and of effects of
    lymphokines "in vivo" reinforce the view that lymphokines 'are'
    mediators and regulators of (cellular) immune responses.

---

* for references see Dumonde, 1970; Cohen et al., 1979; De Weck et
  al., 1980.

inflammatory responses (Dumonde et al., 1969). In the case of endocrine and neurotransmitter substances, and certain factors in
acute inflammation, comprehensive evidence was available (in the
formof "Dale criteria") to implicate them as mediators of given
physiological processes. These criteria were : 1) identification
of the proposed mediator by biological or pharmacological tests
which could measure its amount or activity; 2) known mechanisms
for production, destruction or inactivation of the proposed mediator; 3) satisfactory mimicry of the physiological process by application of the proposed mediator; 4) release of the proposed mediator during appropriate function of the physiological process;
5) specific depletion of the proposed mediator from the system
should prevent the physiological process from being elicited;
6) substances that specifically potentiate the effects of the proposed mediator should also enhance the physiological response.

In the field of cellular immunity, a number of different
acronyms were being used ("factors") in describing the biological
activities of non-antibody lymphocyte products, in different
aspects of cellular immunity, but whose status as physiological
mediators was far from established. Against this background the
term "lymphokine" was proposed also to indicate the general source
of these materials ("factors"), i.e. lymphocyte activation; and to
indicate the physiological process within which they might exert
their principal biological activities, i.e., the control of lymphocyte activation.

Work on lymphokines escalated during the 1970's. By the end
of the decade, two international conferences on lymphokines had
been held and two major symposium volumes had been published
(Cohen et al., 1979; De Weck et al., 1980). A special journal was
established to publish short review articles on lymphokines (Pick,
1980) and it is now an acceptable view that lymphokines are mediators and regulators of interactions between antigen-activated lymphocytes and other cells participating in the immunological response. Although the critical investigators will appreciate that
for the majority of lymphokine activities, the "Dale criteria" are
far from fulfilled, an overview of lymphokine research in the
1970's is presented in Table 1.

Table 2. Lymphokines in the early 1980's*.

1. Attempts to generate neutralizing antibodies are becoming more
   successful.

2. Analysis of mitogenic lymphokines (interleukins) has revealed
   cell cycle effects whereby expansion of specific T cell clones
   "in vitro" is now being undertaken.

3. Mass culture techniques for maintaining lymphoid cell lines
   (100 - 300 litre fermenters) may circumvent some problems of
   lymphokine (LK) production, LK purification, cell and gene cloning.

4. Hybridoma technology is being applied to LK production as well
   as to the production of antibodies to lymphokines.

5. Improvements in design and precision of bioassays of lymphokine
   activity are required to provide a foundation for the development
   of immuno-assays.

6. Material standards of lymphokine activities are required to help
   clarify nomenclature, classification and biochemical characterization.

7. Concept of lymphokines as 'biological response modifiers' in
   cancer (Goldstein and Chirigos, 1981) adds a further dimension
   to the clinical significance of mediators of cellular immunity
   (see Dumonde and Maini, 1971).

---

* for recent references see Hadden and Stewart, 1981, Paetkau; 1981.

1.2. Current "State of the Art"

     Attempts are now being made to re-classify lymphokine activi-
ties according to their characterizable effects on isolated cell
populations (ie motility; proliferation; activation; viability:
see Cohen, 1980), according to the type of cell target (lymphocyte, macrophage, polymorph, fibroblast, osteoclast, eosinophil, vascular endothelium, etc: see Waksman, 1980) and according to the
extent to which lymphokine activities appear to require specific

antigen for their expression and/or appear to be "restricted" to containing or interacting with identifiable MHC or V gene products (Waksman, 1980). Table 2 summarizes the principal directions in which lymphokine research is proceeding in the early 1980's and which encompasses biochemical,biological and clinical approaches to the role of lymphokines as intrinsic regulators of immunological responses.

Illustrative biochemical approaches are: (a) whether monoclonal antibodies may be used to separate one lymphokine activity from another; (b) whether single-activity ("monoclonal") lymphokines can be prepared for characterization studies; (c) whether selected lymphoid cell lines may facilitate recognition and transfer of genes controlling specified lymphokines; and (d) whether lymphokines consist structurally of polypeptide subunits with superimposed molecular variations (eg the extent of glycosylation). References to the recent literature are to be found in Hadden and Stewart, 1981, and Paetkau, 1981.

Illustrative biological problems are: (a) that parallel-line and parallel bioassays still need further development; (b) that the role of lymphokines in pharmacologically-induced immunomodulation and in natural surveillance awaits clarification and (possibly) further experimental models; and (c) that the concept of a molecular pharmacology of cell-mediated immunity (Dumonde, et al., 1973) requires investigation of lymphokine receptors, agonists and antagonists, against the background of increasing knowledge of functional lymphoid cell subpopulations.

Illustrative clinical questions are: (a) whether application of lymphokine assays to human disease reveals evidence of a "molecular pathology" of the lymphokine system; (b) whether abnormalities in lymphokine production, action or response can be used to assist the understanding of human immunopathology; (c) whether lymphokine agonists or antagonists might be of therapeutic value; and (d) whether lymphokines themselves might emerge as useful "biological response modifiers" in neoplasia and host defence (Dumonde et al., 1981a).

The status of lymphokines as intrinsic mediators of immunoregulatory networks is now firmly established. Although attempts are being made to study lymphokine production "in vivo" (Neta and Salvin, 1981), much lymphokine research still takes place "on the walls of test tubes". In contrast, it might be said that much lymphokine action probably takes place "on the walls of small blood vessels". In the remainder of this paper we shall speculate on how extrinsic (neuroendocrine) mechanisms may contribute to immunoregulation "in vivo" by interacting with cells producing and responding to lymphokines in the vascular microenvironment of lymphoid and non-lymphoid tissues.

2. LYMPHOCYTE-ENDOTHELIAL INTERACTIONS AND IMMUNOREGULATION

Alongside the growth of research into lymphokines as "cell cooperators" in intrinsic immunoregulatory networks there is a recent regrowth of interest in mechanisms which govern the compartmentation of lymphocytes between blood and tissues (Butcher and Weissman, 1980; Gowans and Steer, 1980) and in mechanisms which might determine the control of lymphocyte activation during lymphocyte positioning (de Sousa, 1981). There is a physiologically significant recirculation of lymphocytes through non-lymphoid organs in the absence of antigen, which can be increased by antigenic exposure (Trevella and Morris, 1980) and the biological value of lymphocyte recirculation through both lymphoid and non--lymphoid tissues is viewed as fundamental to maintenance of adaptive immunity. Vascular endothelium constitutes the ultimate blood-tissue barrier and interactions between recirculatory lymphocytes and vascular endothelium take place in microenvironments with lymphoid and non-lymphoid tissues where control of lymphocyte activation during physiological diapedesis is presumably obligatory. The question arises as to the nature of these lymphocyte--endothelial interactions and of whether these may be governed by intrinsic and extrinsic factors with resultant homeostatic effects on the immunological response.

2.1. Mechanisms of Lymphocyte-Endothelial Interaction

Four main theories have been proposed to explain cell positioning and patterning, by the control of cell movement in multicellular animals, which seem relevant to mechanisms of lymphocyte--endothelial interaction. There are : (a) specific adhesion (due to mutual receptor recognition); (b) differential or random adhesion (ie no specific recognition); (c) chemotaxis; and (d) an interaction-modulation theory (Curtis, 1978) in which a degree of specific cell-cell interaction is modulated locally by diffusible agents. Because peripheral blood lymphocytes selectively adhere to high endothelial venules of lymph node sections "in vitro" (Stamper and Woodruff, 1976) it is inferred that receptors on recirculatory lymphocytes simply "recognise" endothelial cell ligands (Butcher et al., 1979) and that a differential distribution of ligand density across or between adjacent endothelial cells governs directional lymphocyte diapedesis. Accordingly, random cell--cell adhesion seems to be an unlikely explanation of the interaction of lymphocytes with high endothelium in lymphoid tissue, and by implication, with microvascular endothelium in non-lymphoid tissues.

This section summarises five experimental approaches which we have undertaken that suggest that lymphocyte-endothelial interactions, and microenvironmental aspects of immunity, may be influenced by diffusable substances produced both by lymphocytes and by endothelial cells. These experiments are : (i) study of the effects of injecting lymphokines into afferent lymphatics of the guinea pig auricular lymph node; (ii) study of the effects of endothelial cell culture supernatants on the transformation of peripheral blood lymphocytes "in vitro"; (iii) study of the effects of lymphocyte activation upon the ability of lymphocytes to adhere to, and integrate into, confluent monolayers of cultured vascular endothelial cells; and (iv) histopathological studies of the effects of injecting human lymphoblastoid cell line lymphokine intradermally in man. In addition, we have undertaken a fifth set of experiments which show that vascular endothelial cells in culture can present antigen for lymphocyte sensitisation and recall.

2.2. Lymphokine Injection into Guinea Pig Lymph Nodes

Experiments consisted of injecting preformed lymphokine into the afferent lymphatics of the guinea pig ear by micromanipulation and of assessing the nature and time course of cellular changes in the regional (auricular) lymph node (Dumonde et al., 1973).

Intralymphatic injection of only 17 guinea pig lymphokine (estimated to be produced by only 250 antigen-sensitive lymphocytes) resulted in a five-fold increase in lymph node weight and lymphocyte content within 24 hours. This represented an overall retention of twice the number of recirculating lymphocytes that

normally pass through the node in that time. It was concluded that
introduction of lymphokines into a resting node could double the
rate of lymphocyte entry across the microvasculature; and that
generation of small quantities of lymphokine within the microenvironment of an antigen-stimulated node might help to recruit and
activate additional recirculatory lymphocytes during immune induction (Kelly et al., 1972; Kelly and Wolstencroft, 1974; Kelly et
al., 1975).

2.3. Modulation of Lymphocyte Transformation by Products of
     Cultured Endothelial Cells

     Experiments consisted of culturing pig aortic vascular endo-
thelial cells to confluence on glass surfaces and of determining
the ability of the prostaglandin-rich culture supernatants (Dumonde et al., 1977; Jose et al., 1981) to affect the transformation of porcine peripheral blood lymphocytes.

     Endothelial culture supernatants inhibited PHA- and perioda-
te-induced lymphocyte transformation in partial concordance with
their content of prostaglandin E_2; and these suppressive effects
were preferentially exerted on weakly-transforming lymphocytes.
When endothelial cell prostaglandin production was abolished by
indomethacin, some endothelial supernatants actually stimulated
lymphocyte transformation. Neither 'regular' or 'indomethacin'
endothelial supernatants were able to modulate strongly-transfor-
ming lymphocytes to the same extent. It was concluded that endothelial cells have the capacity to produce diffusible products
(including prostaglandins) which might exert controlling effects
upon lymphocyte function within the microenvironment of lymphocyte-endothelial interactions (Kasp-Grochowska et al., 1982a).

2.4. Formation of Lymphoendothelial Aggregates "In Vitro"

     Experiments consisted of co-culturing resting or periodate-
-stimulated pig peripheral blood lymphocytes with confluent monolayers of pig aortic endothelium and of assessing the degree of
cellular interaction by phase-contrast microscopy and by examination of fixed and stained preparations and by the use of [111]In-
-labelled lymphocytes. Periodate activation of lymphocytes was
undertaken by pulsing with 5 - 10mM $NaIO_4$ followed by washing and

reincubation for 24 - 30 hours when the cells were judged to be in
a state of lymphokine production (see also Bressler et al., 1980).

        After co-culture for up to 24 hours, two populations of asso-
ciated (^{111}In-) lymphocytes could be identified : 'adherent' and
'integrated'. Adherent lymphocytes lay on top of the endothelial
cells whilst integrated lymphocytes lay between the endothelial
cells in the same phase-contrast plane. Prior activation of lymphocytes had a marked effect on their interaction with endothelium: there was increased adherence in the first two hours of
co-culture followed by an even more intimate association of the
two cell populations. After overnight incubation, these two different cell types formed interwoven lymphoendothelial layers in
which both lymphocytes and endothelial cells appeared to be in a
state of cytoplasmic enlargement (Dumonde, 1978; Kasp-Grochowska
et al., 1982b). We knew that bradykinin could stimulate prostaglandin production by endothelial cell cultures (Dumonde et al.,
1977; Jose et al., 1981); and in some experiments, integration of
activated lymphocytes also led to increased PGE production by
the endothelial cells (Kasp-Grochowska et al., 1982b).

        It was inferred that an increased avidity of activated
lymphocytes for endothelium (Ford, 1975) might also be accompanied
by modulatory effects of lymphocytes upon the metabolism of
adjacent endothelial cells in the microenvironment of lymphocyte-
-endothelial interactions, in such a way as to attempt to suppress
activation of the traversing lymphocytes themselves (Dumonde,
1978; Kasp-Grochowska et al., 1982b).

2.5. Endothelial Activation and Lymphoendothelial Tissue Formation
     following Intradermal Injection of Lymphokines in Man

        As part of a study on the clinical effects of injecting
RPMI-1988 lymphoblastoid cell line lymphokine (LCL-LK) into tu-
mour-bearing patients (Dumonde et al., 1981a) skin biopsies were
obtained, from .patients receiving intradermal injections of 100 -
500   g, quantities of partially purified LCL-LK, for histological
and ultrastructural examination. After an early polymorph response
(30 min - 4 hours) the skin became infiltrated with mononuclear
cells.

        At 24-48 hours after lymphokine injection, skin reactions showed a prominent lymphoendothelial inflammation consisting of perivascular positioning of small lymphocytes around subepidermal and dermal capillaries with hypertrophic endothelium. In the more severe reactions there were areas of dermis that resembled the paracortex of a lymph node and which were also closely similar to a classical tuberculin skin reaction. It was concluded that lymphokines have the capacity to induce lymphoendothelial inflammation in tissues outside the lymphoid system and that extravascular lymphokine can act as a chemotactic stimulus for lymphocyte emigration with concomitant endothelial cell activation in a tissue microenvironment (Dumonde et al., 1981b).

2.6. Antigen-presenting Properties of Cultured Endothelial Cells

Experiments consisted of determining the ability of endothelial cells dissociated from human umbilical vein to replace cultured peripheral blood monocytes in presenting antigen to syngeneic and allogeneic human lymphocytes in primary sensitization and 'recall' experiments (Burger et al., 1981).

In brief, a mixed endothelial cell-lymphocyte culture reaction (MELC) was first suppressed by a monoclonal anti DR serum directed against the endothelial cell phenotype. When an antigen (Keyhole limpet haemocyanin or horseshoe crab haemocyanin) was then added to DR-compatible cocultures, lymphocytes harvested at 14 days were as reactive in antigen-specific lymphocyte transformation as 14 day lymphocytes primed by syngeneic macrophages. Furthermore, antigen on DR-compatible endothelial cells was able to elicit lymphocyte transformation as effectively as antigen on DR-compatible macrophages (Burger et al., 1981). It was concluded that endothelial cells have the capacity for presenting antigen to lymphocytes in association with DR determinants and that this accessory cell function could provide the signal for antigen-specific T cells to localize at appropriate sites in the microvasculature (Burger et al., 1981).

2.7. Implications of Experimental Approaches:
   a 'Lymphoendothelial' Hypothesis of Immunoregulation

Taken together, these five experimental approaches draw attention to the likelihood that vascular endothelial cells may play an important function in effecting the compartmentation and activation of recirculatory lymphocytes; and that the microenvironment of lymphocyte-endothelial interaction is a critical site at which the induction and regulation of T cell-mediated immunity is normally governed. It seems plausible that endothelial cells should actively present antigen to T cells "in vivo" and that their metabolic products should influence the fact, nature and kinetics of specific T cell activation during the processes of lymphocyte-endothelial interaction that ensue. We therefore, introduce the concept of a 'lymphoendothelial' hypothesis of immunoregulation and explore some of its implications in the context of this symposium.

A 'lymphoendothelial' hypothesis of immunoregulation is compatible with an interaction:modulation theory of lymphocyte-endothelial positioning (Curtis, 1978). This would accommodate a degree of molecular specificity of receptor:ligand interaction, between recirculatory (? T-derived) lymphocytes and certain (? specialised) microvascular endothelial cells, which would be intrinsically modulated by locally-diffusible metabolic products of both cell families in the microenvironment of lymphoid and non-lymphoid tissues. Biological flexibility inherent in the involvement of two distinct cell families (Willmer, 1960) in any such regulatory process would allow for second-order modulation of an extrinsic nature. In this second-order modulation, physiological stimuli generated at a distance from these microenvironments could well affect vascular endothelial cells, recirculatory lymphocytes or both cell families. The fact that endothelial cells are competent to present antigen for T-cell activation implies that they may also fulfil the dual immunological requirements of antigen processing in association with MHC (Ia)-dependent signal recognition. Both endothelial cells and lymphocytes can generate autopharmacological products (eg prostaglandins and lymphokines respectively) which can modulate both metabolic and biological activities of the reciprocal cell type (Sidky and Auerbach, 1975; Polverini et al., 1977). It therefore seems likely that feedback homeostatic mechanisms exist which may control this critical element involved in lymphocyte recirculation (Anderson and Anderson, 1976), and hence in the maintenance of adaptive immunity.
A logical corollary of this reasoning is to propose the existence of a body system concerned with the operation of these homeostatic mechanisms: and the simplest descriptive term which would seem to be appropriate is the 'lymphoendothelial system'.

3. CONCEPT OF A LYMPHOENDOTHELIAL SYSTEM

3.1. Definition and Semantics

Let us now propose the existence of a body system which is involved in regulating the traffic and activation of recirculatory lymphocytes in relation to their transmural passage across microvascular endothelium, which governs those homeostatic interactions between lymphocytes and endothelial cells fundamental to the maintenance of adaptive immunity, and which can be functionally modulated by intrinsic (eg immunopharmacological) and extrinsic (eg neuroendocrine) signals.

Semantic explorations. The Oxford English Dictionary uses the term 'system' in four distinct ways : a) a connected set of things forming a complex whole in accordance with some scheme or plan; b)a group of bodies moving rapidly round one another in space; c)a set of parts of similar structure or function; and d) the scheme/plan/belief ...itself.

Hazards of systematization are well recognised in scientific philosophy (see Rather, 1972) where the exploration may be presented colloquially as follows : a) it's easier to accumulate facts than to reduce them to order; b) how do we know when we have gathered enough facts? c) how can we gather meaningful facts without a system of thought? and d) yet the system of scientific thought determines the character of facts to be accumulated (Rather, 1972).

Against this background of reflection of systematics and on the hazards of systematization, the term 'lymphoendothelial system' is offered without further qualification or apology.

3.2. Physiological and Pathological Implications

A fuller review is in preparation and only a few illustrative points are presented here.

Physiology, developmental biology and genetics. In terms of normality, a lymphoendothelial system controlling compartmentation and metabolic activity of recirculatory lymphocytes would be expected to operate homeostatically by means of intrinsic and extrinsic signals affecting cell movement and cellular interactions.

Thus corticosteroids are illustrative of a variety of extrinsic signals which can modulate the metabolism of both endothelial cells (Jose et al., 1981) and lymphocytes (Smith et al.,
1977; Distelhorst and Benutto, 1981). In developmental terms there
may well be a natural 'affinity' between lymphocytes and endothelial cells. Willmer (1960) has argued that they may share a common
'mechanocyte' ancestor concerned with metabolic (muco-substance)
excretion and ion regulation; and it seems likely that the two
cell types may have developed together as blood took over coordi-
nation from coelomic fluid (Manning and Turner, 1976).
Genetic considerations are implied by Weissman's group who view
the act of lymphocyte:endothelial interaction as being phyloge-
netically conserved whilst its detailed molecular biology is subject to species variation (Butcher et al., 1979).

Immunology, autopharmacology and reactive pathology. Antigen-
-presenting properties of endothelial cells (Hirschberg et al.,
1980) for T-lymphocyte sensitization and recall display genetic
restriction and clonal expression at the DR (Ia) locus (Burger et
al., 1981). Auto-pharmacological mechanisms involved in immunological and inflammatory responses may well modulate this accessory
cell function; and a pathology of intrinsic or extrinsic feedback
mechanisms can be envisaged whereby something 'wrong' with the
behaviour of endothelial cells or lymphocytes to environmental
stimuli or endogenous signals could underlie chronic inflammatory
disease. An impressive number of 'quasi-immune' human diseases
share the common features of widespread lymphoendothelial inflammation (Dumonde, 1978) and linkage to MHC phenotypes, including DR
types. It seems likely that a variety of stimuli, acting via the
lymphocyte, the endothelial cell or the plasma milieu, could precipitate reactive lympho-endothelial dysfunction at a distance
from the primary site of action of the initiating stimulus on the
(genetically) susceptible host. Uncontrolled local production of
lymphokines may arise from a failure of local feedback regulation
of lymphocyte activation. An extension of this reasoning to certain lymphoproliferative diseases (eg angio-immunoblastic lymphadenopathy;cutaneous T-cell lymphomas) invites early investigation.

Lymphokines and the lymphoendothelial system. Lymphokines
therefore emerge, not only as intrinsic mediators of lymphoid cell
cooperation in the immune response (Smith et al., 1980) but also

as potentially important regulators of lymphocyte-endothelial interaction. The events occurring after T-cell-endothelial inter-action are now of great investigative interest (Ford, Smith and Andrews, 1978) in their relevance to the further understanding of self-regulation of the adaptive immune system.

4. LYMPHOKINES AND IMMUNE-NEUROENDOCRINE INTERACTIONS

This concluding section cites recent independent work from our group and Sorkin's group which indicates that lymphokines may affect neuroendocrine function and thereby activate extrinsic immunoregulatory mechanisms.

4.1. Introduction

In 1977 Besedovsky and Sorkin published an important review in which they proposed the existence of two-way interactions between the immunological response and the neuroendocrine appara-tus (Besedovsky and Sorkin, 1977; see also Sorkin, this Sympo-sium). In the knowledge that lymphokines can be detected in the blood in human disease (Adelman et al., 1979) and during systemic reactions of experimental delayed hypersensitivity (Neta and Salvin, 1981) it seemed that lymphokines might act as signals to the neuroendocrine system of the state of lymphoid cell activa-tion. Evidence supporting this was provided by Besedovsky, Del Rey and Sorkin (1981) who showed that intraperitoneal injection into rats of Con A- induced human or rat lymphokines resulted in a rise in plasma cortisol which peaked at 1 -2 hours after injection.

4.2. Hormonal, Haematological and Biochemical Responses to the Intravenous Injection of Lymphokine in Man

Beginning in 1976 our group has been studying the clinical effects of injecting human lymphoid cell line lymphokines (LCL-LK) intravenously into advanced cancer patients without attributable long-term toxicity (Dumonde et al., 1980; 1981a). Constant featu-res of the short-term clinical response in about 20 such patients are a pyrexia and a neutrophil leucocytosis maximal at 2-4 hours after injection, with a lymphopenia maximal at about 4 hours. Patients usually become apyrexial after 6-8 hours and the peripheral white count is usually restored to normal at 24 hours. We wondered whether the lymphopenia could be cortisol-mediated (Thomson et al., 1980) or whether other biochemical mechanisms (eg acute phase proteins: see Pepys, 1981) might be involved.

We undertook a study of hormonal, haematological and biochemical responses of six advanced cancer patients to the intravenous injection of a LCL-LK preparation (Pulley et al., 1981). In addition to the pyrexia, polymorph leucocytosis and lymphopenia previously described (see above) there was a marked rise (up to 7 fold) in plasma cortisol, peaking at 2-4 hours (on all occasions except twice, when steroids were being given). Growth hormone levels were measured in three patients: all showed a 4-8 fold increase also peaking at 2-3 hours. In the one patient studied, an 8 fold increase in plasma ACTH was observed at 3 hours, one hour before the cortisol peak. These hormonal and haematological changes were followed by a marked decrease in plasma levels of zinc and iron (at 6-12 hours) and a subsequent rise in acute phase proteins (C-reactive protein:α_1 acid glycoprotein) maximal between 24-48 hr. These effects were not obtained with a culture medium protein control preparation processed in the same way as the active lymphokines; nor could they be ascribed to the presence of endotoxin or interferon in the lymphokine preparations (Pulley et al., 1981).

These results therefore, extend the work of Besedovsky, Del Rey and Sorkin (1981) and support their view that lymphokines might act as mediators of an immune-neuroendocrine network (see also Sorkin, this Symposium). On this basis small smounts of lymphokines released into the circulation during an immune response would induce hormonal and biochemical effects that could be expected to wind down the immune response itself. Thus, sustained inhibitory effects on T-cell function "in vivo" could well result from a rise in plasma cortisol (Gillis, Crabtree and Smith, 1979) followed by a fall in plasma levels of zinc (Rao and Schwartz, 1980) and iron (De Sousa, 1981), and then followed by a rise in acute phase protein levels (Mortensen et al., 1977). Studies are in progress to determine whether these sequential hormonal and biochemical responses run parallel with the extent and time course of lymphopenia and with alterations in peripheral blood lymphocyte function.

4.3. Mechanisms involved in Host Responses
     to Intravenous Lymphokine

It seems likely that lymphokine-induced lymphopenia is mediated by the rise in plasma cortisol (Thomson et al., 1980) and recent evidence suggests that alteration in lymphocyte traffic patterns is an important factor in corticosteroid-induced lymphopenia. Both T and B small lymphocytes are known to leave the intra-
vascular compartment, principally in lymph nodes, gut-associated
lymphoid tissue, spleen and bone marrow, by migrating between
adjacent vascular endothelial cells within lymphoid tissue (Ford,
1975). Increasing evidence points to the role of selective lymphocyte-endothelial interaction in lymphocyte compartmentation (Ford,
Smith and Andrews, 1978; De Sousa, 1981). Recently, Ford's group
have shown that infusion of prednisolone into rats causes a tempo-
rary sequestration of recirculatory lymphocytes on the extravascu-
lar side of high endothelial venules of lymph nodes as well as
facilitating the extraction of lymphocytes from the blood by vascular endothelium of bone marrow (Cox, 1981; Cox and Ford, 1982).

Prostaglandins (PGE2) have been implicated as local mediators
affecting lymphocyte traffic through lymph nodes (Hopkins et al.,
1981) and steroids are known to suppress PGE2 production by endothelial cells in culture (Jose et al., 1981). Within lymphoid
tissue, cortisol-induced modulation of endothelial cell metabolism, mediated via the cytoskeleton (Blackwell et al., 1980),
might well alter cell surface composition and product secretion
(Thorgeirsson and Robertson, 1978) in such a way as to perturb
cell traffic areas of the 'lymphoendothelial system'. On this
basis, lymphokine-induced lymphopenia would be ascribed to alterations of cell traffic through lymphoid tissues, which could be
initiated by cortisol-mediated effects on endothelial cell function rather than on the lymphocytes directly.

The nature of other responses to intravenous LCL-LK is compatible with an important effect of injected lymphokine on macrophage regulatory networks (see Moore, 1981). Lymphokine-induced
release of macrophage-derived molecules would include endogeneous
pyrogen (Atkins and Francis, 1978), interleukin-1 (LAF) (Murphy et
al., 1980) and factors regulating granulopoiesis and metabolism of
zinc and iron (see also Moore, 1981). Within the hypothalamus
there may be at least two response mechanisms; for on abolishing
the pyrexia with paracetamol there was still a rise in plasma

cortisol (Pulley et al., 1981). On this basis the pyrexia would be prostaglandin-mediated (Dinarello et al., 1977) whilst selective activation of hormone-releasing factors could be mediated via altered neuropeptide/catecholamine levels in the hypothalamus (see also Besedovsky, this Symposium).

The sequence of events which follow intravenous injection of LCL-LK into man are indeed compatible with the view that lympho-kines act as mediators of immune-neuroendocrine interactions by both direct and indirect (eg IL-1 induced) effects on the hypotha-lamus. The net result of these interactions could well contribute to homeostasis of the immunological response, not only by 'feed-back' inhibition of glucocorticoids on lymphokine production it-self (see Besedovsky et al.,1981) but also by mediator effects on lymphocyte compartmentation and macrophage networks. Amongst the anatomical sites on which endocrine and other 'extrinsic' homeo-static agents may take effect, we draw particular attention to the lymphoendothelial system and its lymphocyte-endothelial inter-actions as providing sensitive microenvironments for expression of regulatory mechanisms.

5. CONCLUSIONS

We concur that there is growing experimental evidence impli-cating lymphokines as providing a link between immunological and neuroendocrine responses to environmental stimuli (Besedovsky et al., 1981) and we cite evidence from our clinical investigations which supports and extends this view. Lymphokines themselves share many attributes with hormones (see Martin, 1976) and it seems appropriate that lymphokines seem to affect cell and tissue phy-siology in ways very similar to the actions of 'classical' hormo-nes (see Hadden and Stewart, 1981). We cite experimental evidence supporting a role for lymphokines as local mediators of lymphocy-te-endothelial interaction which we view as an obligatory compo-nent in the self-regulation of immunological responses. We infer that 'lymphoendothelial' micro-environments are sites not only for the action of intrinsic immunoregulatory networks but also for the physiological action of extrinsic (ie neuroendocrine) factors modulating the immune response. We propose the term 'lymphoendo-thelial system' to communicate this concept of an interactive physiological system governing the compartmentation and activation of recirculatory lymphocytes and which itself is regulated homeostatically by lymphokines, hormones and doubtless other products of cell and tissue metabolism. The concept of immune-neuroendocrine interactions, so elegantly illustrated by this Symposium as a whole, will add impetus to these explorations.

6. ACKNOWLEDGEMENTS

We thank the Medical Research Council, The Wellcome Trust, the Arthritis and Rheumatism Council, the Prevention of Blindness Research Fund, the Sir Halley Stewart Trust, Organon NV, and the Special Trustees of St. Thomas' Hospital for support of our investigative work.

REFERENCES

Adelman, N.E., Hammond, E., Cohen, S., and Dvorak, D., 1979, Lymphokines as inflammatory mediators, in: "Biology of Lymphokines", S. Cohen, E. Pick and J.J. Oppenheim, eds., Accademic Press, New York, p. 13.

Anderson, A.O., and Anderson, N.D., 1976, Lymphocyte emigration from high endothelial venules in rat lymph nodes, Immunology, 31:731.

Atkins, E., and Francis, L., 1978, Pathogenesis of fever in delayed hypersensitivity: factors influencing release of pyrogen-inducing lymphokines, Infect. Immun., 21:806.

Besedovsky H., and Sorkin, E., 1977, Network of immune-neuroendocrine interactions, Clin. Exp. Immunol., 27:1.

Besedovsky, H.O., Del Rey, A., and Sorkin, E., 1981, Lymphokine-containing supernatants from Con A -stimulated cells increase corticosterone blood levels, J. Immunol., 126:385.

Blackwell, G.J., Carnuccio, R., di Rosa, M., Flower, R.J., Parente, L., and Persico, P., 1980, Macrocortin: a polypeptide causing the anti-phospholipase effect of glucocorticoids, Nature, 287:147.

Bressler, J.P., Thurman, G.B., Krzych, U., Goldstein, A.L., Trivers G., and Strausser, H.R., 1980, Lymphokines secreted from sodium periodate-treated lymphocytes, Cell. Immunol., 54:274.

Burger, D.R., Ford, D., Vetto, R.M., Hamblin, A., Goldstein, A., Hubbard, M., and Dumonde, D.C., 1981, Endothelial cell presentation of antigen to human T cells, Human Immunology, 3:209.

Butcher, E.C., and Weissman, I.L., 1980, Cellular, genetic and evolutionary aspects of lymphocyte interactions with high-endothelial venules, in: "Blood cells and vessel walls: functional interactions", Ciba Foundation Symposium 71, Excerpta Medica, New York,p.265.

Butcher, E., Scollay, R., and Weissman, E., 1979, Evidence of continous evolutionary change in structures mediating adherence of lymphocytes to specialized venules, Nature, 280:496.

Cohen, S., 1980, Lymphokines in delayed hypersensitivity, in: "Immunology 80" M. Fougereau and J. Dausset, eds., Academic Press, New York, p.860

Cohen, S., Pick, E., Oppenheim, J.J., 1979, "Biology of the Lymphokines", Academic Press, New York.

Cox, J.H., 1981, Systemic factors influencing lymphocyte recircula-tion, PhD thesis, University of Manchester.

Cox, J.H. and Ford, W.L., 1982, The migration of lymphocytes across specialised vascular endothelium. IV. Prednisolone acts at several points on the recirculation pathways of lymphocytes, Cell. Immunol., in press.

Curtis, A.S.G., 1978, Cell-cell recognition : positioning and patterning systems, Symp. Soc. Exp. Biol., 32:51.

De Sousa, M., 1981, "Lymphocyte circulation : experimental and clinical aspects" John Wiley, New York.

De Weck, A.L., Kristensen, F., and Landy, M., 1980, "Biochemical Characterization of Lymphokines", Academic Press, New York.

Dinarello, C.A., Renfer, L., and Wolff, S.M., 1977, The production of antibody against human leucocytic pyrogen, J. Clin. Invest., 60:465.

Distelhorst, C.W., and Benutto, B., 1981, Glucocorticoid receptor content of T lymphocytes : evidence for heterogeneity, J. Immunol., 126:1630.

Dumonde, D.C., 1967, The role of the macrophage in delayed hyper-sensitivity, Brit. ed. Bull., 23:9.

Dumonde, D.C., 1970, "Lymphokines": Mediators and regulators of cellular immune responses, Ann. Immunol., II, 3:129.

Dumonde, D.C., 1978, The rheumatological signifance of lymphokines in: "Recognition of anti-rheumatic drugs", D.C. Dumonde and M.K. Jasani, eds., MTP Press Ltd., Lancaster, p. 167.

Dumonde, D.C., and Maini, R.N., 1971, The clinical significance of mediators of cellular immunity, Clin. Allergy, 1:123.

Dumonde, D.C., Howson, W.T. and Wolstencroft, R.A., 1968, The role of macrophages and lymphocytes in reactions of delayed hyper-sensitivity. in: "Mechanisms of inflammation induced by immune

reaction", Vth Internat. Symp. Immunopathol., 1967, P.A. Miescher
        and P. Grabar eds., p. 263. Schwabe, Basel, 278.

Dumonde, D.C., Wolstencroft, R.A., Panayi, G.S., Matthew, M.,
        Morley, J., and Howson, W.T., 1969, "Lymphokines": Non-antibody
        mediators of cellular immunity generated by lymphocyte
        activation, Nature, 224:38.

Dumonde, D.C., Kelly, R.H., and Wolstencroft, R.A., 1973, Molecular
        pharmacology of cell-mediated immunity, in: "Microenvironmental
        aspects of Immunity", B.D. Jankovic and K. Isakovic, eds., p.
        Plenum Press, New York,p.705

Dumonde, D.C., Jose, P.J., Page, D.A., and Williams, T.J., 1977,
        Production of prostaglandins by porcine endothelial cells in
        culture, Brit. J. Pharmacol, 61:504.

Dumonde, D.C., Pulley, M.S., O'Connel, D., Soughcott, B.M., Robinson
        M.R.G., Paradinas, F.J., Rigby, C.C., den Hollander, F.C.,
        Schuurs, A., and de Bruin, R.W., 1980, Local and systemic
        administration of lymphokine in patients with advanced cancer,
        Int. J. Immunopharmacol., 2(3):190.

Dumonde, D.C., Pulley, M.S., Paradinas, F.J., Southcott, B.M.,
        O'Connell, D., Robinson, M.R.G., and den Hollander, F., 1981,
        A histological study of intradermal and intralesional injection
        of human lymphoid cell line lymphokine (LCL-LK) in patients
        with advanced cancer, in: "Proc. 3rd Internat. Symp. on Human
        Lymphokines, A. Khan and N.O. Hill, eds., New York, Academic
        Press, in press.

Ford, W.L., 1975, Lymphocyte migration and immune responses, Prog.
        Allergy, 19:1.

Ford, W.L., Smith, M.E., and Andrews, P., 1978, Possible clues to
        the mechanism underlying the selective migration of lymphocytes
        from the blood, in: "Cell-cell recognition", A.S.G. Curtis, ed.,
        Symp. Soc. Exp. Biol., 32:359.

Gillis, S., Crabtree, G.R. and Smith, K.A., 1979,Glucocorticoid-
        induced inhibition of T-cell growth factor production. II. The
        effect on the "in vitro" generation of cytolytic T cells.,J.
        Immunol., 123:1631.

Goldstein, A.L., and Chirigos, M.A., 1981, "Lymphokines and
        thymic factors and their potential utilization in cancer
        therapeutics". Raven Press, New York.

Gowans, J.L. and Steer, H.W., 1980, The function and pathways of
        lymphocyte recirculation, in: "Blood cells and vessel walls:
        functional interactions", Ciba Foundation Symposium 71,
        Excerpta Medica, New York,p.113.

Hadden, J.W., and Stewart, W.E., 1981, "The Lymphokines:

Biochemistry and biological activity." Humana Press, Clifton, New Jersey.

Hirschberg, H., Berg, O.J. and Thorsby, E., 1980, Antigen-presenting properties of human vascular endothelial cells, J. Exp. Med., 152:180.

Hopkins, J., McConnell, I. and Pearson, J.D., 1981, Lymphocyte traffic through antigen-stimulated lymph nodes. II. Role of prostaglandin E2 as a mediator of cell shut-down, Immunology, 42:225.

Jose, P.J., Page, D.A., Wolstenholme, B.E., Williams, T.J., and Dumonde, D.C., 1981, Bradykinin-stimulated prostaglandin E2 production by endothelial cells and its modulation by anti-inflammatory compounds, Inflammation, 5:375.

Kasp-Grochowska, E., Page, D.A., Povey, J., Dumonde, D.C., Jose, P., and Williams, T.J., 1982a, Modulation of lymphocyte transformation by soluble products of cultured endothelial cells, submitted for publication

Kasp-Grochowska, E., Anderson, R., and Dumonde, D.C., 1982b, Lymphocyte-endothelial interactions "in vitro": enhanced association of periodate-activated lymphocytes with confluent endothelial cell monolayers, submitted for publication.

Kelly, R.H. and Wolstencroft, R.A., 1974, Germinal centre proliferation in response to mitogenic lymphokines, Clin. Exp. Immunol., 18:321.

Kelly, R.H., Wolstencroft, R.A., Dumonde, D.C., and Balfour, B.M., 1972, Role of lymphocyte activation products (LAP) in cell-mediated immunity. II. Effects of lymphocyte activation products on lymph node activation architecture and evidence for peripheral release of LAP following antigenic stimulation, Clin. Exp. Immunol., 10:49.

Kelly, R.H., Harvey, V.S., Sadler, T.E., and Dumonde, D.C., 1975, Accelerated cytodifferentiation of antibody-secreting cells in guinea-pig lymph nodes stimulated by sheep erythrocytes and lymphokines, Clin. Exp. Immunol., 20:141.

Manning, M.J. and Turner, R.J., 1976, "Comparative Immunobiology" Blackie, London.

Moore, M.A.S., 1981, Macrophage regulatory networks, in: "The Lymphokines: Biochemistry and biological activity", J.W. Hadden and W.E. Stewart, eds., Humana Press, p.305. Clifton, New Jersey.

Mortensen, R.F., Osmand, A.P., and Gewurz, H., 1975, Effects of C-reactive protein on the lymphoid system: I. Binding to thymus-dependent lymphocytes and alteration of their functions, J. Exp. Med., 141:821.

Murphy, P.A., Simon, P.L. and Willoughby, W.F., 1980, Endogeneous
    pyrogens made by rabbit peritoneal exudate cells are identical
    with lymphocyte-activating factors made by rabbit alveolar
    macrophages, J. Immunol., 124:2498

Neta, R., and Salvin, S., 1981, Production of lymphokines "in vivo",
    Lymphokines, 2:295.

Paetkau, V., 1981, Lymphokines on the move, Nature, 294:689.

Pepys, M.B., 1981, C-reactive protein fifty years on, Lancet, (i):653.

Pick, E., ed., 1980, "Lymphokine Reports: a forum for non-antibody
    lymphocyte products", Vol. 1, Academic Press, New York.

Polverini, P.J., Cotran, R.S., and Sholley, M.M., 1977, Endothelial
    proliferation in the delayed hypersensitivity reaction: an
    autoradiographic study, J. Immunol., 118:529.

Pulley, M., Dumonde, D.C., Carter, G., Muller, B., Fleck, A.,
    Southcott, B.M., and den Hollander F., 1981, Hormonal, haemato-
    logical and acute phase protein responses of advanced cancer
    patients to the intravenous injection of lymphoid cell lympho-
    kine, in: "International Symposium on Human Lymphokines", A.
    Khan and N.O. Hill, eds., Academic Press, New York, in press.

Rao, K.M.K., and Schwarts, S.A., 1980, Zinc modulates mitogenic
    responses of human lymphocytes by affecting structures
    influenced by cytochalasin B, Clin. Immunol. Immunopathol.,
    16:463.

Rather, L.J., 1972, "Addison and the White Corpuscles: an aspect
    of ninetenth century biology", Wellcome Institute of the
    History of Medicine, London.

Sidley, Y.A., and Auerbach, R., 1975, Lymphocyte-induced angiogenesis:
    a quantitative and sensitive assay of the graft-v-host reaction,
    J. Exp. Med., 141:1084.

Smith, K.A., Crabtree, G.R., Kennedy, S.J., and Munck, A.U., 1977,
    Glucocorticoid receptors and glucocorticoid sensitivity of
    mitogen-stimulated and unstimulated human lymphocytes, Nature,
    267:523.

Smith, K.A., Lachman, L.B., Oppenheim, J.J. and Favata, M.F., 1980,
    The functional relationships of the interleukins, J. Exp. Med.,
    151:1551.

Stamper, H.B., and Woodruff, J.J., 1976, Lymphocyte homing into
    lymph nodes: "in vitro" demonstration of the selective affinity
    of recirculating lymphocytes for high-endothelial venules,
    J. Exp. Med., 144:828.

Thorgeirsson, G. and Robertson, A.L., 1978, The Vascular Endothelium
    - Pathobiologic significance, Amer. J. Pathol., 93:803.

Thomson, S.P., McMahon, L.J., and Nugent, C.A., 1980, Endogeneous
    cortisol: a regulator of the number of lymphocytes in peripheral
    blood, Clin. Immunol. Immunopathol., 17:506.
Trevella, W., and Morris, B., 1980, Reassortment of cell populations
    within the lymphoid apparatus of the sheep, in: "Blood vessels
    and vessel walls: functional interactions", Ciba Foundation
    Symposium, 71:127-139.
Turk, J. L., 1967, "Delayed Hypersensitivity", North-Holland, Amster-
    dam.
Waksman, B. H., 1980, Lymphokine research: a historical review,
    Lymphokine Reports, 1:1-5.
Willmer, E. N., 1960, "Cytology and Evolution", Academic Press,
    New York.

CYCLIC NUCLEOTIDES AND RELATED MECHANISMS

IN IMMUNE REGULATION : A MINI REVIEW

John W. Hadden

Laboratory of Immunopharmacology Memorial Sloan
Kettering Cancer Center,New York, NY 10021, USA

1.INTRODUCTION

Much of the study of immune regulation over the last twenty years has focused on the dissection of cellular function and interactions "in vitro". While clearly "in vivo" studies have supported the models of regulation which have derived, this type of extrapolative approach tells only part of the story of immune regulation. The "in vitro" studies generally employ artificial media containing a drab of serum often from different species; they do not pretend to offer a dynamic fluid environment akin to that which exists "in vivo". It is becoming abundantly clear that the immune system operates "in vivo" within a homeostatic milieu replete with neurologic, neuroendocrine, endocrine and microenvironmental regulatory influences clearly as complex as those regulating the internal network of intercommunication among the cells of the system.

The principal cells to be dealt with in this minireview, the lymphocyte, the macrophage and the granulocyte, all bear receptors for a variety of hormonal influences in addition to those related to inflammatory and immune functions. These hormonal receptors (see Fig. 1) respond to stimulation by neurotransmitter influences derived from the parasympathetic nervous system (acetylcholine-muscarinic) and the sympathetic nervous system (norepinephrine- α adrenergic) and neurohumoral-adrenal system (epi-

nephrine-β adrenergic and corticosteroids). While the cholinergic
and adrenergic receptors may not be acted upon while the cells are
in circulation, they certainly are as the cells percolate through
various organs and as they infiltrate sites of inflammation.
In addition, these receptors are responsive to circulating endocrine influences including insulin, growth hormone, thyroid hormone, probably sex hormones, as well as glucocorticosteroids.
It is clear that deficiency or experimental ablation of the endocrine organs producing these hormones gives rise to immunodeficiency and it seems natural to presume that circadian cycling and
age- and disease-related changes in the function of these organs
contribute in a corresponding way to changes in immune function.

The cells involved also bear receptor for humoral mediators
which develop at the site of inflammation. These include receptors
for prostaglandins (PG) of the E and F series, serotonin and
histamine (H_1 and H_2) and complement components like C_{3a}, C_{3b} and
C_{5a} . Interestingly, these cells are also markedly responsive to
stimulation by exogenous bacterially-derived substances presumably
through receptors similar to those employed for hormones.
A partial list of these substances includes endotoxin, choleratoxin, B. pertusis, and peptidoglycans like muramyl dipeptide
(MDP). Imagine all these receptors in addition to those for
antigen, mitogen, lymphokin, suppressor and helper factors, chemo-
tatractants, activating molecules, growth factors, and chalones.
What is surprising is that with this myriad of receptors, there

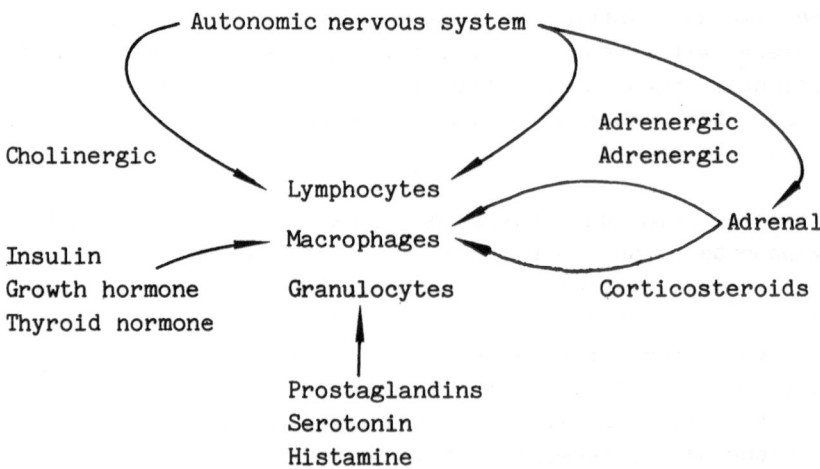

Fig. 1. Neuro-hormonal influences upon lymphoid and accessory cells.

appears at this time to be only a relatively limited repertoire of transmembrane and intracellular mechanisms for translating these influences into changes in cellular functions.

2. CYCLIC NUCLEOTIDE AND OTHER HORMONE TRANSLATING MECHANISMS

The two best studied systems for expressing hormone action are those of intracellular cyclic nucleotide messengers, cyclic 3':5' adenosine and guanosine monophosphate (cyclic AMP and cyclic GMP, respectively) and a number of hormonal influences have been linked to these systems (Hadden, et al., 1977). In general, stimuli acting on these systems are restricted to cell surface sites of action. This is particularly true for the cyclic AMP system where adenylate cyclase, the enzyme which makes cyclic AMP, is predominantly restricted to the plasma membrane as evidenced by immunofluorescent techniques. Lymphocytes hold some exception to this rule in having a nuclear membrane adenylate cyclase responsive to catecholamines (Wedner and Parker, 1977). Guanylate cyclase, in addition to having cell surface form, it also has a soluble and a possibly granule-associated form (Coffey and Hadden, 1981a); however, the differential regulation of the membrane and cytosol forms is not well understood.

Other translation systems, less well understood, include plasma membrane adenosine triphosphatases (ATPases). In lymphocytes and other tissues these enzymes have been shown to be directly modulated by insulin, growth hormone, adrenergic stimulation and corticosteroids (Hadden et al., 1972; Rubin et al., 1973; Coffey et al., 1974c, 1975) and indirectly by corticosteroids and thyroid hormone (Hellerstrom et al., 1965; Ismai-Beigi and Edelman, 1981). These ATPases are linked to transport processes for both monovalent (Na+ and K+) and divalent (Ca++ and Mg++) cations and also probably for sugars, nucleotides and amino acids.

The steroid hormones including the sex hormones, testosterone, progesterone and estradiol, generally employ intracellular receptors which bind the hormone and transport it to intranuclear acceptor sites involved in the regulation of transcription. It seems likely that others of the above mentioned hormonal influences will ultimately be shown to act via this type of mechanism. The thymic hormones to be discussed in a subsequent section seem likely candidates in this regard.

In addition to these mechanisms, it would appear that the
regulation of calcium availability and its influx into the cells
is central for activating influences for chemotaxis, phagocytosis,
degranulation and proliferation (Hadden et al., 1979; Freedman,
1979). To date, these five types of mechanisms, cyclic AMP, cyclic
GMP, ATPase, nuclear acceptors and calcium regulators, can be
envisioned to be both antagonistic as well as complementary. A
dualistic or Yin Yang notion for the generally antagonistic roles
played by the cyclic nucleotides has been proposed (Goldberg et
al., 1974). ATPases can be viewed as mechanisms linked to cyclic
GMP, as is the case with insulin, perhaps alfa-adrenergics and B.
pertussis, do so directly or through action on competitive systems
such as cyclic GMP or ATPase. To make things even more complex,
certain hormonal influences can act on the two cyclic nucleotide
systems yielding opposing effects through different receptors.
Examples are histamine acting through H_1 (cyclic GMP linked) and H_2
(cyclic AMP linked) and catecholamines like epinephrine acting
through alfa-adrenergic (ATPase, cyclic GMP linked) and beta-
-adrenergic (cyclic AMP linked) receptors. These receptor distri-
butions appear to shift with temperature, diseases like allergic
asthma, age and other factors. The nuclear based mechanisms are
either separate and distinct, as is the case with many steroid
hormone actions, or interactive as with corticosteroids and thyroid hormone. In the latter case, nuclear-derived RNA-dependent
modifications of membrane structure can lead to modified responsiveness of cyclic nucleotide cyclases and ATPases. The calcium
related mechanisms have been linked to both cyclic AMP and cyclic
GMP in mediating different functions and a simplified view is not
available at this time.

It is apparently then that the many hormonal, inflammatory
and immunologic stimuli mentioned play their music on lymphocytes,
macrophages and granulocytes with 5 sets of keys. While many
combination signals can be envisioned, particularly with activating influences as with chemotactic influences (Ca++, cyclic GMP
and/or cyclic AMP), phagocytic signals (Ca++, cyclic GMP and
cyclic AMP) mitogens (CA++ and cyclic GMP), knowledge of the
relationships of signal mechanisms to function provides a repertoire which is insufficient to account adequately for differential regulation. The yet unanswered questions of specificity of
action (as with thymic hormones) in relation to nonspecificity (as
with prostaglandins, catecholamines and cholinergics) and of intensity and duration of action will probably provide the half

tones necessary to complete a score which would allow adequate
interpretation of the actions of the many signals involved in
differential regulation of the immune system.

Although it is premature to present such a complex musical
score, this mini-review attempts to set the general scene and to
catalogue some of the many influences which have been demonstrated
to act on the lymphocyte, macrophage and granulocyte, emphasizing
those with physiologic import. Due to limited space, the reader is
referred to previously published reviews for more complete referencing of these influences and their related functions (Hadden,
1977; Strom and Carpenter, 1977; Watson, 1977; Hadden and Englard,
1977; Ignarro, 1977; Parker, 1976). The referencing of this review
will focus on developments of the last few years. The reader is
left to his imagination to envision the myriad of actions and
interactions of substances acting on each of these cells and the
resultant feedback reactions and intercommunications both positive
and negative which occur all within a dynamic scenario of varying
phases of maturation, proliferation and differentiation.

3. LYMPHOCYTE DIFFERENTIATION

The prothymocyte and pre B cell have been shown to be
sensitive to a variety of cyclic AMP raising agents including
endotoxin, isoproterenol, PGE_1 (Scheid et al., 1978; Hammerling et
al., 1976), and adenosine (Ikehara and Hadden, unpublished) which
induce nonspecifically the appearance of surface markers characteristic of the more mature phenotype (θ, TL, LY, C', Fc, and Pc).
Agents which increase cyclic GMP such as insulin, imidazole and
carbamacholine antagonize the induction (Sheid et al., 1978; Hammerling et al., 1976). The natural inducers are though to be the
thymic hormones in the case of prothymocytes and bursapoietin for
pre B cells. They have been hypothezized to act directly via cyclic AMP (Scheid et al., 1975); however, intensive efforts by
experienced laboratories to confirm this hypothesis have failed to
show that thymosin fraction V (Naylor et al., 1976), thymopoietin
(Sunshine et al., 1978) and facteur thymique serique (FTS) (Bach,
1977) do increase cyclic AMP levels in prothymocytes. The probable
interpretation is that thymic hormones act in prothymocytes in a
cyclic AMP-linked fashion, perhaps in a manner like steroid hormones, and they do not act to stimulate directly membrane adenylate
cyclase. No data are available for interpreting the mechanism of
action of bursapoietin.

At the level of the thymus and in the periphery, T cells continue to be sensitive to thymic hormone influences and respond with enhanced proliferation, receptor display (active rosetting), and secretion of soluble mediators. In this context the hormonal influences appear to be mediated by cylclic GMP as thymopoietin and thymosin fraction V have both been shown to increase cyclic GMP levels in mature T cell in association with the modulation of various functions (Sunshine et al., 1978; Naylor et al., 1976).

Two putative thymic hormones, serum factor (SF) and thymic humoral factor have been reported to increase cyclic AMP levels of thymocytes (Astaldi et al., 1976; Kook and Trainin, 1974). One of these, SF, has been shown to be adenosine, therefore while not a hormone, it may be a cofactor. The other remains to be chemically defined. It is of note that thymic epithelial supernatants contain a factor (S) which increases cyclic AMP levels in thymocytes (Kruisbeek et al., 1978; confirmed by us).
The possibility exists that there are thymic hormones which increase cyclic AMP. These need to be confirmed and chemically defined. The relationship of such hormones to thymic chalone which has been hypothesized to act via cyclic AMP (Attallah and Houck, 1977) and inhibitor of DNA synthesis (IDS), which has been shown to act via cyclic AMP (Wagshal et al., 1978), remains to be determined. In any case, the hormones, the chalone(s) and IDS, all of which have been linked to cyclic AMP, are antiproliferative in their action on thymocytes as is, of course, cyclic AMP itself when added directly to the thymocytes. It is only following removal of the hormone or factor that the cells appear to be more responsive to subsequent stimulation by mitogen. Whether this effect derives from an induction of mitogen receptors, an enhancement of their display or by other mechanisms is not clear.
Our own experience and that of a number of colleagues (personal communication) studying the action of various thymic hormones on immature, peanut agglutinin positive (PNA+) thymocytes is that they have failed to show marked effects on induction of receptors or functions. A lymphocyte produced factor, T cell growth factor (TCGF - interleukin II) and two macrophage produced factors, T cell activating factors (TAF) and lymphocyte activating factor (LAF), probably equal to interleukin I, both have more demonstrable effects to promote thymocyte proliferation induced by mitogens (Smith, 1980; Katz et al., 1978). Both LAF and TAF have been shown to increase cyclic GMP levels (Katz et al., 1978; Waksman et al.,

1980) and we have experiments in progress to determine if TCGF also does so.

A variety of other substances which have been described to act non specifically on thymocytes including insulin, PGE_1, epinephrine, acetylcholine, growth hormone, parathormone, thyrocalcitonin, antidiuretic hormone, vasopressin, testosterone, estradiol (Whitfield et al., 1976; MacManus et al., 1975; Whitfield, 1980; Morgan et al., 1975; Morgan, 1978). An elaborate hypothesis has been proposed which links both 1) those active on cyclic AMP with magnesium and 2) those active on cyclic GMP with calcium to the promotion of the intracycle proliferative behavior of a thymocyte subpopulation (about 15%). The effects observed may relate to the G_1-S boundary-defined selection of distinct daughter subsets; if so, cyclic AMP would promote one type of subset selection, helper cell and cyclic GMP would promote another, e.g., suppressor cell. In the above system testosterone inhibit the first reaction (cyclic AMP-related) and estrogen inhibits the second, or cyclic GMP-related, reaction. "In vivo" effects of sex hormones have been observed which suggest that estrogen promotes helper and testosterone suppressor function of T cells; however, it is notable that the effects of those sex hormones may not be directly on thymocytes but mediated by effects on thymic epithelial cells (Talal et al., 1981).

The action of hydrocortisone on thymocytes, particularly murine thymocytes, has been extensively studied (Munck and Leung, 1977; Munck and Young, 1975) and it is generally thought that immature thymocytes in contrast to mature T cells are particularly sensitive to the lytic effects of hydrocortisone. The mechanism of this action remains unclear since the immature and mature cells are apparently equisensitive to glucocorticoid effects "in vitro" (Triglia and Rothemberg, 1981). Of all the effects described on developing thymocytes, it would appear that thymic hormones act most obviously on prothymocytes and mature T cells while interleukin I and II and IDS may be more active on the cells at an intermediate stage of development, presumably on the PNA+ thymocyte population. The nonspecific influences like prostaglandins and catecholamines probably are not sufficient to induce T cell differentiation, rather they provide the background humoral milieu which makes possible and accentuates induction by the more specific factors.

Table 1. Agents and mechanisms in lymphocyte modulation

Cyclic GMP	Cyclic AMP	ATPase/other
Mitogens	Beta-adrenergics	Alfa-adrenergics
Acetylcholine	Prostaglandins PGE	Corticosteroids
Insulin	Histamine (H_2)	Insulin
Serotonin	Endotoxin	Growth hormone
Endotoxin	Choleratoxin	Thyroid hormone
Thymosin	B. Pertussis	
Thymopoietin	Adenosine	
Imidazole-Histamine(?H_1)	Thymic humoral factor	
Interleukin I (LAF)	Inhibitor of DNA synthesis (? Chalone)	
	(Parathormone,ADH,thyrocalcitonin and vasopressin)	

4. LYMPHOCYTE FUNCTION

Since the initial description of adrenergic receptors on mature lymphocytes (Hadden et al., 1970), the responses of lymphocytes to a large variety of modulating influences linked to cyclic nucleotides and related mechanisms have been described (Table 1; for review see Hadden, 1977, and Wedner and Parker, 1976). Agents linked to cyclic AMP include beta adrenergics, choleratoxin, adenosine, histamine (H_2) and prostaglandin E_1 (Table 1); the effects of several of these are potentiated by hydrocortisone. Agents linked to cyclic GMP include insulin, acetylcholine, imidazole (and thus presumably histamine H_1), serotonin, thymosin and thymopoietin. Where function has been correlated with the cyclic nucleotide change it is apparent that agents which increase cyclic GMP have been associated with the promotion of lymphocyte proliferation, lymphokine production, cytotoxic activity and receptor display (active rosetting) and agents which increase cyclic AMP levels have been associated with inhibition of these processes (Table 2). Cyclic AMP has also been linked to induction of suppressor cell function by histamine and paradoxically to the inhibition of suppressor cell action as well (Teh and Paetkau, 1976; Johnson et al., 1977; Webb and Jamieson,

Table 2. Cyclic nucleotides in lymphocyte regulation

Cyclic GMP		Cyclic AMP
+	Proliferation	-
+	Killing (Also NK and ADCC)	-
+	Lymphokine production	-
+	Motility	-
+	Active rosetting	-
-	Differentiation	+

1976; Rocklin, 1977). Recent observations in this series include a similar type of cyclic nucleotide regulation of lymphocyte motility (Schreiner and Unanue, 1975), of colony formation (Eckels and Gershwin, 1981),of subset receptor display (Gupta, 1979), of the production of lymphotoxin (Prieur and Granger, 1975) and leukocyte migration inhibitor factor (Bendtzen and Klysner, 1979; Bendtzen et al., 1981), and of natural killer cell activity (Roder and Klein, 1979). Recent evidence indicates that insulin and growth hormone effects, while not obviously directly modulating lymphocyte function, are critical in allowing and sustaining lymphocyte activation (Snow et al., 1980, 1981; Kumagai et al., 1981; Eckels and Gershwin, 1981).

5. LYMPHOCYTE PROLIFERATION

This rather controversial topic has been previously reviewed by us and other in detail (Hadden et al, 1979a; Wedner and Parker, 1976; Strom et al., 1977; Resch, 1976). The sum of the evidence points to a central role for calcium and cyclic GMP in the process of induction of lymphocyte proliferation. A variety of mitogens including phytohemaglutinin, concanavalin A, calcium ionophore, endotoxin, dextran sulphate, periodate and pokeweed mitogen have been shown by more than a dozen laboratories to increase lymphocyte levels of cyclic GMP (see Hadden et al., 1979a). These cyclic nucleotide responses as well as the proliferative responses following mitogen stimulation have been shown to be defective in aging, malnutrition, and cancer (Tam and Walford, 1978, 1980; Spach and Aschkenasy, 1979; Schumm et al., 1974).

Recently, low density lipoproteins have been shown to inhibit the
PHA-induced cyclic GMP increase and proliferation which may
indicate a mechanism of dysfunction in lipid disorders related to
arteriosclerotic cardiovascular disease (Hui and Harmony, 1980a,
b). A variety of studies indicate that mitogens require extracellular calcium to induce lymphocyte proliferation and induce
calcium influx as part of the initiation event (see Hadden et al.,
1979, for referencing). Our recent studies (Coffey and Hadden,
1981; Coffey et al., 1977; Coffey et al., 1978; Ananthakrishnan et
al., 1981), extend the observation that lymphocyte activation by
phytohemagglutinin is a calcium-dependent process by showing the
necessity for calcium in the increases of cyclic GMP, of guanylate
cyclase, and of early nuclear RNA synthesis.

Hirata et al. (1980) and Parker et al. (1979) have shown that
PHA induces phospholipid methylation and arachidonic acid release.
We have demonstrated that guanylate cyclase activation by PHA
depends on the production of hydroxy and hydroperoxy eicosa-
tetraenoic acids (HPETE's and HETE's) via the lipoxygenase pathway

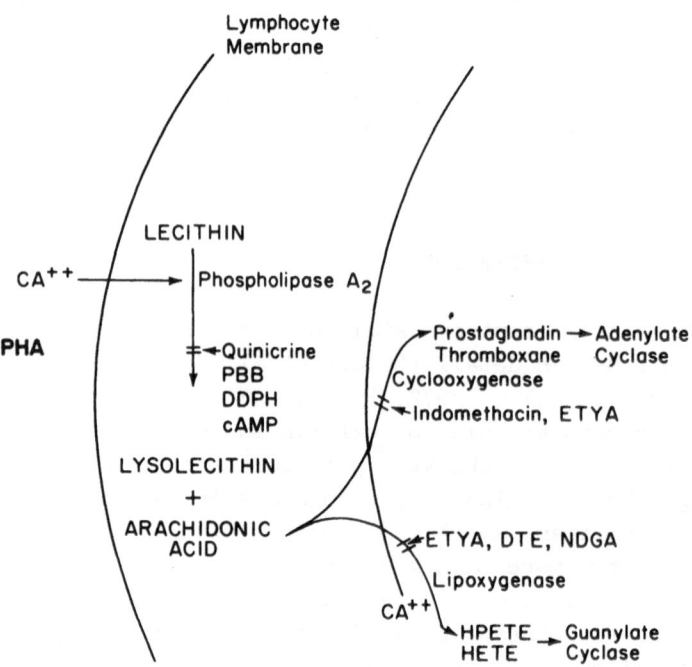

Fig. 2. Hypothetical mechanism of guanylate cyclase activation
by PHA.

(Coffey et al., 1977, 1978). Fig. 2 depicts our current hypothesis of the mechanism by which PHA activates guanylate cyclase in lymphocytes. Release of archidonic acid by PHA produces little by way of prostaglandin synthesis and inhibition of the cycloxygenase pathway has minor effects of lymphocyte activation. On the other hand, inhibition of the lipoxygenase pathway prevents both guanylate cyclase activation and lymphocyte proliferation (Coffey and Hadden, 1981a,b). In addition, HETE's directly stimulate guanylate cyclase (Coffey and Hadden, 1981a,b). It is the activation of this pathway in conjunction with calcium influx that is directly related to early nuclear events (Ananthakrishnan et al., 1981).

Mitogens have only inconsistently been shown to induce early increases of cyclic AMP levels, in relation to high concentrations which are inhibitory (see Hadden et al., 1979 for review). This effect when observed is not apparently mediated by prostaglandins. The fact that certain mitogens do not need to induce early increases in cyclic AMP supports the notion that the effect when it occurs is an epiphenomenon. Agents which increase cyclic AMP levels inhibit mitogen activation, the degree of this effect appears to vary according to the type of mitogen, in part relating to accessory cell function (Novogrodsky et al., 1979).
Mitogen-induced prostaglandin production and the resultant activation of adenylate cyclase of lymphocytes is probably dependent on adherent accessory cells and is restricted to the early phases of the activation process.

It is apparent that following the initial events of lymphocyte activation (Goodwin et al., 1981), an increase in cyclic AMP takes place (Hui and Harmony, 1980a) in the G_1 phase of the cell cycle, which may be dependent on PG synthesis and is certainly important to the initiation of DNA synthesis (Carpentieri et al., 1980; Wang et al., 1978). A role of TCGF (interleukin II) as a co-mitogen acting later in the cell cycle (probably the G_1-S boundary) has recently been elaborated (Smith, 1980) and an action via cyclic GMP would seem likely. It is clear, therefore, that a series of biochemical events involving calcium influx and both cyclic GMP and cyclic AMP generation are required to initiate lymphocyte proliferation.

The antiproliferative effect of glucocorticoids on lymphocytes would appear in part to derive from direct actions and in part from their actions to accentuate responses of agonists like

Table 3. Cyclic nucleotides in macrophage regulation

Cyclic GMP	Cyclic AMP
Mitogenic factors (MMF, PMA)	Beta-adrenergics
Activating factors (MAF, MDP, DMWF)	Prostaglandin PGE
Prostaglandin F_2 Serotonin Fc receptor activation Ascorbate Transfer factor	

epinephrine, PGE_1, histamine which increase cyclic AMP and to inhibit calcium influx and cyclic GMP generation (Hadden et al., 1975), perhaps through action to inhibit phospholipase mediated release of arachidonic acid.

6. MACROPHAGE FUNCTION AND ACTIVATION

To date, hormonal regulation of the macrophage has been studied less extensively than the lymphocyte (Hadden and Englard, 1977; Pick, 1977; Hadden, 1978). The macrophage has been shown to be sensitive to agents increasing cyclic AMP such as epinephrine, PGE_1, choleratoxin, muramyl dipeptide and agents which increase cyclic GMP like $PGF_{2\alpha}$, ascorbate, serotonin, insulin, carbamyl-choline, transfer factor and muramyl dipeptide (Table 3).

Elevations of cyclic AMP by prostaglandin have been linked to inhibition of proliferation of macrophage precursors induced by colony stimulating factor (CSF) (Kurland et al., 1978; Taetle and Koessler, 1980) and of proliferation of mature macrophages induced by macrophage mitogenic factor (Hadden et al., 1978). Cyclic AMP and agents which increase cyclic AMP in macrophages, including prostaglandins, have been similarly linked to inhibition of phagocytosis, chemiluminescence, and enzyme release (Weissman et al., 1971; Gemsa et al., 1975; Rossi et al., 1972; Welscher and

Cruchaud, 1976, 1978; Smith and Weidemann, 1980), of locomotion (Pick, 1972; Gallin et al., 1978; Oropeza-Rendon et al., 1979), of aggregation (Rouveix et al., 1980), of fusion (Papadimitriou, and Sforcina, 1975), of migration inhibition induced by lymphokines (Pick, 1977; Koopman et al., 1973), of macrophage plasminogen activator production (Vassili et al., 1976; Foster, 1980) and of macrophage tumoricidal activity (Schultz et al., 1978). On the positive side, increases in cyclic AMP mediated by prostaglandin production have been linked to induction of collagenase production by macrophages (Wahl and Wahl, 1979; McCarthy et al., 1980).

The effect of muramyl dipeptide on macrophages is particularly interesting in that this substance increases both cyclic AMP and cyclic GMP levels of macrophages (Wahl et al., 1979; Hadden and Englard, 1977). The effect to increase cyclic AMP levels results from the action of MDP to induce prostaglandin metabolism. The biological effects of muramyl dipeptide to induce collagenase production and to inhibit lymphokine-induced macrophage proliferation can be blocked by indomethacin which inhibits prostaglandin synthesis (Chedid et al., 1979). The effect of MDP to induce macrophage activation to kill Listeria monocytogenes is unaffected by indomethacin and appears to be related to the increases of cyclic GMP levels (Hadden and Englard, 1979; Englard Ph.D. Thesis, 1981, Cornell Graduate School of Medical Sciences). It is notable that the effects of MDP to act "in vivo" as an immunoadjuvant and to protect animals from bacterial challenge is unaffected by treatment with indomethacin. Only the effect of muramyl dipeptide to induce fever is blocked by this treatment. It appears then that MDP's main action as a macrophage activator is mediated by cyclic GMP and its inhibitory side effects to induce fever (pyrogen induction) and collagen production, and to inhibit macrophage proliferation as a result of cyclic AMP production derived from prostaglandin synthesis.

Other agents which increase cyclic GMP levels in macrophages have been related to increased chemotaxis (Gallin et al., 1978), Fc receptor display (Rhodes, 1975), aggregation (Rouveix et al., 1980), proliferation (Kurland et al., 1977) and phagocytosis and killing of bacteria (Hadden and Englard, 1979). Insulin, an agent linked to cyclic GMP in other cells, has shown variable effects on macrophages including increased fusion (Papadimitriou and Sforcina, 1975), reduced Fc receptor display and impaired antibody--dependent cytotoxicity (Rhodes, 1975; Bar and Kahn, 1977).

On the other hand, corticosteroids have been shown to inhibit a number of macrophage functions (see Parrillo and Fauci, 1979) including migration inhibitory factor (MIF) action (Balow and Rosenthal, 1973), plasminogen activator release(Vassalli et al., 1976), and proliferation in response to lymphokine stimulation (Duncan et al., 1981).

The discussion so far has referred to the modulation by hormones of macrophage functions already triggered by lymphokine, phagocytic stimulus, or other activating influences. The issue of the mechanisms of macrophage regulation by these factors and influences is not at all clear. The first factor to be analyzed in its effect on macrophages is migration inhibitory factor (MIF). A number of laboratories have noted that MIF does not increase macrophage levels of cyclic AMP (Pick, 1972; Block et al., 1978; Koopman et al., 1973). Gordon, et al. (1976) reported that lymphokine-rich supernatants induce increases in prostaglandin levels of macrophages; however, we have had difficulty in repro-ducing this observation when partially purified lymphokines were compared to control fractions similary processed (Hadden et al., 1979). Phagocytic stimuli and a variety of inflammatory stimuli have been reported to induce the release of arachidonic acid and production of prostaglandins by macrophages (Humes et al., 1977; Brune et al., 1978; Stenson and Parker, 1980). Reports on accom-panying increases in cyclic AMP induced by these stimuli have been sparse; Smith et al. (1980) have recently shown that one phago-cytic stimulus, zymosan, induced an increase in cyclic AMP which, if blocked by indomethacin, does not impair phagocytosis or the production of chemiluminescence. A similar effect was observed with the calcium ionophore A23187. These data indicate that the increases in macrophage prostaglandin levels and cyclic AMP levels are not part of the initiation processes and may rather be invol-ved in feedback inhibitory mechanisms.

It seems more likely that calcium and/or cyclic GMP are involved in the triggering mechanisms. Bromberg and Pick (1980) have reported that lymphokine fractions containing MIF (and other lymphokines such as the mitogenic and chemotactic factor) and the calcium ionophore do not increase macrophage levels of cyclic GMP. On the other hand, we have observed that similar lymphokine fractions increase cyclic GMP in macrophages and have noted that a number of macrophage activators including macrophage activating factor, muramyl dipeptide, listeria factor, the calcium ionophore, and phorbol myristate acetate, also increase macrophage levels of cyclic GMP (Hadden and Englard, 1979; Hadden et al., 1979b; Hadden and Coffey, unpublished observations). Smith et al. (1980) have also observed that macrophage levels of cyclic GMP are increased by both the calcium opnophore and zymosan. These increases were further shown to be dependent on calcium and were not inhibited by indomethacin. Pick et al. (1979) have observed that lympho-kine-rich fractions induce calcium influx and it seems likely that both the ionophore and phagocytic stimuli will be shown to be associated with calcium influx and/or mobilization in the macro-phage, as they are in the granulocyte. While the discrepancy between Pick's data and those of us and Smith et al., are not easily resolvable, they most likely rest upon technical problems involved in the measurement of cyclic GMP levels in macrophages.

Chemiluminescence following zymosan ingestion and beta glucuronidase release following IgE Fc receptor binding to macrophages have also both been shown to be calcium-dependent and to be associated with cyclic GMP increases (Smith et al., 1980; Dessaint et al., 1980). Both the chemiluminescence response and enzyme release are generally closely associated with the process of phagocytosis. A variety of phagocytic as well as non-phagocytic stimuli are associated with arachidonic acid release of macro-phages (see Stenson and Parker, 1980).
Smith and coworkers (Smith and Weidemann, 1980; Smith et al., 1980) have linked the release of arachidonic acid to the production of chemiluminescence via the lipoxygenase pathway, so it seems likely that the variety of activators linked to cyclic GMP in the macrophage will involve the same type of pathway involved in lymphocyte triggering depicted in Fig. 2.

It is tempting to speculate that cyclic GMP and calcium will be involved in the initiation of macrophage proliferation and activation as is the case for the lymphocyte and in the initiation of phagocytosis as appears to be the case with the granulocytes (reviewed in the next section). One question obviously derives and that is if the signal for both processes are the same, why don't macrophages replicate as a result of phagocytosis? A logical but unproven answer is that the induction of prostaglandin metabolism by phagocytic stimuli (Humes et al., 1977) yields increases of cyclic AMP which then block the proliferative response.

Table 4. Cyclic nucleotides in granulocyte regulation

Cyclic GMP	Cyclic AMP	ATPase/Other
Phagocytic stimuli	Beta-adrenergics	Insulin
Chemotactic stimuli	Prostaglandin	Glucocorticoids
Tuftsin, HETE		
Acetyl cholin	Choleratoxin	
Insulin		
Serotonin		
Ascorbate		

7. NEUTROPHIL FUNCTION AND ACTIVATION

The neutrophil has been shown to respond to a variety of agents linked to cyclic AMP including prostaglandin, beta adrenergics, histamine and choleratoxin and the effects are potentiated by hydrocortisone (Ignarro, 1977; Weissman et al., 1980; Marone et al., 1980); however, the responses are small compared to the lymphocyte and other cells (Marone et al., 1980). Hormonal agents linked to cyclic GMP include serotonin ascorbic acid and acetylcholine, and $PGF_2\alpha$ (see Ignarro, 1977) (Table 4).

The effect of agents which increase cyclic AMP in granulocytes have been related to the inhibition of phagocytosis, zymosan-induced enzyme release and of chemotaxis. While the effect of agents which increase cyclic GMP have been linked to increased degranulation and chemotaxis (see Ignarro, 1977; Weissman et al., 1980, for references).

It was originally shown by Park et al. (1971), that phagocytosis resulted in an increase in cyclic AMP in granulocytes; however, this observation could not be confirmed by Manganiello et al. (1971). A lack of effect of ingested zymosan on cyclic AMP levels of granulocytes was also shown by Ignarro et al. (1974). These workers (Smith and Ignarro, 1975) also showed a calcium influx-related increase in cyclic GMP with zymosan ingestion by PMN's. Weissmann and coworkers (Weissmann et al., 1979; Weissmann et al., 1980; Smolen and Weissmann, 1981) were unable to confirm these observations about cyclic GMP elevations and instead found early increases (less than 2 min) in cyclic AMP with agents both particulate (Ag-Ab complexes and zymosan)and soluble which promote the release of enzymes by granulocytes.

Using immunofluorescent techniques, Pryzwansky et al. (1981) have shown localized cyclic AMP formation in granulocytes associated with phagosome formation around zymosan or latex particles; cyclic GMP which was associated with the granular cytoplasmic region could not be evaluated quantitatively. It remains to be clarified whether the cyclic AMP changes observed are related to the activation process or more likely to feed back inhibitory mechanisms; it is clear that agents which increase cyclic AMP or preserve it from catabolism inhibit ingestion and degranulation.

It also remains to be determined if the cyclic GMP changes are reproducible early events, which are related to the activation process. The application to the granulocyte of the rigorous cyclic AMP purification procedures found by us to be critical in making accurate measurements in the lymphocyte seems to be important in resolving this controversy.

The activation of granulocytes by chemoattractants is a complex process involving directed movement, calcium influx, oxygen radical production with chemiluminescence and primary granule release (see Weissmann et al., 1979, for review). Hatch et al., (1977) have described the effects of a number of chemoattractants which activate this process to increase neutrophil levels of cyclic GMP. Correspondingly, Hagmann and Fishman (1980) found that one chemoattractant, N-formyl methionyl-lucyl-phenylalanine (F-met leu Phe), decreases adenylate cyclase activity of granulocytes and Najjar and Schmidt (1980) have observed that Tuftsin, which increases chemotaxis as well as other leukocyte functions, elevates levels of cyclic GMP. To the converse, Simchowitz et al., (1980) have failed to find increases in cyclic GMP with the complement fragment C5A instead, they observed small, transient increases in cyclic AMP within the first 5 minutes of stimulation. It has not been determined whether, as the macrophage, this cyclic AMP increase is dependent on prostaglandin metabolism. It is known that inhibition of PG synthesis by indomethacin does not prevent the chemotactic response.

Leukocyte activation by the calcium ionophore A 23187 yields modifications of mobility, oxygen consumption and hexose monophosphate shunt activity, and degranulation which are similar to those induced by phagocytosis and activation by chemotactic influen-

ces. This type of activation is associated with arachidonic acid
release and production of products of both the cyclo-oxygenase and
the lipoxygenase pathway including in the latter case production
of hydroeicosatetraenoic acids (HPETEs, HETEs) and leukotrienes
(Goldstein et al., 1978; Stenson and Parker, 1979).
Inhibition of cyclo-oxygenase by lipoxygenase pathway inhibits the
chemotactic and chemiluminescence responses (Showell et al., 1980;
Weissmann et al., 1980). Products of the lipoxygenase pathway such
as HETE have recently been shown to be involved in the chemotactic
response (Goetzl and Sun, 1979; Goetzl and Pickett, 1980), in the
degranulation response (Stenson and Parker, 1980), in hexose
transport (Bass et al., 1980) and in cyclic GMP increases (Goetzl
et al., 1980). It seems likely then that the pathway depicted in
Fig. 2 is also involved in granulocyte activation and that cyclic
GMP and calcium influx are central issues.

Bendtzen et al., (1981) have observed that LIF induced
neutrophil migration inhibition is modulated by cyclic nucleotides
such that agents which increase cyclic GMP promote and agents
which increase cyclic GMP inhibit LIF action. LIF itself increases
granulocyte cyclic GMP levels without effect on cyclic AMP levels.
It remains to be determined what effects LIF has relevant to the
processes of chemotaxis, phagocytosis and degranulation.

To complete the list, insulin has been linked in granulocytes
to the maintenance of normal chemotaxis (Mowat and Baum, 1971) and
to glycogen synthesis (Stossel et al., 1970) and glucocorticoids,
at high concentrations, to inhibition of phagocytosis movement and
degranulation (see Parillo and Fauci,1979).

8. CONCLUSION

The lymphocyte, macrophage and granulocyte are exposed "in
vivo" to a variety of environmental and humoral influences including neurotransmitters, hormones, and inflammatory mediators which
modulate their functions in response to immunologically specific
stimuli, including both antigen and soluble mediators.
It appears that one way or another the mechanisms of hormone
action, i.e. the cyclic nucleotides, membrane ATPases, nuclear
processes and calcium influx are involved in the expression of
both the nonspecific and the specific stimuli. Recent studies into
the mechanisms of activation of each of these cells point to a

central role for release and conversion to prostaglandins, via the cyclo-oxygenase pathway as acting in negative feedback mechanisms via cyclic AMP, and to HETE's, via the lipoxygenase pathway as acting in positive activating mechanisms via cyclic GMP. Calciuminflux and mobilization appears to be central to lymphocyte activation, for proliferation, and granulocyte activation, for movement and degranulation. As a general rule, these and related processes appear to be modulated in a positive way by cyclic GMP related mechanisms and in a negative way by cyclic AMP. Such hormones as thymic hormones, insulin, growth hormones and thyroid hormone are more complicated in their actions and appear to provide the background miliéu which allows and supports the actions of immunologic stimuli. These nonspecific influences and their mechanisms are perhaps far more critical than suspected in the maintenance and regulation of in vivo immune responses.

REFERENCES

Ananthakrishman, R., Coffey, R.G., and Hadden, J.W., 1981, Cyclic GMP and Calcium in lymphocyte activation by phytohemagglutinin, Lymphocyte Differentiation, in press.

Astaldi, A., Astaldi, G.C.B., Schellekens, P.T.A., and Eijsvoogel, V.P.,1976, Thymic factor in human sera demonstrable by a cyclic AMP assay, Nature, 260:713.

Attallah, A.M., and Houck, J.C., 1977, Tentative mechanisms of lymphocyte chalone action, Exp. Cell Res., 105:137.

Bach, M.A., 1977, Lymphocyte-mediated cytotoxicity: effects of ageing, adult thymectomy and thymic factor, J. Immunol., 119:641.

Balow, J.E., and Rosenthal, A.S., 1973, Glucocorticoid suppression of macrophage migration inhibitory factor, J. Exp. Med., 137:1031.

Bar, R.S., and Kahn, R.C., 1977, Insulin inhibition of antibody-dependent cytotoxicity and insulin receptors in macrophages, Nature, 265:632.

Bass, D.A., O'Flaherty, J.T., Szejda, P., De Chatelet, L.R., McCall, C.E., 1980, Role of arachidonic acid in stimulation of hexose transport by human polymorphonuclear leukocytes, Proc. Natl. Acad. Sci., USA , 77:5125.

Bendtzen, K., and Klysner, R., 1979, Increased polymorphonuclear leukocyte cGMP levels induced by the human lymphokine, leukocyte migration inhibitory factor (LIF), Immunopharmacol., 1:323.

Bendtzen, K., Mahoney, R., and Rocklin, R.E., 1981, Production of human leukocyte migration inhibitory factor (LIF) by lymphocytes stimulation with phytohemagglutinin. II. Effects of cyclic nucleotides, Clin. Immunol. Immunopathol., 18:221.

Block, L.H., Aloni, B., Biemesderfer, D., Kashgarian, M., and Bitensky, M.W., 1978, Macrophage migration inhibition factor: interactions with calcium, magnesium, and cyclic AMP, J. Immunol., 121:1416.

Bromberg, Y., and Pick., E., 1980, Cyclic GMP metabolism in macrophages. I. Regulation of cyclic GMP levels by calcium and stimulation of cyclic GMP synthesis by NO-generation agents, Cell. Immunol., 52:73.

Brune, K., Glatt, M., and Kalin, H., 1978, Pharmacological control of prostaglandin and thromboxane release from macrophages, Nature, 274:261.

Carpentieri, U., Monahan, T.M., and Gustavson, L.P., 1980, Observations of the level of cyclic nucleotides in three populations of human lymphocytes in culture, J. Cyc. Nucl. Res., 4:253.

Chedid, L., Carelli, C., and Audibert, F., 1979, Recent developments concerning muramyl dipeptide, a synthetic immunoregulating molecule, J. Reticuloendothel. Soc., 26 (Supp.):631.

Coffey, R.G., and Hadden, J.W., 1981a, Arachidonate and metabolites in mitogen activation of lymphocyte guanylate cyclase, in: "Advances in Immunopharmacology," J. Hadden, L. Chedid, P. Mullen and F. Spreafico, eds., Pergamon Press, Oxford, p. 365.

Coffey, R.G., and Hadden, J.W., 1981b, Phytohemagglutinin stimulation of guanylate cyclase in human lymphocytes, J. Biol. Chem., 256:4418.

Coffey, R.G., Hadden, J.W., and Middleton, E., J.R., 1974, Increased adenosine triphosphatase in leukocytes of asthamatic children, J. Clin. Invest., 54:138.

Coffey, R.G., Hadden, E.M., and Hadden, J.W., 1975, Norepinephrine stimulation of membrane ATPase in human lymphocytes, Endocrinol. Res. Comm., 12:179.

Coffey, R.G., Hadden, E.M., and Hadden, J.W., 1977, Evidence of cyclic GMP and calcium mediation of lymphocyte activation by mitogens, J. Immunol., 119:1387.

Coffey, R.G., Hadden, E.M., Lopez, C., and Hadden, J.W., 1978, Cyclic GMP and calcium in the initiation of cellular proliferation, Adv. Cyclic Nucl. Res., 9:66.

Dessaint, J., Waksman, B.H., Metzger, H., nad Capron, A., 1980, Cytophilic binding of IgE to the macrophage. III. Involvement of cyclic GMP and calcium in macrophage activation by dimeric or aggregated rat myeloma IgE, Cell. Immunol., 51:280.

Duncan, M.R., Sadlik, J.R., and Hadden, J.W., 1981, Glucocorticoid modulation of lymphokine-induced macrophage proliferation, J. Immunol., submitted.

Eckels, D.D., and Gershwin, M.E., 1981, Pharmacologic and biochemical modulation of human T-lymphocyte colony formation:hormonal influences, Immunopharmacol., 2:259.

Foster, S., 1980, Cyclic nucleotides and cellular secretion. Cyclic nucleotides, possible intracellular mediators of macrophage activation and secretory processes, Agents and Actions, 10:556.

Freedman, M.H., 1979, Early biochemical events in lymphocyte activation. I. Investigations on the nature and significance of early calcium fluxes observed in mitogen induced T and B lymphocytes, Cell. Immunol., 44:290.

Gallin, J., Sandler, J.A., Clyman, R.I., Manganiello, V.C. and Vaughan, M., 1978, Agents that increase cyclic AMP inhibit accumulation of cGMP and depress human monocyte locomotion, J. Immunol., 120:492.

Goetzl, E.J., and Pickett, W.C., 1980, The human PMN leukocyte chemotactic activity of complex hydroxy-eicosatetraenoic acids (HETEs), J. Immunol., 125:1789.

Goetzl, E.J., and Sun, F.F., 1979, Generation of unique mono-hydroxy-eicosate-traenoic acids from arachidonic acid by human neutrophils, J. Exp. Med., 150:406.

Goetzl, E.J., Hill, H.R., and Gorman, R.R., 1980, Unique aspects of the modulation of human neurophil function by 12-L-lydroperoxy-f, 8,10,14-eicosategraenoic acid, Prostaglandins, 19:71.

Goldberg, N.D., Hadden, M.K., Durham, E., Lopez, C., and Hadden, J.W., 1974, Evidence for opposing influences of cyclic GMP and cyclic AMP in the regulation of cell proliferation and other biological processes. Cold Spring Harbor Symposium "Control of proliferation in Animal Cells," Cold Spring Harbor Press, New York, p. 609.

Goldstein, I.M., Malmsten, C.L., Kindahl, H., Kaplan, H.B., Radmark, O., Samuelsson, B., and Weissman, G., 1978, Thromboxane generation by human peripheral blood polymorphonuclear leukocytes, J. Exp. Med., 148:787.

Goodwin, J.S., Bromberg, S., and Messner, R.P., 1981, Studies on the cyclic AMP response to prostaglandin in human lymphocytes, Cell. Immunol., 60:298.

Gordon, D., Bray, M.A., Morley, J., 1976, Control of lymphokine secretion by prostaglandins, Nature, 262:401.

Gupta, S., 1979, Subpopulations of human T lymphocytes. XII. In vi-

tro effect of agents modifying intracellular levels of cyclic
nucleotides on T cells with receptors for IgM (Tμ), IgG (Tγ),
or IgA (Tα), J. Immunol, 123:2664.

Hadden, J.W., 1977, Cyclic nucleotides in lymphocyte proliferation
and differentiation. in:"Immunopharmacology," Hadden, J.W.,
Coffey, R.G., and Spreafico, F., eds., vol 3, Plenum Publishing
Corp., New York, p. 1.

Hadden, J.W., 1978, The action of immunopotentiators in vitro on
lymphocyte and macrophage activation, in:"The Pharmacology of
Immunoregulation," Werner, G.H. and Floc'h, F., eds., Academic
Press, New York, p. 369.

Hadden, J.W., and Englard, A., 1977, Molecular aspects of macropha-
ge activation and proliferation, in: "Immunopharmacology,"
Hadden, J.W., Coffey, R.G. and Spreafico, F., eds., vol. 3,
Plenum Publishing Corp., New York, p. 87.

Hadden, J.W., and Englard, A., 1979, Molecular aspects of macrophage activation and proliferation, in:"10th Int. Course on Transplantation and Clinical Immunology," Excerpta Medica, Amsterdam, p. 279.

Hadden, J.W., Hadden, E.M., and Middleton, E., jr, 1970, Lymphocyte
blast transformation. I. Demonstration of adrenergic receptors
in human peripheral lymphocytes, J. Cell. Immunol., 1:583.

Hadden, J.W., Hadden, E.M., Wilson, E.E., Good, R.A., and Coffey,
R.G., 1972, Direct action of insulin on plasma membrane ATPase
activity in human lymphocytes, Nature, New Biol., 235:174.

Hadden, J.W., Hadden, E.M., Coffey, R.G., Johnson, E.M., and John-
son, L.D., 1975, Cyclic GMP and lymphocyte activation, in:
"Immune Recognition," A. Rosenthal.,ed., Academic Press, New
York, p. 359.

Hadden, J.W., Coffey, R.G., and Spreafico, F.,1977, Immunopharmacology, vol. 3, Plenum Publishing Corp, New York.

Hadden, J.W., Sadlik, J.R., and Hadden, E.M., 1978, The induction
of macrophage proliferation in vitro by a lymphocyte produced
factor, J. Immunol., 121:231.

Hadden, J.W., Sadlik, J.R., Englard, A., Warfel, A., and Hadden,
E., 1979a, Lymphokine-induced macrophage proliferation, ac-
tivation, and fusion, in:"Biochemical Characterization of the
Lymphokines," A. DeWeck, ed., Academic Press, New York, p. 235.

Hadden, J.W., Englard, A., Sadlik, J.R., and Hadden, E., 1979b, The
comparative effects of isoprinosine, levamisole, muramyl dipeptide and SM1213 on lymphocyte and macrophage proliferation and
activation in vitro, Int. J. Immunopharmacol., 1:17.

Hadden, J.W., Coffey, R.G., Ananthakrishnan, R., and Hadden, E.M.,

1979c, Cyclic nucleotides and calcium in lymphocyte regulation and activation, Proc. N.Y. Acad. Sci., 332:241.

Hagmann, J., and Fishman, P.H., 1980, Modulation of adenylate cyclase in intact macrophages by microtubulues. Actions of colchicine and chemotactic factor, J. Biol. Chem., 255:2659.

Hammerling, U., Chin, A.F., Abbot, J., Goldstein, G., Sonnenberg, M., and Hoffmann, M.K., 1976, Ontogeny of B-lymphocytes. 3. Opposite signals transmitted to B-lymphocyte precursor cells by inducing agents and hormones, Eur. J. Immunol., 6:868.

Hatch, G.E., Nichols, W.K., and Hill, H.R., 1977, Cyclic nucleotide changes in human neutrophils induced by chemoattractants and chemotactic modulators, J. Immunol., 119:450.

Hellerstrom, C., Taljedal, I., and Hellman, B., 1965, Quantitative studies on isolated pancreatic islets of mammals. 5' nucleotidase and adenosine triphosphate activities in normal and cortisone-treated rats, Endocrinol., 76:315.

Hirata, F., Toyoshima, S., Axelrod, J., and Waxdal, J., 1980, Phospholipid methylation: a biochemical signal modulating lymphocyte mitogenesis, Proc. Natl. Acad. Sci., USA, 77:862.

Hui, D.Y., and Harmony, J.A., 1980a, Inhibition of CA^{2+} accumulation in mitogen-activated lymphocytes: role of membrane-bound plasma lipoproteins, Proc. Natl. Acad. Sci., USA, 77:4764.

Hui, D.Y., and Harmony, J.A., 1980b, Inhibition by low density lipoproteins of mitogen-stimulated cyclic nucleotide production by lymphocytes, J. Biol. Chem., 255:1413.

Humes, J.L., Bonney, R.J., Pelus, L., Dahlgren, M.E., Sadowski, S.J., Kuehl, F.A., Jr., and Davies, P., 1977, Macrophages synthetize and release prostaglandins in response to inflammatory stimuli, Nature, 269:149.

Ignarro, L.J., 1977, Regulation of polymorphonuclear leukocyte, macrophage, and platelet function, in: "Immunopharmacology," Vol. 3, J.W. Hadden, R.G. Coffey, and F. Spreafico, eds., Plenum Publishing Corp., New York, p. 61.

Ignarro, L.J., Lint, T.F., and Goerge, W.J., 1974, Hormonal control of lysosomal enzyme release from human neutrophils. Effects of autonomic agents on enzyme release, phagocytosis and cyclic nucleotide levels, J. Exp. Med., 139:1395.

Ismai-Beigi, F., and Edelman, I.S., 1971, The mechanism of calorigenic action of thyroid hormone, J. Gen. Physiol., 57:710.

Johnson, H.M., Blalock, J.E., and Baron, S., 1977, Separation of mitogen-induced suppressor and helper cell activities during inhibition of interferon production by cyclic AMP, Cell. Immunol., 33:170.

Katz, S.P., Kierszenbaum, F., and Waksman, B.H., 1978, Mechanisms of action of "lymphocyte-activating factor," (LAF). III. Evidence that LAF acts on stimulated lymphocytes by raising cyclic GMP in G_1, J. Immunol., 121:2386.

Kook, A., and Trainin, N., 1974, Hormone-like activity of a thymus humoral factor on the induction of immune competence in lymphoid cells, J. Exp. Med., 139:193.

Koopman, W.J., Gillis, M.H., and David, J.R., 1973, Prevention of MIF activity by agents known to increase cellular cyclic AMP, J. Immunol., 110:1609.

Mowat, A.G., and Baum, J., 1971, Chemotaxis of polymorphonuclear leukocytes from patients with diabetes mellitus, New Engl. J. Med., 284:621.

Novogrodsky, A., Rubin, A.L., and Stenzel, K.H., 1979, Selective suppression by adherent cells, prostaglandin, and cyclic AMP analogues of blasto-genesis induced by different mitogens, J. Immunol., 122:1.

Kruisbeek, A.M., Astaldi, G.C.B., Blankwater, M.J., Zijlstra, J.J., Levert, L.A., and Astaldi, A., 1978, The in vitro effect of a thymic epithelial culture supernatant on mixed lymphocyte reactivity and intracellular cAMP levels of thymocytes and on antibody production to SRBC by Nu/Nu spleen cells, Cell. Immunol., 35:134.

Kumagai, J.-I., Akiyama, H., Iwashita, S., Iida, H., and Yahara, I., 1981, In vitro generation of resting lymphocytes from stimulated lymphocytes and its inhibition by insulin, J. Immunol., 126:1249.

Kurland, J.I., Hadden, J.W., and Moore, M.A.S., 1977, Role of cyclic nucleotides in the preparation of committed granulocyte--macrophage progenitor cells, Cancer Res., 37:4535.

MacManus, J.P., Whitfield, J.F, Boynton, A.L., and Rixon, R.H., 1975, Role of cyclic nucleotides and calcium in the positive control of cell proliferation, in: "Advances in Cyclic Nucleotide Research," vol. 5, G.I. Drummond, P. Greengard, P., and Robinson, G.A., eds., Raven Press, New York, p. 719.

Manganiello, V., Evans, W.H., Stossel, T.P., Mason, R.J., and Vaughan, M., 1971, The effect of polystyrene beads of cyclic 3', 5'-adenosine monophosphate concentration in leukocytes, J. Clin. Invest., 50:2741.

Marone, G., Thomas, L.L., and Lichtenstein, L.M., 1980, The role of agonists that activate adenylate cyclase in the control of cAMP metabolism and enzyme release by human polymorphonuclear leukocytes, J. Immunol., 125:2277.

McCarthy, J.B., Wahl, S.M., Rees, J.C., Olsen, C.E., Sandberg, A.L., and Wahl, L.M., 1980, Mediation of macrophage collagenase production by 3'-5'cyclic adenosine monophosphate, J. Immunol., 124:2405.

Morgan, J.I., Hall, A.K., and Perris, A.D., 1975, Requirements for divalent cations by hormonal mitogens and their interactions with sex steroids, Biochem. Biophys. Res. Comm., 66:188.

Morgan, J.I., Hall, A.K., and Perris, A.D., 1978, The ionic dependence and steroid blockade of cyclic nucleotide-induced mitogenesis in isolated rat thymic lymphocytes, J. Cyclic. Nucl. Res., 3:303.

Munck, A., and Leung, K., 1977, Glucocorticoid receptors and mechanism of action, in: "Receptors and Mechanism of Action of Steroid Hormones," Part II. J.R. Pasquatini, ed., Marcel Dekker, Inc., New York, p. 311.

Munck, A., and Young, D.A., 1975, Corticosteroids and lymphoid tissue, in: "Handbook of Physiology," Section 7, Endocrinology, vol. 6, American Physiological Society, Washington, D.C., p. 231.

Najjar, V.A., and Schmidt, J.J., 1980, The chemistry and biology of tuftsin , Lymphokine Reports, 1:157.

Naylor, P.H., Sheppard, H., Thurman, G.B., and Goldstein, A.L., 1976, Increase of cyclic GMP induced in murine thymocytes by thymosin fraction 5, Biochem. Biophys. Res. Comm., 73:843.

Oropeza-Rendon, R.L., Speth, V., Hiller, G., Weber, K., and Fischer, H., 1979, Prostaglandin E reversibly induced morphological changes in macrophages and inhibits phagocytosis, Exp. Cell. Res., 119:365.

Papadimitrious, J.M., and Sforcina, D., 1975, The effects of drugs on monocytic fusion in vivo, Exp. Cell. Res., 91:233.

Parrillo, J.E., and Fauci, A.S., 1979, Mechanisms of glucocorticoid action on immune processes, Ann. Rev. Pharmacol. Toxicol., 19:179.

Park, B.H., Good, R.A., Beck, N.P., and Davis, B.B., 1971, Concentration of cyclic adenosine 3', 5'-monophosphate in human leukocytes during phagocytosis, Nature, New Biol., 229:27.

Parker, C.W., 1976, Control of lymphocyte function, New. Engl. J. Med., 295:1180.

Parker, C.W., Kelly, J.P., Falkenhein, S.F., and Huber, M.G., 1979, Release of arachidonic acid from human lymphocytes in response to mitogenic lectins, J. Exp. Med., 149:1487.

Pick, E., 1972, Cyclic AMP affects macrophage migration, Nature, New Biol., 238:176.

Pick, E., 1977, Lymphokines: physiologic control and pharmacologi-
    cal modulation of their production and action, in: "Immunophar-
    macology," vol. 3,   J.W. Hadden, R.G. Coffey, and F. Spreafico,
    eds., Plenum Publishing Corp., New York, p. 163.

Pick, E., Seger, M., Honig, S., and Griffel, B., 1979, Intracellu-
    lar mediation of lymphokine action: mimicry of migration inhi-
    bitory factor (MIF) action by phorbol myristate acetate (PMA)
    and the ionophore A23187, Ann. N.Y. Acad. Sci., 332:378.

Prieur, A.M., and Granger, G.A., 1975, The effects of agents
    which modulate levels of the cyclic nucleotides on human lym-
    photoxin secretion and activity in vitro, Transplantation,
    20:331.

Pryzwansky, K.B., Steiner, A.L., Spitznagel, J.K., and Kapoor,
    C.L., 1981, Compartmentalization of cyclic AMP during phagocy-
    tosis by human neutrophilic granulocytes, Science, 211:407.

Resch, K., 1976, Membrane associated events in lymphocyte activa-
    tion, in: "Receptors and Recognition Series A," vol. 1,   P.
    Cuatrecasas, and M.F., Greaves, eds., Chapman and Hall, Lon-
    don, p. 61.

Rhodes, J., 1975, Modulation of macrophage Fc receptor expression
    in vitro by insulin and cyclic nucleotides, Nature, 257:597.

Rocklin, R.E., 1977, Histamine-induced suppressor factor (HSF):
    effect on migration inhibitory factor (MIF) production and pro-
    liferation, J. Immunol., 118:1734.

Roder, J.C., and Klein, M., 1979, Target-effector interaction in
    the natural killer cell system. IV. Modulation by cyclic nucleo-
    tides, J. Immunol., 123:2785.

Rossi, F., Romeo, D., and Patriarca, P., 1972, Mechanism of phago-
    cytosis-associated oxidative metabolism in polkymorphonuclear
    leukocytes and macrophages, J. Reticuloendothel. Soc., 12:127.

Rouveix, B., Badenoch-Jones, P., Larno, S., and Turk, J.L., 1980,
    Lymphokine-induced macrophage aggregation: the possible role
    of cyclic nucleotides, Immunopharmacol., 2:319.

Rubin, M.S., Swislocki, N.I., and Sonnenberg, M., 1973, Alteration
    of liver plasma membrane protein conformation by bovin growth
    hormone in vitro, Arch. Biochem. Biophys., 157:243.

Scheid, M.P., Goldstein, G., and Boyse, E.A., 1978, The generation
    and regulation of lympohocyte populations, Evidence from diffe-
    rentiative induction systems in vitro, J. Exp. Med., 147:1727.

Scheid, M.P., Goldstein, G., Hammerling, U., and Boyse, E.A., 1975,
    Induction of T and B lymphocyte differentiation in vitro, in:
    "Membrane Receptors in Lymphocytes" M. Seligman, J.L., Preu-
    dhomme, and F.M., Kourelsky, eds., Elsevier Publishing Co.,

New York, p. 162.

Schreiner, G.F., and Unanue, E.R., 1975, The modulation of spontaneous and anti-Ig-stimulated motility of lymphocytes by cyclic
nucleotides and adrenergic and cholinergic agents, J. Immunol.,
114:802.

Schultz, R.M., Pavlidis, N.A., Stylos, W.A., and Chirigos, M.A.,
1978, Regulation of macrophage tumoricidal function: a role
for prostaglandins of the E series, Science, 202:320.

Schumm, D.E., Morris, H.P., and Webb, T.E., 1974, Early biochemical
changes in phytohemagglutinin-stimulated peripheral blood lymphocytes from normal and tumor-bearing rats, Eur. J. Cancer,
10:107.

Showell, H.J., Naccache, P., Sha'afi, R.I., Becker, E.L., 1980, Inhibition of rabbit neutrophil lysosomal enzyme secretion, non-
-stimulated and chemotactic factor stimulated locomotion by nor-
dihydroguaiaretic acid, Life Sci., 27:421.

Simochowitz, L., Fischbein, L.C., Spilberg, I., and Atkinson, J.P.,
1980, Induction of a transient elevation of intracellular levels of adenosine - 3', 5' -cyclic monophosphate by chemotactic factors: an early event in human neutrophil activation, J.
Immunol., 124:1482.

Smith, K.A., 1980, T-cell growth factor, Immunological Rev., 51:337.

Smith, R.J., and Ignarro, L.J., 1975, Bioregulation of lysosomal enzyme secretion from human neutrophils: roles of guanosine 3'
:5'-monophosphate and calcium in stimulus-secretion coupling,
Proc. Natl. Acad. Sci., USA, 72:108.

Smith, R.L., and Weidemann, M.J., 1980, Reactive oxygen production
associated with arachidonic acid metabolism by peritoneal macrophages, Biochem. Biophys. Res. Comm., 96:973.

Smith, R.L., Hunt, N.H., Merritt, J.E., Evants, T., and Weidemann,
M.J., 1980, Cyclic nucleotide metabolism and reactive oxygen
production by macrophages, Biochem. Biophys. Res. Comm.,
96:1079.

Smolen, J.E., and Weissmann, G., 1981, Stimuli which provoke secretion of azurophil enzymes from human neutrophils induce incre-
ments in adenosine cyclic 3'-5'-monophosphate, Biochem. Biophys. Acta, 672:197.

Snow, C.E., Feldbush, T.L., and Oaks, J.A., 1980, The role of insulin in the response of murine T lymphocytes to mitogenic stimulation in vitro, J. Immunol., 124:739.

Snow, C.E., Feldbush, T.L., and Oaks, J.A., 1981, The effect of
growth hormone and insulin upon MLC responses and the generation of cytotoxic lymphocytes, J. Immunol., 126:161.

Spach, C., and Aschkenasy, A., 1979, Effects of a protein-free diet on the changes in cyclic AMP and cyclic GMP levels induced by immunization in splenic T and B lymphocytes in the rat, J. Nutr., 109:1265.

Stenson, W.F., and Parker, C.W., 1979, Metabolism of arachidonic acid in ionophore-stimulated neutrophils, J. Clin. Invest., 64:1457.

Stenson, W.F., and Parker, C.W., 1980, Prostaglandins, macrophages, and immunity, J. Immunol., 125:1.

Stossel, T.P., Murad, F., Mason, R.J., and Vaughan, M., 1970, Regulation of glycogen metabolism in polymorphonuclear leukocytes, J. Biol. Chem., 245:6228.

Strom, T.B., and Carpenter, C.B., 1977, Regulation of alloimmunity by cyclic nucleotides, in: "Immunopharmacology," Vol. 3, J.W., Hadden, R.G., Coffey, and F., Spreafico, eds., Plenum Publishing Corp., New York, p. 47.

Strom, T.B., Lundin, A.P., III, and Carpenter, C.B., 1977, The role of cyclic nucleotides in lymphocyte activation and function, in: "Progress in Clinical Immunology," Vol. 3, R.S., Schwartz, ed., Grune and Stratton, New York, p. 115.

Sunshine, G.H., Basch, R.S., Coffey, R.G., Cohen, K.W., Goldstein, G., and Hadden, J.W., 1978, Thymopoietin enhances the allogeneic response and cyclic nucleotide levels of mouse peripheral, thymus derived lymphocytes, J. Immunol., 120:1594.

Taetle, R., and Koessler, A., 1980, Effects of cyclic nucleotides and prostaglandins on normal and abnormal human myeloid progenitor proliferation, Cancer Res., 40:1223.

Talal, N., Roubinian, J.R., Dauphinee, M.J., Jones, L.A., and Siiteri, P.K., 1981, Effects of sex hormones on spontaneous autoimmune disease in NZB/NZW hybrid mice, in: "Advances in Immunopharmacology," J.W., Hadden, L., Chedid, P., Mullen, and F., Spreafico, eds., Pergamon Press, Oxford, p. 127.

Tam, C.F. and Walford, R.L., 1978, Cyclic nucleotide levels in resting and mitogen-stimulated spleen cell suspensions from young and old mice, Mech. Age. Develop., 7:309.

Tam, C.F. and Walford, R.L., 1980, Alterations in cyclic nucleotides and cyclase-specific activities in T lymphocytes of ageing normal humans and patients with Down's syndrome, J. Immunol., 125:1665.

Teh, H.S. and Paetkau, 1976, Regulation of immune response. II. The cellular basis of cyclic AMP effects on humoral immunity., Cell. Immunol., 24:220.

Triglia, D. and Rothenberg, E., 1981, "Mature" thymocytes are not glucocorticoid - resistant in vitro, J. Immunol., 127:64.

Vassalli, J.D., Hamilton, J. and Reich, E., 1976, Macrophage plasminogen activator : induction by concanavalin A and phorbol myristate acetate, Cell, 11:695.

Wagshal, A.B., Jegasothy, B.V., and Waksman, B.H., 1978, Regulatory substances produced by lymphocytes. II. Cell cyclic specificity of inhibitor of DNA synthesis action in lymphocytes, J. Exp. Med., 147:171.

Wahl, S.M., and Wahl, L.M., 1979, Lymphokine modulation of connective tissue metabolism, Ann. N.Y. Acad. Sci., 332:411.

Wahl, S., Wahl, L., McCarthy, J., Chedid, L., and Mergenhagen, S., 1979, Macrophage activation by mycobacterial water soluble compounds and synthetic muramyl dipeptide, J. Immunol., 122:2226.

Waksman, B.H., Dessaint, J.-P., and Katz, S.P., 1980, Proteolysis, calcium, and cyclic nucleotides in macrophage T-lymphocyte interaction, in: "Biochemical Characterization of Lymphokines," A.L., deWeck, F., Krinstensen, and M., Landy, eds., Academic Press, New York, p. 435.

Wang, T., Sheppard, J.R., and Foker, J.E., 1978, Rise and fall of cyclic AMP required for onset of lymphocyte DNA synthesis, Science, 201:155.

Watson, J., 1977, Involvement of cyclic nucleotides as intracellular mediators in the induction of antibody synthesis, in: "Immunopharmacology," vol.3, J.W., Hadden, R.G., Coffey, and F., Spreafico, eds., Plenum Publishing Corp., New York, p. 29.

Webb, D.R., and Jamieson, A.T., 1976, Control of mitogen-induced transformation: characterization of a splenic suppressor cell. and its modes of action, Cell Immunol., 24:45.

Wedner, H.J., and Parker, C.W., 1976, Lymphocyte activation, Prog. in Allergy, 20:195.

Wedner, H.J., and Parker, C.W., 1977, Adenylate cyclase activity in lymphocyte subcellular fractions, Characterization of a nuclear adenylate cyclase, Biochem. J., 162:483.

Weissemann, G., Dukor, P., and Zurier, R.B., 1971, Effects of cyclic AMP on release of lysosomal enzymes from phagocytes, Nature, New Biol., 231:131.

Weissmann, G., Korchak, H.M., Perez, H.D., Smolen, J.E., Goldstein, I.M., and Hoffstein, S.T., 1979, The secretory code of the neutrophil, J. Reticuloendothel. Soc., 26 (Supp.):687.

Weissmann, G., Smolen, J., and Korchak, H., 1980, Release of inflammatory mediatory from stimulant neutrophils, New Engl. J. Med., 303:27.

Welscher, H.D., and Cruchaud, A., 1976, The influence of various particles and 3', 5' cyclic adenosine monophosphate on release of lysosomal enzymes by mouse macrophages, <u>J. Reticuloendothel. Soc.</u>, 20:405.

Welscher, H.D., and Cruchaud, A., 1978, Conditions for maximal synthesis of cyclic AMP by mouse macrophages in response to adrenergic stimulation, <u>Eur. J. Immunol.</u>, 8:180.

Whitfield, J.F., 1980, The regulation of cell proliferation by calcium and cyclic AMP, <u>Mol. Cell. Biochem.</u>, 27:155.

Whitfield, J.F., MacManus, J.P., Rixon, R.H., Boynton, A.L., Yondale, T., and Sweirenga, S., 1976, Positive control of cell proliferation by interplay of calcium and cyclic nucleotides, <u>In Vitro</u>, 12:1.

ANATOMICAL AND PHYSIOLOGICAL CONNECTIONS BETWEEN THE CENTRAL NERVOUS AND THE IMMUNE SYSTEMS (NEUROIMMUNOMODULATION)

Novera Herbert Spector

The Neurosciences Program, School of Medecine
University of Alabama in Birmingham, Birmingham
Alabama 35295, U.S.A.

1. A HISTORICAL NOTE

Long ago, "Physiology" included embryology, immunology, neurobiology, cell biology, biophysics, biochemistry, molecular biology, and many other subjects. Today, at a World Congress of Physiology, one can find few papers on immunology: anatomy is even more remote. Specialization and specialists have separated each of these into separate disciplines and even many sub-disciplines.
However, biological entities such as the human organism fail to recognize these artificial divisions, and the best of the specialists in each separate science are being forced to the conclusion that one cannot understand whole-animal functions, or even limited-area stimuli-response mechanisms, without a more integrative approach. To describe the influence of the central nervous system upon immune responses of the entire body, I proposed the term "neuroimmunomodulation" (NIM). We cannot yet rule out neuroimmunogenesis, but the evidence for NIM is overwhelming (Spector 1979, 1980; Spector, and Korneva, 1981).
The earliest experiment that I am aware of in this field was recorded in 1911 (Luk'yanenko, 1961), but anecdotal evidence goes back to ancient times. Nonetheless, until the past few years, neither physiology societies, nor immunology societies, nor neurobiology societies had any regular place in their programs for reports of these experiments. In 1974, at a satellite meeting of

231

the International Union of Physiological Sciences (IUPS), held in
Teheran, entitled "Recent Advances in Physiology", I was asked, at
the last minute, to present a review of NIM. At the IUPS Congress
in Paris in 1977, the first, informal (non-program) meeting on NIM
was convened by this author, and an ad hoc "club" was established,
with 12 charter members, from several countries. This list of
names has now grown to over 200. The first formal recognition by
the IUPS of this critical area of research came at the 1980
Congress in Budapest where a formal symposium on NIM was included
in the program.
Brief reports from this meeting were gathered for a small book,
now in preparation for press.
The (North American) Society for Neuroscience, for the first time
ever, at its 1981 annual meeting, will include a single session
for contributed papers on NIM. Finally, this International Workshop, thanks to Prof. Nicola Fabris and his colleagues, esta-
blishes an historic landmark by including several sessions on NIM,
the first formal recognition by the international community of immunologists, that NIM cannot be ignored, if we are to understand
even the simplest phenomena of immune reactions by any whole
organism.

2. ANATOMICAL CONNECTIONS

    It has been known for more than a century that there are
nerve endings in the various organs and tissues that now are known
to comprise the immune system. However, even today, when one asks
the anatomist or histologist," what are the afferent and efferent
functions of these nerves?", the usual response is a blank stare
or a shrug of the shoulders. Only recently have a small number of
investigators concerned themselves with this problem. In addition,
a few have begun to look at the central connections of these
nerves, and at their embryological origins. I will not attempt
here to present a comprehensive review of these studies, but will
emphasize a few of the recent developments.

2.1. Thymus

    Crotti (1918), Hammar (1935), Sergeeva (1974) and Gordon et
al. (1979), among others, described the autonomic innervation of
the thymus. In addition to the vagus, the phrenic nerve, inferior

laryngeal nerve and the descendens cervicales (ansa hypoglossi) all may contribute fibers. Hammar assumed that vagal innervation is essential for the initiation of thymic development. On the other hand, it has been suggested that the thymus is involved in "normal differentiation of the brain", especially in its endocrine systems (Pierpaoli and Besedovsky, 1975; for further references, see Bulloch and Moore, 1981). Sorkin, Pierpaoli, Besedovsky and Fabris, among others present at this symposium, have emphasized the neuroendocrine connections between thymus and central nervous systems. Chemical and physical sympathectomies of the thymus have yielded profound effects upon various aspects of antigen-antibody responses (e.g. Thoenen and Tranzer, 1968; Besedovsky et al., 1979; Miles et al., 1981; Williams et al., 1981).

These functional aspects of the anatomical connections give strong evidence that there is much more involved in nerve supply to the thymus (as well as to bone marrow, spleen, lymph nodes, etc.) than mere control of vascular tone, although control of the smooth muscles in the blood vessel walls and elsewhere undoubtedly also can indirectly affect overall immune responses. Both adrenergic and cholinergic terminals are present: both types of transmitters affect immunologic responses (Bulloch, 1981).

An elaborate series of investigations by Bulloch and her colleagues has given a clearer picture, not only of the innervation of thymus, in various "normal" and "abnormal" strains of rats and mice, but also of the central nervous system connections, their ontogeny, and their function (Bulloch, 1981; Bulloch and Moore, 1980; Bulloch and Moore, 1981).
Using horseradish peroxidase to label neuronal connections, thymus innervation was traced back to specific neuron perikarya in both the ventral horn of spinal cord and in several specific nuclei of the medulla, most particularly the retrofacial nucleus, and including also the nucleus ambiguous. In the thymus itself, histochemistry revealed nerve endings not only along blood vessels, but also in the parenchyma of the cortex and medulla.
"Staggerer" mice, known to be deficient in certain immune responses, showed aberrant distribution of catecholaminergic nerve endings, again suggesting a functional-anatomical link between the nervous and immune (and, of course, the endocrine) systems.

In studies on human pre- and post-natal thymus, Ghali et al. (1980) found neural connections at 11 weeks of fetal development:

at 20 weeks, nerves were found in the parenchyma of both cortex and medulla, which persist in the post-natal period in individuals at least 15 years. The innervation of the human thymus is not too different from that of rodents (see also, for similar findings: Solov'ev, 1966). Some observations on "accidental" versus "normal" involution led Ghali and his colleagues to an interesting conclusion consistent with our general picture of neuroimmunomodulation. A 2-month old boy who died of pneumonia had an involuted thymus, with nerves restricted to the capsule and some trabeculae. In a 25-year old with "normal" involution, there were again no nerves remaining in the sub-capsular zone. Based on these and other observations Ghali et al., concluded that "involution of the gland, whether physiological or secondary to severe illness, was accompanied by the absence of nerves which indicates that in order to function the gland must be innervated".

Another question is brought to mind which is not asked by Ghali et al., perhaps because their study could not yet give the answer: did the 2-month old boy die of pneumonia because his thymus lacked innervation, or was deinnervation and involution "secondary" (as assumed in the paper) to the pneumonia?

2.2. Bone Marrow

Despite the fact that neural supply to bones was described in 1700 (du Verney) and although there is currently good physiological evidence that brain lesions or brain stimulation can affect bone marrow function (e.g., Baciu, 1962; Hall et al., 1978), it was possible, only recently, for some competent anatomists-physiologists to state that "...convincing evidence is lacking for the direct innervation of parenchyma cells",(Webber et al., 1970). (Their own experiments demonstrated that stimulation of lumbar sympathetic nerves in rats resulted in an outflow of reticulocytes from bone into the blood stream).

Yet, Kuntz and Richins (1945) and Calvo (1968) had already demonstrated that "the necessary anatomical conditions exist permitting a direct influence of the nervous system on the function of the bone marrow", including direct innervation of the parenchyma. Based on studies of mice, rats, rabbits and monkeys, Calvo showed the distribution of both myelinated and unmyelinated fibers within the periosteum and the marrow of femur, tibia and

humerus, including in all cases, the parenchyma and the endothelium of the sinuses. A schematic representation of the various
elements of bone marrow neural supply are shown in Figure 1.

The extensive studies of Calvo and his colleagues continue to
the present day (Calvo, 1981) and continue to lay a solid ground
work in embryology and anatomy for the physiological analysis of
NIM.

Afferent pathways from bone to brain also have been described
(e.g., Orlov et al., 1978 a,b).

2.3. Bursa of Fabricius

Innervation of most organs and tissues may serve at least two
needs: 1) it usually is needed for normal differentiation and
growth, and 2) for normal functioning, in the integration of the
organ's functions with the rest of the body.

Based on experiments with ectopic autologous implants of the
bursa of Fabricius, Thompson and Cooper (1971) suggested that

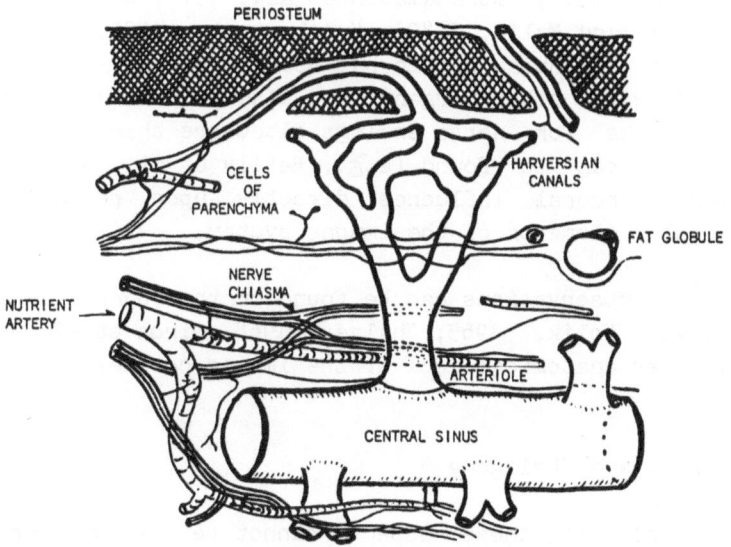

Fig. 1. Schematic representation of the various elements of bone
marrow neural supply (from Calvo, 1978).

"alterations in innervation" could be partially responsible for
the transplanted bursas' failure to develop normally and to continue lymphopoiesis. They also transplanted these bursae, but left
the vascular and neural connections intact, and then, afterwards,
cut them. Finding an unchanged histological appearance and lymphoid cells in various stages of maturation, they concluded that an
intact nerve supply is not necessary for "normal lymphopoiesis".

Without attempting to discuss why the results of these two
experiments were different, we may simply ask: how will the
lymphocytes function upon maturity? Is early innervation required
for later adequate immunocompetence? Perhaps further experiments
are needed to answer this critical question.

2.4. Other Organs and Tissues

There is a growing literature on the innervation, both sympathetic and parasympathetic, of the spleen. In recent years there
has been more attention to the functional, developmental, and
comparative anatomy of these conditions (e.g. Von Euler, 1967;
Livett et al., 1968; Gersbach, 1970; Klein and Lagercrantz, 1971;
Baumgarten et al., 1972; Thureson-Klein et al., 1979; Nahorski et
al., 1979; Blaschke and Uvnas, 1979; Dixon et al., 1979; Sharma
and Banerjee, 1979; Abrahamsson et al., 1979; Besedovsky et al.,
1979, Hidaka and Malik, 1980). Kudoh et al. (1979) clearly demonstrated that the human spleen has both adrenergic and cholinergic
supply. As with other organs and tissues of the immune system,
when one looks for nerve endings elsewhere than in the vascular
system, they can be found (e.g., Reilly et al., 1976), strongly
suggesting a neural influence directly upon reticulocytes and
other cellular elements of the immune system.

Similar observations can be found on the innervation of lymph
nodes (e.g., Volik, 1965; Shalvev, 1968, Giron et al., 1980), and
the many other anatomical loci of the immune complex.

2.5. Ontogeny and Phylogeny

While all of these aspects cannot be reviewed here, it may
confidently be expected, as in other areas of anatomy, that when
we are aware of the historical development of a system or systems,

both in the individual and in the species, that we will understand
better the function. Much of this work will be in the future, but
already, as mentioned above, observations of the embryological
origins, coupled with the relative timing of their respective
functional maturations, give us clues to the interrelationships of
these systems.

3. PHYSIOLOGICAL CONNECTIONS

3.1. Effects of Neural Lesions and Stimulation

Peripheral nerve sectioning as well as central lesions,
especially in the hypothalamus, but also in many other brain
areas, have resulted in both increases and decreases in peripheral
circulating antibodies in response to specific antigens. Lesions
in specific loci in the hypothalamus (which loci may depend on the
species, the conditions of the experiment or the laboratory in
which the experiment is done) or in other regions of the brainstem
may protect an animal against lethal anaphylaxis (for reviews, see
Spector, 1980; Stein et al., 1981).

Recent studies have shown that such lesions (including chemical sympathectomies) also may have profound effects on cell
counts in bone marrow, changes in lymphoid cells in thymus and
spleen, and ability of these cells to divide and to function in
various immunological capacities (e.g., Hall et al., 1978, 1979;
Besedovsky et al., 1979, Cross et al., 1980; Roszman et al., 1981;
Warejka and Levy, 1980; Brooks et al., 1981; Miles et al., 1981).

On the other hand stimulation of peripheral nerves or of the
brain; mechanical (Schulhof and Mathies, 1927), electrical (Psegalinski, 1944; Benetato, 1955; Korneva and Khai, 1967; Webber et
al., 1970) or antigenic (Baciu, 1946), will also have effects upon
peripheral immune responses. In at least one experiment, the
effect upon circulating antibodies was opposite to that of a
lesion in the same area (Korneva and Khai, 1967).

An early and most ingenious experiment was that of Baciu
(1946), using his "isolated head" preparation. In the experimental dog, the only direct neural or vascular connection with the
rest of its body was the spinal cord and presumably the parasym-
pathetics; the blood circulation was maintained by cross-perfusion

Table 1. Summary of neuroendocrines which may be involved in immune functions. Each of the four categories are controlled by the brain and directly or indirectly may provide feedback information to the brain. Based on MacLean and Reichlin (1981). This list is growing by leaps and bounds!

PITUITARY	AUTONOMIC NERVOUS SYSTEM	SENSORY GANGLIA	BRAIN SECRETION
FSH LH - Gonadal Steroids	Acetylcholine	Substance P	Pineal (Melatonin, others)
TSH - Thyroid Hormones	Norepinephrine	Somatostatin	Somatostatin
ACTH	Serotonin	VIP	Fibroblast Growth Factor
Adrenal Cortical Hormones	Somatostatin		Neurotensin
Vasopressin	VIP		Bombesin
Oxytocin	Enkephalins		CCK
Neurophysin	Substance P		Enkephalins
Beta-Lipotropin	Cholecystokinin		
Beta-Endorphin			
Fibroblast Growth Factor			
Thymocyte Growth Factor			
Endothelial Growth Factor			

with a second animal. When typhus bacilli were injected into the brain, peripheral phagocytosis in the same animal was increased. Later, Benetato et al. (1949) reported that the rate of phagocytosis could be increased also by electrical stimulation of the hypothalamus.

3.2. Neuroendocrine Relation

In this symposium, it is hardly necessary to belabor the neuro-endocrine-immune interrelationships. Yet it is still possible for some immunologists to deny the influence of the nervous system (Spector, 1980). Well known to immunologists are the manifold effects of steroids on many immune reactions: perhaps not equally realized are the feedback loops via the vascular system, the dorsomedial and other nuclei in the hypothalamus, median eminence, pituitary and finally the adrenals, gonads and other endocrine-producing tissues. Many other neuroendocrines are involved in immune processes: these are amply treated in this volume and well reviewed by Jankovic and Isakovic (1973), Besedovsky and Sorkin (1981), Hall (1981), Hall and Goldstein (1981), Cohen and Vrnic (1981) and MacLean and Reichlin (1981).

This field is expanding so rapidly that even these latest reviews cannot list all of the recent developments, some of which are important for an understanding of NIM. Table 1, from MacLean and Reichlin, lists some of the neuroendocrines which may modulate immune responses. To these may be added other neurally active polypeptides, the number of which seems to expand almost exponentially each year (Iversen et al., 1978; Guillemin, 1977, 1978) as well as purine nucleotides which also are probably neurotransmitters (Burnstock, 1972, 1979). An interesting sidelight of all of this is that in many extensive reviews and symposia on functions of neuropeptides, neurotransmitters and neuromodulators, even within the past few years (e.g., Liebeskind et al., 1978; Burnstock and Hokfelt, 1979; and many others) no mention is made of their possible roles in immune reactions!

MacLean and Reichlin, in their comprehensive review, state that "that effects of melatonin on the immune process are unknown" and further, that the "physiological role" of beta-enkephalin is unknown, although they suggest that both of these substances may play a role in immunity. However, even as their review goes to

press, there already is evidence that these substances are involved. Pierpaoli and Maestroni (1980) found that immunodeficient
nude mice could regain their ability to reject allogeneic skin
grafts by thymocyte-transfer coupled with injections of melatonin.
This treatment was effective only when melatonin inoculation was
done in the evening. Gilman et al. (1981) found that beta-endor-
phin enhanced the proliferative response of spleen cells, in
vitro, to concanavalin A.

3.3. Receptors on Cellular Elements

In 1970, Hadden et al. reported the presence of adrenergic
receptors on human lymphocytes. Since then, wherever one has
looked, one has found evidence of receptors on the various cells
of the immune system for acetylcholine and many other putative
neurotransmitters, histamines (Roszkowski et al, 1977), and other
neurally-active polypetides and neuromodulators. Some of the
functional consequences of these connections have been briefly
reviewed by Hall (1981). While most of the implications are far
from being explored experimentally, these findings serve further
to suggest the direct influences of the nervous system upon immune
responses at the cellular and "molecular" levels.

3.4. Feedback Loops

In medical schools and in many research laboratories, the
study of complex, multicellular living organisms is divided arbi-
trarily according to "disciplines". Textbooks are written about
"Physiology", "Anatomy", "Endocrinology", "Immunology" and so on.
Review articles are further sub-specialized, and finally,in most
research labs, tunnel vision becomes narrower and narrower.
While all of these divisions and sub-divisions may have heuristic
value, when it comes to understanding the whole organism, they are
counterproductive. The living organism does not function according
to medical school departments, but rather as an integrated whole.
Part of this integration can be studied by looking at feedback
loops: i.e., how does the brain respond to changes in endocrine or
antibody or antigen levels in the periphery?... how do endocrine
and immune organs respond to changes in the brain?....and so on.

It has been known for many years, and will not be reviewed here, that most endocrine systems have negative feedback loops, especially via the hypothalamus, median eminence and pituitary. Information is transmitted in part via the vascular system and also directly ("hard-wired") by nerve fibers, for example, from paraventricular and supraoptic nuclei to the pars nervosa of the pituitary; or via the spinal cord to the adrenals.

Little is known about the hard-wired afferent limbs of the loop. However, single neuron electrical recordings from specific brain areas reveal changes in firing rates as well as in firing patterns in response to changes in peripheral circulating levels of steroids (Ruf and Steiner, 1967) or of antigens and antibodies (Klimenko, 1972; Korneva and Klimenko, 1976; Besedovsky et al., 1977; Spector and Korneva, 1981). Exactly how and by what pathways these neurons in the brain receive and transduce and interpret these signals from the blood is still unknown.

Single neurons, in many loci in the central nervous system, most especially in the medial preoptic nuclei and anterior hypo-thalamus respond by complex changes in firing rates and patterns, to changes in deep body temperature (Nakayama et al., 1961) to local brain temperature and in some cases to both (Wit and Wang, 1967). Some neurons in the same area are exquisitely sensitive to endogenous or exogenous pyrogens (Cooper et al., 1966).
Efferent signals from these neurons may trigger many physiological and behavioral mechanisms that raise or lower whole body tempe-rature (Kahn, 1904; Fusco, 1959; Hammel et al., 1960; Bligh, 1966; Spector et al., 1969; Spector, 1969). Of course local and whole body temperature changes play a role, not only in affecting the rate of any biochemical reaction, but more specifically, in any immune reaction.

The simplest known reflex, the "axon reflex" or "flare" response, involving only one neuron, can account for a local inflammatory response, possibly due to the release of ATP, and/or "substance P" and/or histamine and/or bradykinin. In this case the efferent feedback travels in the same neuronal fiber that trans-mits the afferent signal. The degree of complexity in other NIM loops is far greater but still susceptible to experimental analy-sis and eventual understanding.

3.5. Chronological Factors

The nervous system, the immune system and the endocrine system are all subject to a variety of rhythms, of varying periods: the evolutionary cycle, the lifetime cycle (embryo, development, aging, death), lunar circadian and ultradian cycles. Not to be constantly aware of these and their complex inter--relationships is perilous for the investigator as well as for the unwitting victim of the careless clinical pratictioner.
A drug given at one time of day may cure, at another time, kill (e.g. Halberg, 1976). Much of the confusion in the basic literature stems from a carelessness in controlling for temporal factors. For example, norepinephrine can have opposite effects on feeding behavior and temperature regulation when administered in the day or in the night; it will also have different effects at the same time of day depending on the species used: the rodent is nocturnally active; many primates are the opposite.

With respect to NIM, I have cited above the fascinating finding of Pierpaoli and Maestroni (1980) that melatonin may have an entirely different effect on an immune reaction when given in the morning or in the evening.

It is well known that corticosteroids, growth hormone, sex hormones, and other endocrines under neural control will vary in their blood concentrations according to lunar, circadian and ultradian rhythms. Since all of these are known to affect immune reaction, it should not be surprising that many immune elements are subject to the same cycles. Bartter and Delea (1962) reviewed some of these (circadian) rhythms in terms of numbers of lymphocytes in circulation. Other circadian factors in allograft rejections, antibody formation and so on are reviewed by Abo et al. (1980) as well as by other authors in the same volume (Smolensky et al., 1980). As with feeding and temperature responses, Abo and his colleagues point out that circadian immunological rhythms in mouse and man are out of phase.

Feedback loops governing cyclicity in immune responses will probably be found to include in their circuits, the pineal gland, the superchiasmatic nucleus of the hypothalamus, the pituitary and other, secondary, way-stations in the nervous and endocrine systems.

4. PSYCHONEUROIMMUNOLOGY

In what may be called, loosely, psychological influences upon the immune system, we can find the most voluminous, the most ancient and yet still the most tenous evidence for neuroimmunomodulation. A large part of this body of knowledge is being brought up to date with the publication this year of a compilation of reviews entitled "Psychoneuroimmunology" (Ader, 1981). Several chapters, by leading investigators in this field, deal with such difficult, almost undefinable, factors such as "stress", "emotions", "conditioning" and so on. Because these subjects are so complex and difficult, many choose to ignore thm; however that makes them not less real, only more challenging.

4.1. Stress

Walter B. Cannon, more than 50 years ago defined "stress" by implication, in physiological terms, by referring to the catecholamine response of the adrenal medulla to fright, fight and flight situations. Later, Hans Selye (1936) redefined stress in terms of the response of the adrenal cortex and changes in corticosteroid levels. Other hormones, such as prolactin and growth hormone, have been shown to rase in blood following exposure to assorted stressors. John Mason (1975) looked for an entire spectrum of endocrine responses in response to stressful situations in primates, including humans. Several of these hormones have known effects on immune responses.

Grief and other "stressful" situations, in humans has been reported to significantly increase susceptibility to cancer, to lower lymphocyte cytotoxicity, natural killer cell activity, to change immunoglobulin levels and to depress other aspects of immune competence. Isolation or crowding in mice increases their susceptibility to cancer. Rotation, loud noises, electric shock and many other stressors lead to changes in immune functions in interferon levels, and susceptibility to many diseases, in experimental animals.

What do we mean by "stress"? Each investigator has a different definition. Many reviews have been written on this subject (e.g., Selye, 1936, 1946, 1950, 1975; Solomon and Moos, 1964; Amkraut and Solomon, 1974; Mason, 1975; Palmblad et al., 1976; Palmblad,

1981; Monjan and Collector, 1977; Fox, 1978; Monjan, 1981; Fox, 1981; Riley, 1981; Riley et al., 1981; Cohen and Crnic, 1981), and several journals are devoted largely to this subject (J. Psychosomatic Res.; Psychosomatic Medicine; J. Human Stress; etc. etc.). I will not attempt to cover this vast topic here, except to state that any change in an animal's environment, external or internal, may be considered a stressor: brain, endocrine organs, and the immune system all will respond. The anatomy and physiology of these responses must be analyzed in detail if we are to (a) understand the basic mechanisms, and (b) use this understanding both in clinic and in preventive medicine.

4.2. Environmental Factors and Interferon Production

Among changes in an animal's environment that may be considered stressors, I have mentioned sound levels, which may affect susceptibility to viral or virus-related diseases (e.g. Jensen and Rasmussen, 1963a,b, 1970; Monjan and Collector, 1977; Monjan, 1981) and isolation or crowding (Riley, 1975, 1981; Riley et al., 1981). Rasmussen et al. (1957) found an increased susceptibility to herpes simplex virus in mice following restraint. Placing a mouse in a small restraining box creates, for the animal, a drastic environmental change, one that is likely to raise corticosterone and prolactin levels. Various stressors in different species have been reported to raise or lower interferon (IFN) production. How does restraint affect IFN production, in the presence of a viral infection?

In a pilot experiment, we (Spector et al., 1981) compared the effects of repeated daily injections of polyinosinic-polycytidylic acid ("Poly I:C", a synthetic polyribonucleotide that induces the production of IFN, but which raises little or no antibody) in groups of female mice subjected to different environmental conditions. In addition to four control groups, there were three experimental groups: a) ten animals that were placed in plastic restraining boxes each day from 9.00 to 11:00 h., for 10 successive days; b) 10 animals that were placed in cages with chocolate-chip cookies and saccharin-sweetened water for the same time periods; and c) 5 animals that were kept in their home cages. Each animal in these 3 groups was injected, i.p., daily with $20\,\mu g$ of Poly I:C at 10 h. Control groups had: restraint only; or sweets only; or saline inoculation only; or handling only. On day 1, day 5, and

day 10, at 16 h (6 hr post-inoculation) each animal was bled and
0.1 ml of serum was collected,frozen and sent to Galveston, Texas,
where J. Sabados, in S. Baron's lab, assayed all samples for IFN
activity.

On day 1, almost all animals that were innoculated with Poly
I:C showed an IFN level higher than 200 units, but by day 10, the
Poly I:C-only and sweets groups had IFN levels close to baseline
(lower than 30 units), while the restraint group had a mean level
of 295 units, a 10-fold difference (P<.05). The mean IFN level of
the chocolate-chip group was significantly lower on the 10th day
than on the first or fifth (P<.01),, while the restraint group was
not significantly different (P>.05) on day 10 from day 1. All of
the control groups (saline only or no innoculation) had IFN levels
lower than 30 (= baseline).

These experiments are now being repeated, using larger
numbers. Spleen, adrenals and thymus weights are being measured,
and peripheral blood monitored for thymosine α_1 and corticosterone
levels (with N. Hall and A. Goldstein) and other indices of
immunocompetence. Meanwhile, these preliminary data indicate that
an environmental change such as restraint can alter the mouse's
IFN response to a viral (or at least a pseudo-viral) challenge,
suggesting again the influence of neural and neuroendocrine
factors.

4.3. Conditioning

In the 1920's at the Pasteur Institute in Paris, Metalnikov
(1934) and his colleagues began a series of experiments that have
been repeated and extended in a multitude of variations by a fair
number of investigators in many countries, with many species, and
with varying results. Simply put, Metalnikov (1934) reported that
by using "classical" (Pavlovian) conditioning techniques, an
immune response could be generated by a "conditioned" stimulus
alone, that is, in the absence of an antigen. Today, a very
limited number of investigators have begun again to investigate
these phenomena, encouraged once more by the recent experiments of
Ader and Cohen, reported in part at this symposium. Despite the
many failures reported, it is my opinion that the evidence is now
overwhelming that conditioning can modify immune responses,
including both decreases and increases in resistance to many

diseases, antibody levels, phagocytosis, and many other indices of
immune competence. The most comprehensive, if not the latest,
review of this subject was written by Luk'yanenko (1961). Other
good reviews can be found in Dolin and Dolina (1972), Spector
(1980) and Ader (1981b). Ader does an excellent job of reevalua-
ting some of the data from several of the old and still controversial experiments.

In my laboratory, we are looking for evidence for a conditioning effect upon interferon production. In pilot experiments,
the evidence is so far equivocal, but much more needs to be done to
explore and to explain these phenomena.

4.4. Hypnosis

After more than a century of research in hypnosis and a very
large number of published reports, there is still a great deal of
confusion as to a) what hypnosis does to the brain and to the rest
of the body, and b) how much influence hypnosis can have upon
either immune responses or the disease process. However, there are
certain observations that are easily reproducible: a flare on the
skin can be produced or reduced by hypnosis; allergic responses
can be increased or decreased; many physiological changes can be
produced which have, in turn, known effects upon immunity,
"resistance", and disease. It would be difficult to explain away
these results in any other fashion than to ascribe them to neuro-

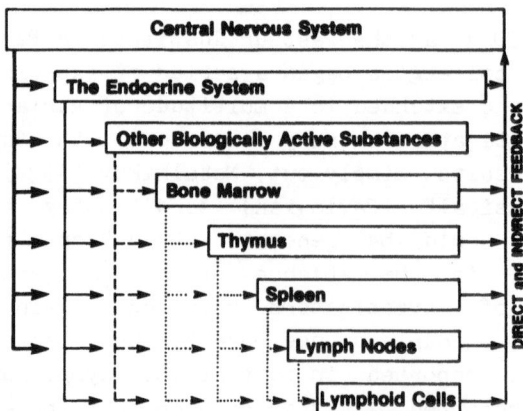

Fig. 2. Neuroimmunomodulation interactions.

immunomodulation (for an interesting footnote on hypnosis and immunity, by a very respectable immunologist, see Good, 1981).

4.5. Witchcraft

I have described elsewhere (Spector, 1980) the legion of anecdotal and circumstantial evidence for NIM, including folklore, shamanism, tales of old wives and/or professors of medicine and psychiatry. A recent example of neuromodulation of a host of somatic illnesses, perhaps better documented than most, appears in, of all places, the Journal of the American Medical Association (Kirkpatrick, 1981). The author describes a severe case of advanced lupus erythematosus, with glomerulonephritis and immune complex disease in a 28 year old woman, very resistant to all conventional medical treatment. Perhaps in desperation, she returned to her native village in the Phillipines, where she was treated for less

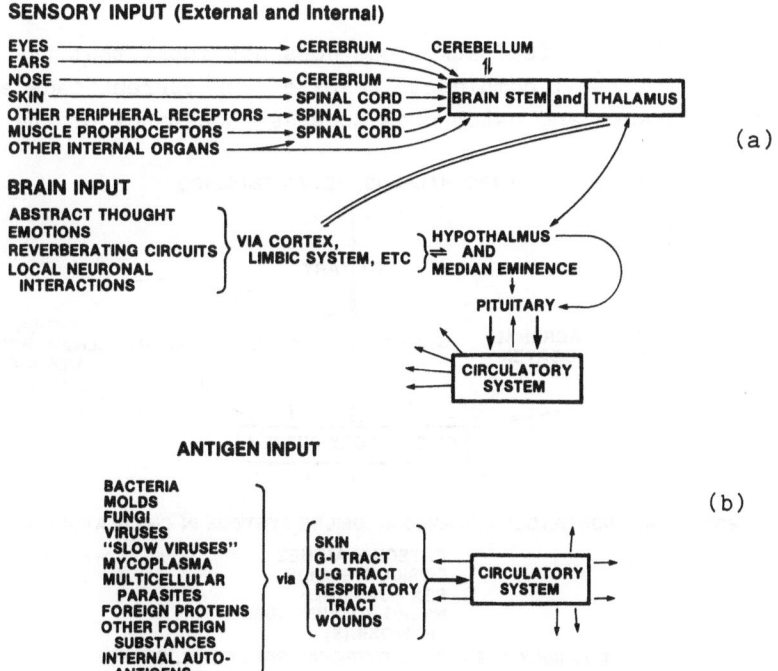

Fig. 3. External and internal inputs to the immune system can be classified under sensory, brain and antigen inputs.

than 3 weeks by a witchdoctor. Upon her return USA, she was "normal".

"...by what mechanisms," asks the physician, "did the machinations of Asian medicine man cure active lupus nephritis, change myxedema into euthyroidism, and allow precipitous with drawal from corticosteroid treatment without symptoms of adrenal insufficiency?" The answers to these perfectly reasonable questions are not yet available, but the type of research needed to provide them is clear.

5. SUMMARY

Figure 2, redrawn from Korneva et al. (1978; also in Spector and Korneva, 1981) diagrams neatly the cascading influences of the central nervous system (CNS) upon the various organs, tissues and cells of the immune system. To the original diagram, should be added, to complete the many anatomic and physiologic loops, the pathways back to the CNS (Figure 2).

A series of feedback loops does not imply that the system is self-sustaining and complete. Despite our current fads and liking for catchphrases and catchwords such as "constancy of the internal

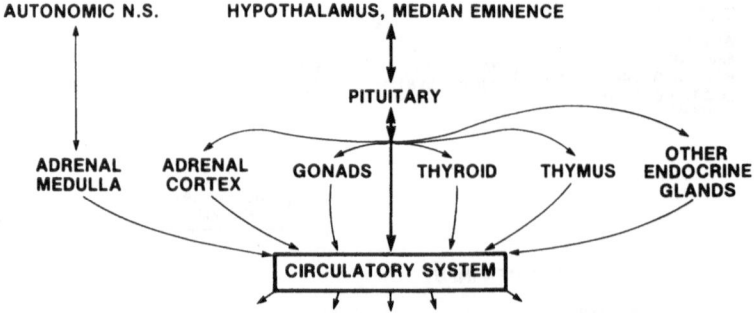

Fig. 4. Endocrine relays in the interactions between the central nervous and the immune systems.

miliéu" and "homeostasis," no biological system is ever constant, or in a state of equilibrium (Spector, 1980). Rhythmic changes, with varying time periods, not always synchronous for all biological factors (e.g., hormone levels, neuronal firing patterns) continually change the internal milieu. External and internal inputs to the system constantly stimulate it into activity. These can be classified roughly as in Figures 3 a and b, under sensory input, and antigen input. All of these interact via neural and vascular pathways at extracellular and intracellular sites as outlined in Figures 4 and 5. If we leave out some of the details shown in Figures 3 through 5, a rough outline of the whole system, which encompasses the 3 subsystems (nervous, endocrine and immune) can be seen as the complicated diagram in Figure 6. Of course the reality is more complex than our cartoons,but these help us to visualize, to ask questions and do the necessary experiments, which will enable us to draw better, more accurate diagrams, and eventually come closer to understanding the reality of the anatomic and physiologic connections between the CNS and the immune systems.

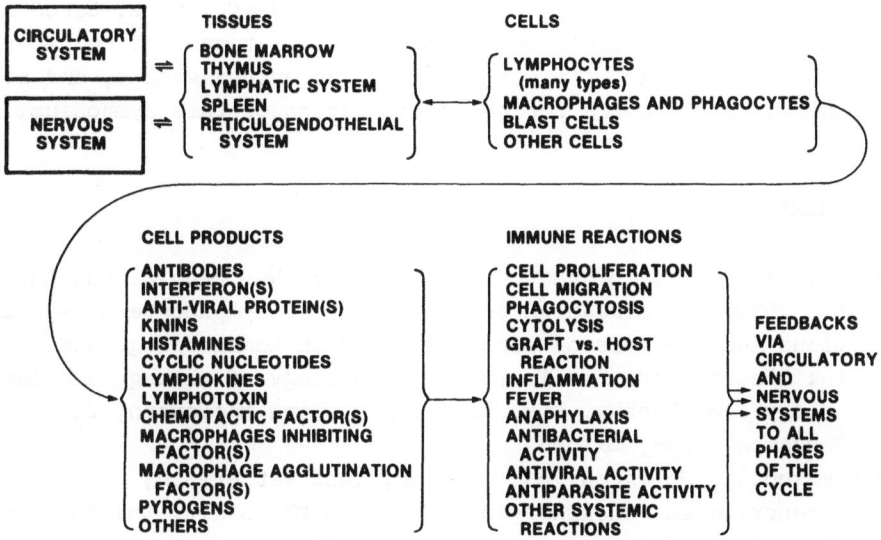

Fig. 5. Neural and vascular pathways of interactions between the central nervous and the immune system: organs and tissues of the immune system recruited in the interactions.

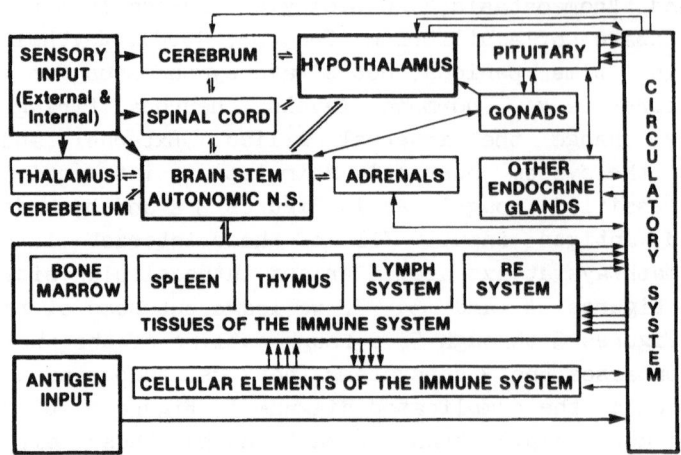

Fig. 6. Schematic representation of the interactions between the
central nervous and immune systems.

ACKNOWLEDGEMENTS

       Thanks   are   due   to   D.   Thompson   and   B. Testasecca for their
cheerful typing and retypings of this manuscript; to D. Dwyer and
C. Gertz for their critical readings of the draft; to S. Baron and
J. Peterson and A. Schlosberg for their assistance and collaboration, to V. Pegram for his support and encouragement, and most
especially, to N. Fabris for the organization of this symposium.

REFERENCES

Abo, T., Kawate, T., Hinuma, S., Itoh,K.Abo, W., Sato,J. and Kumagai,
      K., 1980, The circadian periodicities of lymphocyte sub-popula-
      tions and the role of corticosteroid in human beings and mice,
      in: "Recent advances in the chronobiology of allergy and immu-
      nology", Smolenzky, M.H, Reinberg A., and MecGovern, J.P.,
      Pergamon Press, Oxford.
Abrahamsson,T., Holmgren, S., Nilsson,S.and Pettersson, K., 1979,
      Adrenergic and cholinergic effects on the heart, the lung and
      the spleen of the African lungfish, Protopterus aethiopicus.
      Acta Physiol. Scand., 107(2):141.
Ader, R., ed., 1981a, Psychoneuroimmunology, Academic Press, N.Y.
Ader, R., 1981b, A historical account of conditioned immunobiologic

responses, in: "Psychoneuroimmunology", R. Ader, ed., Academic Press, N.Y., p. 321.

Amkraut, A. and Solomon, G.F., 1974, From the symbolic stimulus to the pathophysiologic response: immune mechanisms, Int. J. Psychiatry Med., 5(4):542.

Baciu, I., 1946, The role of the central nervous system in the inducement of the phagocytic reaction, doctoral dissertation, Inst. of Physiol. and Med. Physics, Univ. of Cluj (Romanian: English translation available).

Baciu, I., 1962, La régulation nerveuse et humorale de l'erythro-poièse, J. Physiol., (Paris), 54:441.

Bartter, F.C. and Delea, C.S., 1962, A map of blood and urinary changes related to circadian variations in adrenal cortical function in normal subjects, Ann. N. Y. Acad. Sci., 98:969.

Baumgarten, H.G., Gothert, M., Holstein, A.F. and Schlossberger, H.G., 1972, Chemical sympathectomy induced by 5,6-dihydroxy-tryptamine, Z. Zellforsch. Mikrosk. Anat., 128(1):115.

Benetato, G., 1955, Sur le mécanisme nerveux central de la réaction leucocytaire et phagocytaire. J. Physiol., (Paris) 47:39.

Benetato, G., Oprisiu, C. and Baciu, I., 1949, Sur le role du système nerveux central dans le déclenchement de la réaction phagocy-taire, Recuil d'etudes medicales, Ed. Inst. de Cultura Univer-sala, Bucharest.

Besedovsky, H.O. and Sorkin, E., 1981, Immunologic-neuroendocrine circuits: physiological approaches. in: "Psychoneuroimmunology", R. Ader, ed., Academic Press, N.Y., p.

Besedovsky, H., Sorkin, E., Felix, D. and Haas, H., 1977, Hypotha-lamic changes during the immune response, Eur.J. Immunol., 7(5):323.

Besedovsky, H.O., del Rey, A., Sorkin, E., DaPrada, M. and Keller, H.H., 1979, Immunoregulation mediated by the sympathetic ner-vous system, Cell. Immunol., 48:346.

Blaschke, E. and Uvnas, B., 1979, Effect of splenic nerve stimula-tion on the contents of noradrenaline, ATP and sulphomucopoly-saccharides in noradrenergic vesicle fractions in the cat spleen, Acta Physiol. Scand., 105(4):496.

Bligh, J., 1966, The thermosensitivity of the hypothalamus and ther-moregulation in mammals, Biol. Rev. Cambridge Phil. Soc., 41:317.

Brooks, W.H., Cross, R.J. Roszman, T.L., Markesbery, W.R., 1981, Neuroimmunomodulation: neural anatomical basis for impairment and facilitation, in press.

Bulloch, K., 1981, Neuroendocrine immune circuitry: pathways invol-

ved with the induction and persistence of humoral immunity.
Ph.D. Dissertation, U.C.S.D., San Diego.

Bulloch, K., and Moore, R.Y., 1980, Nucleus ambiguus projections to
the thymus gland: possible pathways for regulation of the immune response and the neuroendocrine network, Anat. Record.,
196:25a (abstr.).

Bulloch, K. and Moore, R.Y., 1981, Thymus gland innervation by
brainstem and spinal cord in mouse and rat, Am. J. Anat., in
press.

Burnstock, G., 1972, The purinergic nervous system, Pharm. Rev.,
24:509.

Burnstock, G., 1979, Past and current evidence for the purinergic
nerve hypothesis, in: "Physiological and regulatory functions
of adenosine and adenine nucleotides", H.P. Baer and G.I.
Drummond, eds., Raven Press, N.Y.

Burnstock, G. and Hokfelt, T., 1979, Non-adrenergic, non-cholinergic
autonomic neurotransmission mechanisms, Neurosci. Res. Program
Bull., 17(3), M.I.T. Press, Cambridge.

Calvo, W., 1968, The innervation of the bone marrow in laboratory
animals, Am. J. Anat., 123:(2)315.

Calvo, W., 1981, Bone marrow hemopoiesis in the human fetus. in:
"Genetics, structure and function of blood cells", Adv. Physiol.
Sci. Vol. 6, S.R. Hollan, G. Gardos, B. Sardaki, eds., Akade-
miai Kiado, Budapest.

Cohen, J.J. and Crnic, L.S., 1981, Glucocorticoids, stress and the
immune response, in: "Immunopharmacology", D.R. Webb, ed.,
Marcel Dekker, N.Y., in press.

Cooper, K.E., Cranston, W.I. and Honour, A.J., 1966, The site of
action of leucocyte pyrogen in the rabbit brain, J. Physiol.
(London), 186:22.

Cross, R.J., Markesbery, W.R., Brooks, W.H. and Roszman, T.L., 1980,
Hypothalamic-immune interactions. I. The acute effect of anterior hypothalamic lesions on the immune response, Brain Res.,
196:79.

Crotti, A., 1981, Thyroid and Thymus. Lea and Febiger, Philadelphia.

Dolin, A.O., and Dolina, C.A., 1972, Pathway of higher neural functions, Vysshaya Shkola, Moscow (Russian).

Von Euler, U.S., 1967, Some factors affecting catecholamine uptake,
storage, and release in adrenergic nerve granules, Circ. Res.,
21(6), Suppl. 3:5.

Fox, B.H., 1978, Premorbid psychological factors as related to cancer
incidence, J. Behav. Med., 1(1):45.

Fox, B.H., 1981, Psychosocial factors and the immune system in human cancer, in: "Psyconeuroimmunology", R. Ader, ed., Academic Press, N.Y., p. 103.

Fusco, M.M., 1959, Responses to Local Heating of the Hypothalamus, Doctoral Diss., Univ. of Pennsylvania, Philadelphia.

Gersbach, P., 1970, Contribution to the study of the innervation of the spleen, comparative anatomical study, Arch. Anat. Histol. Embryol. (Strasbourg), 53(5):397.

Ghali, W.M., Abdel-Rahman, S., Nagib, M. and Mahran, Z.Y. (1980), Intrinsic innervation and vasculature of pre- and post-natal human thymus, Acta anat., 108:115.

Gilman, S.C., Schwartz, J.M., Milner, R.J. Bloom, F.E. and Feldman, J.D., 1981, Enhancement of lymphocyte proliferative responses by B-endorphin, Proc. Soc. for Neurosci., (abstr.) in press.

Giron, L.T. Jr., Crutcher, K.A. and Davis, J.N., 1980, Lymph nodes...a possible site for sympathetic neuronal regulation of immune responses, Ann. Neurol., 8(5):520.

Good, R.A., 1981, Forward to psychoneuroimmunology, R. Ader, ed., Academic Press, N.Y.

Gordon, D.S., Sergeeva, V.E. and Zelenova, I.G., 1979, Functional morphology of adrenergic innervation and adreno-containing structures in lymphoid organs, Arkh. Anat. Gistol. Embriol., 77:13 (Russian).

Guillemin, R., 1977, The expanding significance of hypothalamic peptides, or,is endocrinology a branch of neuroendocrinology?, Rec. Progr. Hormone Res., 33:1.

Guillemin, R., 1978, Biochemical and physiological correlates of hypothalamic peptides: the new endocrinology of the neuron, Res. Publ. Assoc. Nerv. Ment. Dis., 56:155.

Hadden, J.W., Hadden, E.M., and Middleton, E., 1970, Lymphocyte blast transformation. I. Demonstration of adrenergic receptors in human peripheral lymphocytes, Cell. Immunol., 1:583.

Halberg, F., 1976, From aniatrotoxicosis and aniatrosepsis toward chronotherapy, Timing and toxicity: the necessity for relating treatment to bodily rhythms. Tempus non solum dosis venenum facit, in: "Chronobiological aspects of endocrinology", J. Ashoff, F. Ceresa and F. Halberg, eds., F.K. Schattauer Verlag, Stuttgart.

Hall, N.R., 1981, Behavioral and neuroendocrine interactions with immunogenesis. in: "Behavioral neuroendocrinology", C.B. Nemeroff and A.J. Dunn, eds., Spectrum, N.Y., p.

Hall, N.R. and Goldstein, A.L., 1981, Neurotransmitters and the immune system, in: "Psychoneuroimmunology", R. Ader, ed., Academic, N.Y.

Hall, N.R., Lewis, J.K. Schimpff, R.D., Smith, R.T., Trescot, A.M.,
    Gray, H.E., Wenzel, S.E., Abraham, W.C. and Zornetzer S. F.,
    1978, Effects of diencephalic and brainstem lesions on haemo-
    poietic stem cells, Soc. Neurosci., 4:20, Abstr.
Hammar, J.A., 1935, Innervations-verhaltnisse der krelorgane der
    thymus bis in den 4 Fetalmont, Z. Microskanst. Forsch., 8:253.
Hammel, H.T., Hardy, J.D. and Fusco, M.M., 1960, Thermoregulatory
    responses to hypothalamic cooling in unanesthetized dogs, Am.
    J. Physiol., 198:481.
Hidaka, T. and Malik, K.U., 1980, Release of prostaglandins evoked
    by neurohormonal stimuli in the isolated spleen of rabbit, Eur.
    J. Pharmacol., 62(1):97.
Iversen, L.L., Nicoll, R.A. and Vale, W.W., 1978, Neurobiology of
    Peptides, Neurosci. Res. Prog. Bull., 16(2), M.I.T. Press,
    Cambridge.
Jankovic, B.D. and Isakovic, K., 1973, Neuro-endocrine correlates
    of immune response. I. Effects of brain lesions on antibody
    production, Arthus reactivity and delayed hypersensitivity
    in the rat, Int. Arch. Allergy, 45:360.
Jensen, M.M. and Rasmussen, A.F. Jr., 1963a, Stress and suscepti-
    bility to viral infection. I. Response of adrenals, liver,
    thymus, spleen and peripheral leukocyte counts to sound stress,
    J. Immunol., 90:17.
Jensen, M.M. and Rasmussen, A.F. Jr., 1963b, Stress and susceptibi-
    lity to viral infection. II. Sound stress and susceptibility
    to vesicular stomatitis virus, J. Immunol., 90:21.
Jensen, M.M. and Rasmussen, A.F. Jr., 1970, Audiogenic stress and
    susceptibility to infection, in: "Physiological Effects of
    Noise", B.L. Welch and A.S. Welch, eds., Plenum Press, N.Y.
Kahn, R.H., 1904, Uber der Erwarmung des carotidblutes, Arch. Anat.
    Physiol., 28 (Suppl.):81.
Kirkpatrick, R.A., 1981, Witchcraft and lupus erythematosus,
    J.A.M.A, 245(19):1937.
Klein, R.L. and Lagerkrantz, H., 1971, Unidirectional fluxes in
    isolated splenic nerve vesicles measured by a millipore filter
    technique: effects of noradrenaline and competitive reversal
    of reserpine inhibition, Acta Physiol. Scand., 83(2):179.
Klimenko, V.M., 1972, The study of some neuronal mechanisms of
    hypothalamic regulation of immune reactions in rabbits, Avto-
    ref. Kand. Diss. Inst for Exper. Med., Leningrad (Russian).
Korneva, E.A. and Kahai, L.M., 1967, Effect of stimulation of va-
    rious structures of the mesencephalon on the course of immuno-
    logical reactions, Fiziol. Zh. SSSR I.M., Sechenova 53(1):42

(Russian).

Korneva, E.A. and Klimenko, V.M., 1976, Neuronale hypothalamusaki-
    vitat and homoostatische reactionen, Ergeb. Exp. Med., 23:373.

Korneva, E.A., Klimenko, V.M. and Shkhinek, E.K., 1978, Neurohumoral
    maintenance of immune homeostasis, Nauka, Leningrad (Russian).

Kudoh, G., Hoshi, K. and Murakami, T., 1979, Fluorescence microsco-
    pic and enzyme histochemical studies of the innervation of the
    human spleen, Arch. Histol. Jap., 42(2):169.

Kuntz, A. and Richins, C.A., 1945, Innervation of the bone marrow,
    J. Comp. Neur., 83:213.

Liebeskind, J.C. and Dismukes, R.K., 1978, Peptides and behavior: a
    critical analysis of research strategies, M.I.T. Press,
    Cambridge.

Livett, B.G., Geffen, L.B. and Austin, L., 1968, Axoplasmic trans-
    port of 14C-noradrenaline and protein in splenic nerves, Na-
    ture, 217(125):278.

Luk'yanenko, V.I., 1961, The problem of conditioned-reflex regula-
    tion of immunologic reactions, Usp. Sovrem. Biol., 51(2):170
    (Russian).

Lupetti, M. and Dolfi, A., 1980, A contribution to the study of
    lymphopoiesis in the bursa of Fabricius in Gallus domesticus,
    Transplantation, 29(1):67.

MacLean, D. and Reichlin, S., 1981, Neuroendocrinology and the
    immune process, in: "Psychoneuroimmunology", R. Ader, ed.,
    Academic, N.Y.

Mason, J.W., 1975, A historical view of the stress field, J. Human
    Stress, 1:6.

Metalnikov, S., 1934, Role du systéme nerveux et des facteurs bio-
    logiques et psychiques dans l'immunité, Masson, Paris.

Miles, K., Quintans, J., Chelmicka-Schorr, E. and Arnason, B.G.W.,
    1981, The sympathetic nervous system modulates antibody re-
    sponse to thymus-independent antigens, J. Neuroimmunol., 1:101.

Monjan, A.A., 1981, Stress and immunologic competence: studies in
    animals, in: "Psychoneuroimmunology", R. Ader, ed., Academic
    Press, N.Y.

Monjan, A.A. and Collector, M.I., 1977, Stress-induced modulation of
    the immune response, Science, 196:307.

Nahorski, S.R., Barnett, D.B., Howlett, D.R. and Rugg, E.L., 1979,
    Pharmacological characteristics of beta-adrenoreceptor binding
    sites in intact and sympathectomized rat spleen, Naunyn-
    -Schmiedebergs Arch. Pharmocol., 307(3):227.

Nakayama, T., Eisenman, J.S. and Hardy, J.D., 1961, Single unit
    activity of anterior hypothalamus during local healing,

Science, 134:560.

Orlov, V.P., 1979, Evoked potentials of Deiters' nucleus upon sti-
    mulation of neural elements of bones, cutaneous and muscular
    nerves of decerebrate and cerebellectomized animals, Fiziol.
    Zh. SSSR, 65(10):1487 (Russian).

Orlov, V.P., Merten, A.A., Iankovskii, G.A. and Taivan, I.L., 1978a,
    Pathways participating in conducting osteroreceptive signaling
    into Deiters' vestibular nucleus, Fiziol. Zh. SSSR, 64(3):271
    (Russian).

Orlov, V.P., Merten, A.A., Ianovskii, G.A. and Taivan, I.L., 1978b,
    Evoked potentials in Deiters' nucleus upon stimulation of neu-
    ral elements of bones, cutaneous and muscle nerves, Fiziol. Zh.
    SSSR, 64 (2):155 (Russian).

Palmblad, J., 1981, Stress and immunologic competence: studies in
    man, in: "Psychoneuroimmunology", R. Ader, ed., Academic
    Press, N.Y., p. 229.

Palmblad, J., Cantell, K., Strander, H., Froberg, J., Karlsson, C.G.,
    Levi, L., Granstrom, M. and Unger, P., 1976, Stressor expo-
    sure and immunological response in man: interferon-producing
    capacity and phagocytosis, J. Psychosom. Res., 20:193.

Pierpaoli, W. and Besedovsky, H.O., 1975, Role of the thymus in
    programming of neuroendocrine functions, Clin. Exp. Immunol.,
    20:323.

Pierpaoli, W. and Maestroni, G., 1980, Hormonal circadian periodi-
    city and the immune response, Proc. Int. Union of Physiol.
    Sci., 14:218 (abstr.).

Psegalinski, N., 1944, Polyglobulia hipotalimica, medical thesis,
    Cluj (Romanian), Cited in Baciu, 1962.

Rasmussen, A.F. Jr., Marsh, J.T. and Brill, N.Q., 1957, Increased
    susceptibility to herpes simplex in mice subjected to avoidance-
    -learning stress or restraint, Proc. Soc. Exper. Biol. Med.,
    96:183.

Reilly, F.D., McCuskey, R.S. and Meineke, H.A., 1976, Studies of the
    hemopoietic microenvironment. VIII. Adrenergic and cholinergic
    innervation of the murine spleen, Anat. Rec., 185:109.

Riley, V., 1975, Mouse mammary tumors: alteration of incidence as
    an apparent function of stress, Science, 189:465.

Riley, V., 1981, Psychoneuroendocrine influences on immunocompe-
    tence and neoplasia, Science, 212:1100.

Riley, V., Fitzmaurice, M.A. and Spackman, D.H., 1981, Psychoneuro-·
    immunologic factors in neoplasia: studies in animals, in:
    "Psyconeuroimmunology", r. Ader, ed., Academic Press, p. 31.

Roszkowski, W., Plaut, M. and Lichtenstein, 1977, Selective display of histamine receptors on lymphocytes, Science, 195:683.

Roszman, T.L., Cross, R.J., Brooks, W.H., and Markesbery, W.R., 1981, Hypothalamic-immune interactions. II. Neuroimmunomodulation of suppressor cell function, in Press.

Ruf, K. and Steiner, F.A., 1967, Steroid-sensitive single neurons in rat hypothalamus and midbrain: identification by microelectrophoresis, Science, 156:667.

Schulhof, K. and Mathies, M.M., 1927, Polyglobulia induced by cerebral lesions, J.A.M.A.,89:2093.

Selye, H., 1936, Thumus and adrenals in the response of the organism to injuries and intoxications, Brit. J. Exp. Pathol., 17:234.

Selye, H., 1946, The general adaptation syndrome and the diseases of adaptation, J. Clin. Endocrinol., 6:117.

Selye, H., 1950, The physiology and pathology of exposure to stress, Acta Inc., Montreal.

Selye, H., 1975, Stress in health and disease, Butterworth, London.

Sergeeva, V.E., 1974, Histotopography of catecholamines in the mammalian thymus, Bull. Exper. Biol. Med., 77:456.

Sharma, V.K. and Banerjee, S.P., 1979, Regeneration of ^{3}H-ouabain binding to ($Na^+ + K^+$)-ATPase in chemically sympathectomized cat peripheral organs, Mol. Pharmacol., 15(1):35.

Shavlev, V.N., 1968, On the innervation of lymph nodes, Arkh. Anat. Gist. Embriol., 54(2):96 (Russian).

Smolenzky, M.H., Reinberg, A. and McGovern, J.P., 1980, Recent advances in the chronobiology of allergy and immunology, Pergamon Press, Oxford.

Solomon, G.F., and Moos, R.H., 1964, Emotions, immunity and disease, Arch. Gen. Psychiatry, 2:657.

Solomon, G.F., Amkraut, A.A. and Kasper, P., 1974, Immunity, emotions and stress, Ann. Clin. Res., 6:313.

Solov'ev, V.N., 1966, On the sources of innervation of the thymus gland, Arkh. Anat. Gistol. Embriol., 51(9):76 (Russian).

Spector, N.H., 1969, Thermodes and theories, MCV Quarterly 5(1):20.

Spector, N.H., 1979, Can hypothalamic lesions change circulating antibody or interferon responses to antigens? in: "The pathogenesis of allergic processes in experiment and in the clinic", A.M. Chernukh and V.I. Pytskii, eds., Meditsina, Moscow (Russian)

Spector, N.H., 1980, The central state of the hypothalamus in health and disease: Old and new concepts, in: "Physiology of the hypothalamus", P. Morgane and J. Panksepp, eds., Dekker, N.Y.

Spector, N.H., and Korneva, E.A., 1981, Neurophysiology, immunophysiology and neuroimmunomodulation, in: "Psychoneuroimmunology", R. Ader, ed., Academic Press, N.Y.

Spector, N.H., Brobeck, R. and Hamilton, C.L., 1968, Feeding and core temperature in albino rats: changes induced by preoptic heating and cooling, Science, 161:286.

Spector, N.H., Koob, G.F. and Baron, S., 1977, Hypothalamic influence upon interferon and antibody responses to Newcastle disease virus infection: preliminary report, Proc. Int. Union Physiol. Sci., 13:711 (abstr.).

Spector, N.H., Peterson, J., Schlosberg, V.A. and Baron, S., 1981, Environmental influences upon interferon production in response to Poly I:C, in preparation.

Stein, M., Schleifer, S.J., and Keller, S.E., 1981, Hypothalamic influences on immune responses, in: "Psychoneuroimmunology", R. Ader, ed., Academic Press, N.Y.

Thoenen, H. and Transer, J. P., 1968, Chemical sympathectomy by selective destruction of adrenergic nerve endings with 6-hydroxydopamine, Naunyn-Schmiedebergs, Arch. Pharmak. U. Exp. Path., 261:271.

Thompson, J.H. and Cooper, M.D., 1971, Functional deficiency of autologous implants of the bursa of Fabricius in chickens, Transplantation, 2(1):71.

Thureson-Klein, A., Klein, R.L., and Johansson, O., 1979, Catecholamine-rich cells and varicosities in bovine splenic nerve: vesicle contents and evidence for exocytosis, J. Neurobiol., 10(3):309.

Du Verney, J.G., 1700, De la structure et du sentiment de la moelle, Mem. Acad. R. Sci. Paris, Années (cited in Webber, et al., 1970).

Volik, V. Ia, 1965, Development of the neural apparatus of inguinal lymph nodes in man, Arkh. Anat. Gistol. Embriol., 45(5):34 (Russian)

Warejka, D.J. and Levy, N.L., 1980, Central nervous system control of the immune response: effect of hypothalamic lesions on PHA responsiveness in rats, Fed. Proc., 39(3):914 (abstr.).

Webber, R.H., de Felice, R., Ferguson, R.J. and Powell, J.P., 1970, Bone marrow response to stimulation of the sympathetic trunk in rats, Acta Anat., 77:92.

Williams, J.M., Peterson, R.G., Shea, P.A., Schmedtje, J.F., Bauer, D.C. and Felton, D.L., 1981, Sympathetic innervation of murine thymus and spleen: evidence for a functional link between the nervous and immune systems, Brain Res. Bull., 6:83.

Wit, A. and Wang, S.C., 1967, Effects of increasing ambient temperature on unit activity in the preoptic-anterior hypothamus region, Fed. Proc., 26:555 (abstr).

IMMUNOENDOCRINOLOGY : ENDOCRINE ASPECTS OF AUTOIMMUNE DISEASE

Norman Talal

Medical Centre, Clinical Division
Immunology, 151-T., San Francisco
California

1. SEX STEROID HORMONES

There are important bidirectional relationships between the immune and endocrine systems (Talal, 1978). Our laboratory became interested in these relationships through investigations seeking an explanation for the marked female predominance of autoimmune disorders such as systemic lupus erythematosus (SLE). The female to male ratio in SLE is 15:1 during the childbearing ages and decreases to 2:1 after menopause (Talal, 1979). Furthermore, in Klinefelter's syndrome (XXY) in which genetic males develop gynecomastia and sparse body hair, there is an increased incidence of autoimmune disorders such as SLE and myasthenia gravis (Michalski et al., 1978). These clinical observations led us to speculate that sex hormones might play an important role in the pathogenesis of autoimmune disease.

Five years ago, we undertook a series of investigations in NZB/NZW F_1 (B/W) mice to study this question. These mice develop a lupus-like syndrome characterized by the formation of antibodies to nucleic acids, immune complex glomerulonephritis and death from uremia (Talal et al., 1981). Female mice develop this illness several months earlier than males. Our studies, reported in the literature (Roubinian et al., 1977, 1978, 1979) clearly demonstrate that androgens suppress and estrogens accelerate murine SLE. These actions of sex steroid hormones were shown by monitoring several disease parameters including autoantibody levels, immune

259

complex deposits in the kidney and survival. The ability of male hormone to prolong survival was observed even in older mice with already established disease (Roubinian, et al., 1979).

Synthetic attenuated androgens do not ameliorate B/W disease (Roubinian et al., 1979) although anti-estrogens have a beneficial effect (Shear et al., 1981). Adequate controlled trials attempting to treat human SLE with sex hormone modification have not been reported.

In more recent years, we have concentrated our efforts in trying to define the mechanisms by which sex steroid hormones modulate murine lupus. Because immunological reactivity in general is greater in females that in males (Besedovsky and Sorkin, 1977), both for humans and for mice, we have felt from the beginning that the sex hormone effects in B/W mice represented physiologic actions of hormones manifest on an aberrant system of disordered immunologic regulation.

In collaboration with dr. P.K. Siiteri, the thymus glands of B/W and other murine strains were studied for the presence of classical sex steroid hormone receptor. We observed estrogen receptor-like binding in the cytoplasm prepared from thymus glands obtained from both male and female mice of several strains including Balb/c, C57BL, NZB, NZW and B/W (Talal et al., 1980). The observed binding was of high affinity ($K_D = 10^{-10}\underline{\,}10^{-9}M$) and low capacity and was specific, as is characteristic of receptor binding. Furthermore, estradiol binding was inhibited by diethyl-stilbesterol but not by dihydrotestosterone, progesterone, or cortisol. Treatment of castrated B/W mice with estradiol resulted in translocation of the cytoplasmic receptor to the nucleus. We also found specific binding of dihydrotestosterone in thymic cytoplasm from Balb/c, NZB and B/W mice. Thus, there appear to be receptors for sex steroid hormones in the thymus glands from several strains of mice, both normal and autoimmune. The binding affinity and steroid specificity of these receptors are consistent with tissue estrogen receptors found in the uterus of rats and other species. These receptors suggest that sex hormones could influence immune mechanisms by acting on thymic epithelium or on thymocytes. There is autoradiographic evidence for nuclear concentration of ^{3}H-estradiol in thymic reticular cells of rats (Stumpf and Sar, 1976).

The thymus may not be the only site of sex steroid hormone

action, however. There is evidence for estrogen stimulation of the reticuloendothelial system (Nicol et al., 1966). In recent studies with Dr. Hannah Shear (1981), we have found that sex hormones modulate the clearance of IgG-coated autologous mouse erythrocytes in B/W mice. Estrogen delays clearance from the circulation, whereas androgen promotes more rapid removal. These results probably reflect sex steroid hormone effects on the reticuloendothelial system.

It is interesting that major sites of action for sex steroid hormones may be reticuloendothelium and thymic epithelium. These are two target tissues that are enormously influential in regulating immune function, although they are not themselves lymphoid. Thymic epithelium expresses Ia antigens which are important in directing lymphocyte specificity and in inducing helper-T cell activity. Thymic epithelium also produces thymic hormones which are intimately involved in peripheral T cell differentiation. Thus, by influencing the expression of Ia or the production of thymic hormones, sex steroid could exert influence on the immune response at several levels. Likewise, immune complexes combine with lymphocyte or macrophage Fc receptors, fix complement and induce inflammatory events. Effects of sex steroid hormones on immune complex clearance by cells of the reticuloendothelial system would also have important immunoregulatory actions.

These observations in murine lupus have great relevance for human illness. SLE is a multifactorial disease in which genetic, immunologic, possibily viral and hormonal influences, all contribute to pathogenesis. Evidence is accumulating for a sex hormone factor in human SLE. Lupus patients, like Klinefelter patients, are under a hyperestrogenic influence as a result of an alteration in estrogen metabolism. Women, with SLE have elevations in both 16-α-hydroxyesterone and estriol, while men with this disease have elevation in the former only (Lahita et al., 1979). The 16-hydroxylated metabolites of estradiol retain substantial estrogenic activity and generally behave as active estrogens. This extended estrogenic activity may contribute to the greater prevalence of SLE in women.

2. INTERLEUKINS

The interleukins are polypeptide products of mature or

immature lymphocytes or macrophages that control immune reactivity. As such, they may be considered immune system hormones. We
have recently become interested in Interleukin-2 (IL-2), also
known as T Cell Growth Factor. IL-2 is a lymphokine produced by
mitogen or antigen stimulated T cells (Gillis et al., 1978). IL-2
has significant T cell regulatory function (Farrar et al., 1978;
Watson et al., 1979; Watson, 1979; Shaw et al., 1978; Kruisbeek et
al., 1980). It stimulates thymocyte proliferation, provides
helper activity for antibody production, facilitates the induction
of cytotoxic T cells, and promotes the proliferation of helper and
cytotoxic T lymphocytes in long-term culture (Watson et al., 1979;
Gillis et al., 1978; Wofsy et al., 1981). We find a deficiency of
IL-2 in several autoimmune-susceptible strains of mice. In two
strains (MRL and C57BL6), this deficiency is associated with the
presence of an autoimmune gene called lpr.

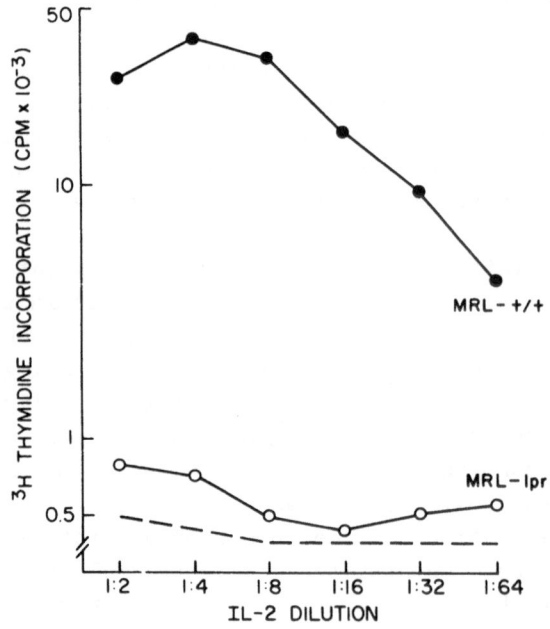

Fig. 1. IL- activity in culture supernatants derived from 5 month
       old MRL-1pr (o——o) and MRL-+/+ (●——●) spleen cells.
       The MRL-1pr gene, hence normal IL-2 activity. Each point
       represents the mean value of six individual mice. The dotted
       line shows the stimulatory effect of Con A (10 μg/ml) alone
       in the assay.

MRL-lpr mice spontaneously develop autoimmune disease characterized by antibodies to nucleic acids, immune complex glomerulonephritis, and death from renal failure (Murphy and Roths, 1978; Andrews et al., 1978). They have certain unique features which make them particularly interesting murine models for SLE. First, they develop massive generalized lymphadenopathy associated with proliferation of Lyt-1$^+$23$^-$ T cells (Theofilopoulos et al., 1980). Second, they exhibit excessive T-helper function (Sawada and Talal, 1979; Theofilopoulos et al., 1980). Finally, a single autosomal recessive gene, lpr, is responsible for both the lymphoproliferation and severe autoimmunity of MRL-lpr mice (Murphy and Roths, 1978). Several immunoregulatory abnormalities which might contribute to autoimmunity in MRL-lpr mice have been indentified (Murphy and Roths, 1978; Andrews et al., 1978; Theofilopoulos et al., 1980; Sawada and Talal, 1979; Watson et al., 1979; Gershon et al., 1978; Creighton et al., 1979; Izui and Eisenberg, 1980; Steinberg et al., 1980; Hom and Talal, in press; Glimcher et al., 1980).

To clarify the molecular basis for abnormal immunoregulation in MRL-lpr mice, we examined the ability of spleen cells to produce and respond to IL-2. MRL-lpr mice had a marked defect in Con A-induced IL-2 production which was present as early as 2 months prior to the onset of clinical disease. By 5 months of age, the defect in IL-2 production was virtually absolute (Fig. 1). The reduction in IL-2 activity was independent of the duration of culture or the dose of Concanavalin A (Con A) used to stimulate IL-2 production. The defect was not related to suppressor cells. We suspected that this IL-2 defect was related in some way to the lpr gene. To test this hypothesis, we studied C57BL6 mice into which the lpr gene was transferred by eight cycles of cross--intercross mating. These C57BL6-lpr mice develop an autoimmune disease similar to that of the MRL-lpr characterized by lymphadenopathy, anti-nuclear antibodies, and early mortality (Wofsy et al.,1981). Like MRL-lpr mice, C57BL6-lpr mice developed a defect in IL-2 activity early in life which became progressively more severe with age. Although spleen cells from 2 month old C57 BL6--lpr mice produced IL-2 normally in response to Con A, spleen cells from 3 month old mice showed a marked reduction in IL-2 activity (Fig. 2). There was virtually no IL-2 activity at 6 months of age.

Con A stimulated spleen cells from MRL-lpr and C57BL6-lpr

mice also proliferated significantly less in response to standard IL-2 preparations than did spleen cells from age-matched congenic controls. This failure of spleen cells to respond to IL-2 normally was not due to absorption of IL-2 by MRL-lpr spleen cells.

Thus, there is an early in life deficiency of IL-2 in two murine strains which subsequently develop SLE. This relationship between IL-2 deficiency and autoimmune disease is intriguing. It suggests that IL-2 is required for normal immunoregulation and for the prevention of autoantibody formation. How IL-2 deficiency leads to autoimmunity, and whether IL-2 administration can ameliorate disease in a manner similar to androgen, are questions for future investigation.

On this point, however, we have found that NZB and B/W mice also manifest IL-2 deficiency but later in life when autoimmune disease is already present (Dauphinee et al., submitted). The

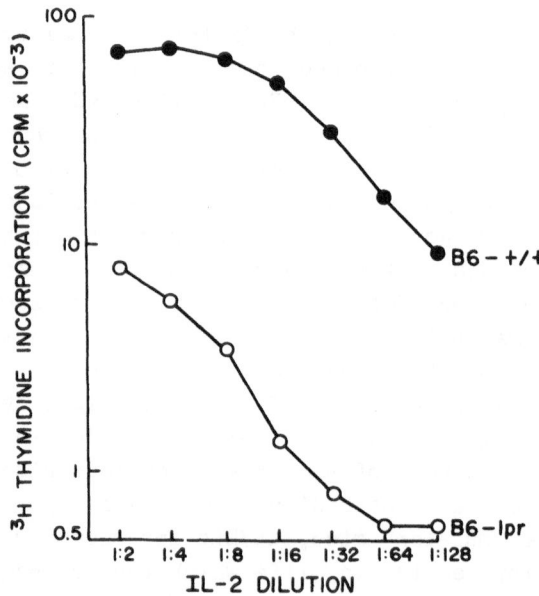

Fig. 2. IL-2 activity in culture supernatants derived from 3 month old C57BL-lpr (o———o) and C57BL6-+/+ (●———●) mice. The C57BL-lpr mice are identical to C57BL6-+/+ (●———●) mice, but having the lpr gene, are deficient in IL-2. Each line represents the mean value of IL-2 activity in four individual mice.

therapeutic effect of androgen is associated in B/W mice with the maintenance of normal IL-2 activity (Dauphinee et al., 1980). This result suggests a relationship between sex hormones and IL-2 activity.

3. DISCUSSION

Our studies should be seen in the broad context of a field that I have called immunoendocrinology (Talal 1976), representing an interface between the twin disciplines of immunology and endocrinology. We have focused attention on two aspects of that overlap: 1) the modulation of autoimmune disease by classical sex steroid hormones, and 2) the association of autoimmunity with a deficiency of an immune hormone called IL-2 (T Cell Growth Factor).

In this report, we have presented recent data on the possible mechanisms whereby sex hormones influence autoimmune disease. The non-lymphoid elements that control immune responses, such as thymic epithelium and cells of the reticuloendothelial system, may be important target sites for sex hormone action. Of course, this does not preclude additional direct effects of these hormones on lymphocytes.

The deficiency of IL-2 opens up an important line of investigation relating lymphokines (immune hormones) to disease processes. We suspect that the decreased autologous mixed lymphocyte response, a common feature of several human and murine autoimmune and lymphoproliferative diseases (Talal et al., 1980), is related to IL-2 deficiency. In all likelihood, many reports relating interleukins to human illness will appear in the near future.

Interactions between the immune and endocrine systems are not limited to endocrine influences on immunity but include immunologic modulation of hormone receptors (e.g. insulin receptors), lymphocytic regulation of osteoclast activity and bone metabolism, and thymic activity as an endocrine organ. The presence of steroid-sensitive receptors in the hypothalamus raises the possibility that neuroendocrine pathways also interact with the immune system. Neuroendocrine influences might be superimposed upon the immune and endocrine systems, creating pathways by which the brain could control vital immune and endocrine mechanisms.

Evidence is accumulating to support a role for neuroendocrine factors in immunity (Cohn, 1979; Pierpaoli and Maestroni, 1978; Rogers et al., 1979).

The lymphocyte surface contains receptors for insulin, histamine, E-prostaglandins, acetylcholine and β-adrenergic catecholamines. These substances influence lymphocyte function.
The existence of cholinergic and β-adrenergic receptor sites suggests a possible link between immune reactivity and the central nervous system. There may also be receptors for morphine and methionine-enkephalin on human T lymphocytes (Wofsy et al., 1981). This observation raises the possibility that brain peptide neurotransmitters could modulate such T cell activities as suppression, help and cytotoxicity. Can neurotransmitters also influence cells such as the natural killer polulation which is though to play an important role in host defense against malignancy? Would such studies elucidate problems well known to psychiatry such as the association of stress with the development of autoimmune and malignant diseases?

Our studies on immune-endocrine interactions in autoimmune disease have certainly not simplified matters. The multifactorial nature of autoimmune disease may at times seem complicated and confusing. However, these many factors also offer opportunities for new therapeutic approaches based on mechanisms which, although outside the classical immune system, may nevertheless restore immune regulation and ameliorate disease.

4. SUMMARY

Two aspects of immunoendocrinology have been studied in murine models for human autoimmune disease. The modulation of murine lupus by sex steroid hormones demonstrates the ability of androgen to suppress and estrogens to accelerate several disease parameters. These effects may be mediated through hormone receptors on thymic epithelium, and by the ability of sex steroid hormones to influence the clearance of particulate immune complexes.

Autoimmune-susceptible mice have a deficiency of interleukin-2 (IL-2), also known as T Cell Growth Factor. In two strains (MRL and C57BL6), the IL-2 deficiency is associated with the presence of the lpr gene which is responsible for autoimmunity and lymphoproliferation.

These studies on immune-endocrine interactions in relation to disease may be seen in a broader context that also involves the central nervous and neuroendocrine systems. The multifactorial nature of human illness offers opportunities for new therapeutic approaches based on mechanisms which, although outside the classical immune system, may nevertheless be favorably manipulated to restore host control over aberrant immunoregulatory networks.

REFERENCES

Andrews, B.S., Eisenberg, R.A., Theofilopoulos, A.N., Izui, S., Wilson, C.B., McConahey, P.J., Murphy, E.D., Roths, J.B., and Dixon, F.J., 1978, Spontaneous murine lupus-like syndromes: I. Clinical and immunopathological manifestations in several strains, J. Exp. Med., 148:1148.

Besedovsky, H., and Sorkin, E., 1977, Network of immune-neuroendocrine interactions, Clin. Exp. Immunol., 27:1.

Cohn, D.A., 1979, High sensitivity to androgen as a contributing factor in sex differences in the immune response, Arthritis Rheum., 22:1218.

Creighton, W.D., Katz, D.H., and Dixon, F.J., 1979, Antigen-specific immunocompetency, B cell function, and regulatory helper and suppressor T cell activities in spontaneously autoimmune mice, J. Immunol., 123:2627.

Dauphinee, M.J., Kipper, S.B., Wofsy, D., and Talal, N., Interleukin-2 deficiency is a common feature of autoimmune mice, manuscript submitted.

Dauphinee, M.J., Kipper, S.B., Roskos, K., Wofsy, D., and Talal, N., 1980, Androgen treatment of autoimmune NZB/W mice enhances IL-2 production, Arthritis Rheumatism Association Meeting, Boston, MA, abstr.

Farrar, J.J., Simon, P.L., Koopman, W.J., and Fuller-Bonar, J., 1978, Biochemical relationship of thymocyte mitogenic factor and factors enhancing humoral and cell-mediated immune responses, J. Immunol., 121:1353.

Gershon, R.K., Horowitz, M., Kemp, J.D., Murphy, D.B., and Murphy, E.D., 1978, The cellular site of immunoregulatory breakdown in the lpr mutant mouse, in: "Genetic Control of Autoimmune Disease," N.R. Rose, P.E. Bigazzi, and N.L. Warner, eds, Elsevier,

North Holland, New York, p. 223.

Gillis, S., Ferm, M.M., Ou, W., and Smith, K.S., 1978, T cell growth factor parameters of production and a quantitative microassay for activity, J. Immunol., 120:2027.

Gillis, S., Baker, P.E., Ruscetti, F.W.,and Smith, K.A., 1978, Long--term culture of human antigen-specific cytotoxic T-cell lines, J. Exp. Med., 148:1093.

Glimcher, L.H., Steinberg, A.D., House, S.B., and Green, I., 1980, The autologous mixed lymphocyte reaction in strains of mice with autoimmune disease, J. Immunol., 124:1832.

Hom, J.T., and Talal, N., Disordered immunologic regulation, in: "Immuno-Dynamics," III. R.S. Krakauer, ed., Elsevier, North Holland/NY, in press.

Izui, S., and Eisenberg, R.A., 1980, Circulating anti-DNA rheumatoid factor complexes in MRL/1 mice, Clin. Immunol. Immunopathol., 15:535.

Kruisbeck, A.M., Zijlstra, J.J., and Krose, T.J.M., 1980, Distinct effects of T cell growth factors and thymic epithelial factors on the generation of cytotoxic T lymphocytes by thymocyte sub-populations, J. Immunol., 125:995.

Lahita, R.G., Bradlow, H.L., Kunkel, H.., and Fishman, J., 1979, Alterations of estrogen metabolism in systemic lupus erythema-tosus, Arthritis Rheum., 22:1195.

Michalski, J.P., Synder, S.M., McLeod, R.L., and Talal, N., 1978, Monozygotic twins with Klinefelter's syndrome discordant for systemic lupus erythematosus and symptomatic myasthenia gravis, Arthritis Rheum., 21:306.

Murphy, E.D., and Roths, J.B., 1978, Autoimmunity and lymphoprolife-ration: Induction by mutant gene lpr, and acceleration by a male-associated factor in strain BXSB, in: "Genetic Control of Autoimmune Disease," N.R. Rose, P.E. Bigazzi, and N.L. Warner, eds., Elsevier, North Holland/New York, p. 207.

Nicol, T., Vernon-Roberts, B., and Quantock, D.C., 1966, Estrogenic and anti-estrogenic effect of estriol, 16-epioestriol, 2-metho-cytosterone and 2-hydroeyoestradiol, 17-beta on the reticuloen-dothelial system and reproductive tract, J. Endocrinol., 35:119.

Pierpaoli, W., and Maestroni, J.M., 1978, Pharmacologic control of the hormonally modulated immune response. III. Prolongation of allogeneic skin graft rejection and prevention of runt disease by a combination of drugs acting on neuroendocrine functions, J. Immunol., 120:1600.

Rogers, M.P., Dubey, D., Reich, P., 1979, The influence of psyche and the brain on immunity and disease susceptibility: A critical review, Psychosom. Med., 41:147.

Roubinian, J.R., Papoian, R., and Talal, N., 1977, Androgenic hormones modulate autoantibody responses and improve survival in murine lupus, J. Clin. Invest., 59:1066.

Roubinian, J.R., Talal, N., Greenspan, J.S., Goodman, J.R., and Siiteri, P.K., 1978, Effect of castration and sex hormone treatment on survival, anti-nucleic acid antibodies, and glomerulonephritis in NZB/NZW F mice, J. Exp. Med., 147:1568.

Roubinian, J.R., and Talal, N., Greenspan, J.S., Goodman, J.R., and Siiteri, P.K., 1979, Delayed androgen treatment prolongs survival in murine lupus, J. Clin. Invest, 63:902.

Roubinian, J.R., Talal, N., Greenspan, J.S., Goodman, J.R., and Nussenzweig, V., 1979, Danazol's failure to suppress autoimmunity in NZB/NZW F mice, Arthritis Rheum., 22:1399.

Sawada, S., and Talal, N., 1979, Evidence for a helper cell promoting anti-DNA antibody production in murine lupus, Arthritis Rheum., 22:655, abstr.

Shaw, J., Monticone, V., Mills, G., and Paetkau, V., 1978, Effects of costimulator on immune responses in vitro, J. Immunol., 120:1974.

Shear, H.L., Roubinian, J.R., Gil, P., and Talal, N., 1981, Clearance of sensitized erythrocytes in NZB/NZW mice. Effects of castration and sex hormone treatment, Eur. J. Immunol., in press.

Steinberg, A.D., Melez, K.A., Raveche, E.S., Reeves, J.P., Boegel, W.A., Smathers, P.A., Taurog, J.D., Weinlein, L., and Duvic, M., 1979, Approach to the study of the role of sex hormones in autoimmunity, Arthritis Rheum., 22:1170.

Steinberg, A.D., Roths, J.B., Murphy, E.D., Steinberg, R.T., and Raveche, E.S., 1980, Effects of thymectomy or androgen administration upon the auto-immune disease of MRL/Mp-lpr/lpr mice, J. Immunol., 125:871.

Stumpf, W.E., and Sar, M., 1976, Receptors and mechanism of action of steroid hormones, in: "Modern Pharmacology-Toxicology," J. Pasqualini, ed., Marcel Dekker, New York, p. 41.

Talal, N., 1978, Autoimmunity and the immunologic network, Arthritis Rheum., 21:853.

Talal, N., 1979, Systemic lupus erythematosus, autoimmunity, sex and inheritance, N. Engl. J. Med., (editorial), 301:838.

Talal, N., 1976, Disordered immunologic regulation and autoimmunity. Transplant. Rev., 31:240.

Talal, N., Roubinian, J.R., Daupinee, M.J., Jones, L.A., and Siiteri, P.K., 1981, Effects of sex hormones on spontaneous autoimmune disease in NZB/NZW hybrid mice, in: "Advances in Immunopharmaco-

logy," J. Hadden et al., eds., Pergamon Press, Oxford and New
    York, p. 127.
Talal, N., Roubinian, J.R., Shear, H., Hom, J.T., Miyasaka, N., 1980,
    Progress in the mechanisms of autoimmune disease, in: "Immunolo-
    gy-1980," M. Fougereau, ed., Academic Press, Inc., London
    Ltd., p. 889.
Theofilopoulos, A.N., Eisenberg, R.A., Bourdon, M., Crowell, J.S.,
    Jr., and Dixon, F.G., 1979, Distribution of lymphocytes identi-
    fied by surface markers in murine strains with systemic lupus
    erythematosus-like syndromes, J. Exp. Med., 149:516.
Theofilopoulos, A. N., Shawler, D.L., Eisenberg, R.A., and Dixon,
    F.J., 1980, Splenic immunoglobulin-secreting cells and their
    regulation in autoimmune mice, J. Exp. Med., 151:446.
Watson, J., Gillis, S., Marbrook, J., Mochizuki, D., amd Smith, K.A.,
    1979, Biochemical and biological characterization of lymphocyte
    regulatory molecules, I. Purification of a class of murine lym-
    phokines, J. Exp. Med., 150:849.
Watson, J., Aarden, L.A., Shaw, J., and Paetkau, V., 1979, Molecular
    and quantitative analysis of helper T cell-replacing factors on
    the induction of antigen-sensitive B lymphocytes, J. Immunol.,
    122:1633.
Watson, J., 1979, Continuous proliferation of murine antigen-speci-
    fic helper T lymphocytes in culture, J. Exp. Med., 150:1510.
Wofsy, D., Dauphinee, M.J., Kipper, S.B., Roths, J.B., Murphy, E.D.,
    and Talal, N., 1981, Deficient Interleukin-2 activity in MRL/Mp
    and C57BL/6J mice bearing the lpr gene, manuscript submitted.
Wybran, J., Apperboom, T., Famaey, J-P., and Govaerts, A., 1979, Sug-
    gestive evidence for receptors for morphine and methionine-en-
    kephalin on normal human blood T lymphocytes, J. Immunol.,
    122:1068.

PROSTAGLANDINS AND IMMUNOREGULATION

Bernard M. Jaffe, M. Gabriella Santoro
Peter Le Port, Cartesio Favalli,
David Hofer, and Enrico Garaci

The Department of Surgery, S.U.N.Y. Downstate Medical
Center, Brooklyn, New York
The Institute of Microbiology, University of Rome
Rome, Italy

1. INTRODUCTION

Although numerous recent studies have implicated prostaglandins in the control of the immune response, both suppressive
and stimulatory effects have been reported. While our earlier
studies dealing with transplantation suggested PGE compounds have
potent immunosuppressive actions, our later studies, which have
focused on tumor-bearing animals, have demonstrated that these
compounds stimulate the immune response. This chapter will review
our work on prostaglandins and immunoregulation and clarify this
apparent paradox.

2. TRANSPLANTATION STUDIES

Our studies have dealt with three transplantation models, he-
terotopic rat heart allografts, and dog and mouse skin allografts.

In the first group of studies, the technique of Ono and
Lindsey (1969) was utilized. In this model, the donor heart is
placed as an accessory in the abdomen with the donor aorta sutured
to the recipient abdominal aorta and the donor pulmonary artery is
anastomosed to the inferior vena cava. At the time of rejection,

271

Table 1. Tissue contents of PGE after rat heart allografting.

Day Numbers	1-3 / 4	4 / 7	5 / 3	6 / 9	7 / 3	8-9 / 3	10 / 6
Spleen							
PGE (ng/gm)	3.46±1.07	1.68±0.38	2.02±0.68	2.91±0.87	2.60±0.76	2.16±0.68	1.87±0.399
Organ Weight	0.50±0.05	0.83±0.03	0.77±0.14	0.88±0.08	1.28±0.09	1.44±0.09	1.12±0.15
Thymus							
PGE (ng/gm)	3.61±1.30	6.65±1.56	8.17±3.98	5.54±1.97	3.69±0.38	1.88±0.30	4.20±2.03
Organ Weight	0.13±0.02	0.16±0.05	0.16±0.05	0.22±0.03	0.16±0.04	0.13±0.05	0.21±0.02
Heart							
PGE (ng/gm)	2.02±0.59	2.23±0.37	2.68±0.38	2.99±0.95	4.02±2.44	1.37±0.29	1.61±0.35
Organ Weight	0.84±0.03	0.79±0.05	0.76±0.05	0.77±0.05	0.78±0.07	0.84±0.04	0.74±0.07
Allograft							
PGE (ng/gm)	2.34±0.69	2.37±0.31	3.73±0.97	9.16±6.41	3.96±2.80	3.07±2.24	3.10±1.63
Organ Weight	1.04±0.06	1.13±0.11	1.71±0.29	1.46±0.03	1.97±0.10	2.15±0.29	2.06±0.36

Table 2. Effect of di-M-PGE$_2$ and indomethacin on murine skin allograft survival.

Group	Number of animals	Skin graft survival (days + S.E)
Control	59	13.6+0.3
Di-M-PGE (5 g)	32	16.7+0.6
Di-M-PGE plus		
Indomethacin (100 g)	21	16.0+0.6
Indomethacin (100 g)	39	12.7+0.2
Indomethacin (150 g)	12	11.8+0.2
Indomethacin (200 g)	9	10.9+0.4

cardiac function ceases. In our studies, 35 heart transplants were
performed from donor Brown Norway to recipient Lewis rats. No
immuno-suppression was utilized. Rats were sacrificed at intervals
and the spleen, thymus, native heart, and transplant heart excised
and weighed. Concentrations of prostaglandin E_2 (PGE_2) were
measured by radio-immunossay (Jaffe et al., 1972; 1973) in one
hundred mg tissue samples. The results of these studies (Jaffe et
al., 1975; Moore and Jaffe, 1974) are presented in Table 1.
Although there were slight increases in the spleen and native
heart PGE_2 concentrations, PGE_2 levels in the transplanted hearts
peaked at the time of rejection (6-7 days). In the allografts, the
mean PGE contents on days 5-7, 12.98 + 6.86 ng, were significantly
higher than comparable data on days 1-4 (2.47 + 0.35 ng). In 16
additional rats, coronary sinus blood was collected and PGE levels
measured (Jaffe and Moore, 1974). On day 7, plasma PGE levels
peaked at 1697 + 577 pg/ml; this value was 3.2 times the basal
levels of 528 + 62 pg/ml (p 0.05).

This release of PGE by allograft tissue at the time of
rejection stimulated an attempt to correlate prostaglandin levels
with a measure of the immune response, the lymphocytotoxic
antibody titers. In this study, (Anderson et al., 1975) five pairs
of dogs were sensitized by undirectional skin allografts over a
6-week period. Lymphocytotoxic antibody titers were measured using
the technique of Mittal et al., (1968) (Jaffe et al., 1972).

Table 3. The effect of di-M-PGE$_2$ and indomethacin on hemagglutinin titers (1/Log$_2$).^{2}

	4 days	7 days
Tumor + diluent	3.25+0.45 (8)[a]	3.13+0.55 (8)
Tumor + di-M-PGE$_2$	4.86+0.40 (7)	4.67+0.21 (6)
Tumor + indomethacin	1.50+0.50 (4)	2.00+0.81 (4)
Normal + diluent	5.83+0.31 (6)	5.25+0.16 (8)
Normal + di-M-PGE$_2$	5.75+0.25 (8)	4.50+0.22 (6)
Normal + indomethacin	5.50+0.70 (2)	6.00

[a] In breackets = no. of animals

Basally, none of the animals had cytotoxic antibodies and PGE levels averaged 1.8 $\pm$ 0.4 ng/ml. Lymphocytotoxic antibody titers peaked (at 1:512) two months after completion of skin allografting; at this time there was a 12-fold increase in PGE to 21.5$\pm$7.5 ng/ml. After this peak, lymphocytotoxin titers fell, reaching 1:8 at 4 months and becoming undetectable at 2 years. PGE levels fell in parallel; concentrations averaged 12.1 $\pm$ 4.0 and 1.6 $\pm$ 0.3 ng//ml at 4 months and 2 years, respectively. The correlation coefficient for these two variable averaged 0.76 (p<0.001).

Having demonstrated that the rejection phenomenon and its immunologic manifestations were associated with a dramatic increase in PGE levels, it became important to determine if the released prostaglandin was protective or destructive. This question was clearly answered in a study (Anderson et al., 1977), in which skin allografts were performed between B10.D female mice (recipient) and (B10.BR x B10.D$_2$) F1 donors. The mice were divided into six groups : control - i.p. diluent; 16,16-dimethyl-PGE$_2$-methyl ester (di-M-PGE$_2$), a long-acting synthetic analog of PGE - 5μg i.p. daily; di-M-PGE$_2$ plus indomethacin - 100μg i.p. thrice weekly; indomethacin alone - 100μg i.p. thrice weekly; indomethacin - 150 μg i.p.; and indomethacin, 200μg i.p. All doses of indomethacin caused significant inhibition of PGE$_2$ biosynthesis, and the effect was dose-related. The results are displayed in table 2.

Table 4. The effect of di-M-PGE$_2$ and indomethacin on plaque-
forming cells (PFC/10^7 spleen cells).

	4 days	7 days
Tumor + diluent	0.20±0.01[a](5)[b]	0.33±0.05 (8)
Tumor + di-M-PGE$_2$	1.01±0.23 (5)	0.81±0.06 (7)
Tumor + indomethacin	0.31±0.04 (4)	0.26±0.04 (4)
Normal + diluent	0.80±0.08 (5)	0.95±0.08 (5)
Normal + indomethacin	0.99±0.07 (2)	1.01

[a]Data represent the ratio of PFC at the time and experimental
condition specified to control PFC from normal mice.
[b]In breackets = no. of animals.

The PGE$_2$ analog clearly prolonged skin allograft survival,
suggesting that the exogenous prostaglandin was immunosuppressive.
On the other hand, indomethacin-induced inhibition of endogenous
prostaglandin biosythesis resulted in significant and dose-related
shortening of graft survival; their viability was shorter than
those of control grafts. This observation suggested that endogenous PGE played a role in allograft survival and that endogenous-
ly synthesized PGE was protective and immuno-suppressive.

3. STUDIES WITH TUMOR-BEARING MICE

We have previously reported that di-M-PGE$_2$ inhibited the rate
of B-16 melanoma and Friend erythroleukemia growth both "in vivo"
and "in vitro" (Santoro et al., 1976, 1977, 1979) and that this
drug potentiated the effects of a number of chemotherapy regimens
(Hofer et al., 1980). Although we documented a dose dependent
inhibition of the mitotic index (Santoro et al., 1977) one
possible mechanism of this tumor inhibitory action was thought to
be an effect on immunoregulation. Consequently, a number of
studies were initiated to evaluate this possibility (Santoro et
al., 1976).

Table 5. The effect of Di-M-PGE$_2$ and indomethacin on the delayed hypersensitivity response (mm).

Treatment	4 days	7 days	10 days
Tumor control	0.2+0.1	0	0.1+0.1
Di-M-PGE$_2$	0.2+0.1	0.1+0.1	0
Indomethacin	0.6+0.2	1.1+0.3	0.7+0.2
Positive control	1.7+0.2 mm		

Fifty mice were inoculated with 10^5 viable B-16 cells and a comparable number were injected with cell-free diluent.The tumor-bearing and normal animals were randomized into di-M-PGE$_2$ ($10\mu g$/day i.p.) or control groups. Mice were challenged with 10^8 sheep erythrocytes (sRBC) in 0.2 ml saline i.p. and hemagglutinin titers (Sever, 1962), plaque-forming cells (Cunningham and Szenberg, 1968) and delayed hypersensitivity (Bonta and de Vos, 1965) measured using standard techniques. The results of these studies are summarized in Tables 3-5. There were consistent observations for each of these determinations of immunologic parameters: 1) the presence of tumor alone resulted in significant immunosuppression; 2) di-M-PGE$_2$ restored immunoresponsiveness in the tumor-bearing animals while indomethacin either was further suppressive or had no effect at all; and 3) in the normal animals di-M-PGE$_2$ was mildly suppressive while indomethacin was totally inactive.

In order to attempt to separate the immunologic effects of di-M-PGE$_2$ from the tumor-inhibitory ones, a series of pretreatment experiments were performed. Ten mice were treated with di-M-PGE$_2$ on the day before inoculation with 10^5 B-16 melanoma tumor cells subcutaneously. A similar control group was pretreated with control diluent. After inoculation, none of the mice were treated. The rates of tumor appearance, of tumor growth (measured by calipers) and of survival were monitored. The pretreated mice fared remarkably well; pretreatment delayed the mean tumor appearance time (12 days vs. 3 for control), slowed growth (90% of the tumors were to small to be measured, and improved median survival (35 vs. 27 days). Since these changes were induced before the ani-

Table 6. The effect of PGA_1 on the immune response of B-16 melanoma-bearing mice.

	Plaque-forming cells ($PFC/10^7$ spleen cells)	Hemagglutinin titers($1/Log_2$)	Delayed hypersensitivity response(mm)	
			24 hours	48 hours
Normal mice				
Control	92.19+1.50	6.29+0.48	2.2+0.2	2.3+0.1
PGA_1	89.70+1.25	6.75+0.36	2.0+0.3	2.1+0.2
Tumor-bearing mice (7 days)				
Control	41.27+4.18	6.17+0.33	0.6+0.2	0.9+0.2
PGA_1	68.32+8.3	6.17+0.42	1.0+0.2	1.5+0.1
Tumor-bearing mice (11 days)				
Control	2.15+0.16	1.60+0.54	–	–
PGA_1	10.60+1.45	3.60+0.54	–	–

mals were inoculated with the tumor, the data strongly suggested that the "in vivo" effects of di-M-PGE_2 were modulated by the immune system.

Since we demonstrated that PGA_1 caused antitumor effects similar to those described above for di-M-PGE_2, we also characterized the effects of this prostaglandin on the immune response in mice bearing B-16 melanoma tumors (Sever, 1962). The results, identical to those for di-M-PGE_2, are displayed in Table 6.

We also used the skin allograft model to characterize tumor--immuno-suppressed animals. In normal mice, PGA_1 (10 μg i.p. daily for seven days) did little to alter mean graft survival (Table 7). As anticipated, the presence of tumor (animals were inoculated 7 days earlier with 10^5 B-16 cells) induced immunosuppression manifest by a prolongation of mean graft survival; this effect was partially overcome by treatment with PGA_1 (Favalli et al., 1980).

These studies suggested that prostaglandins were slightly suppressor in normal mice, but restored the immune response in

Table 7. The effect of PGA_1 on skin allograft survival.

	Number of animals	Median graft survival
Normal mice		
Control	7	9.00 ± 0.82
PGA_1	7	8.63 ± 0.23
Tumor-bearing mice		
Control	6	10.33 ± 1.24
PGA_1	7	9.57 ± 1.17

animals that were already immunosuppressed. Two additional experiments have confirmed the difference in PGE_2 effect, in immunological suppressed mice.

In the first of these studies, adriamycin (7.5 mg/kg) was utilized as immunosuppressive agent. The effects of di-M-PGE_2-treatment of these mice are characterized in Table 8. As anticipated, adriamycin was potently immunosuppressive and this effect was substantially reversed by the simultaneous treatment with di-M-PGE_2. In contrast, in the control mice, di-M-PGE_2 alone had a mild intrinsic immunosuppressive effect.

Table 8. The effect of di-M-PGE_2 on adriamycin-treated mice.

	$PFC/10^6$ spleen cells	Hemagglutinin $(1/Log_2)$
Control (n=5)	680 ± 147	3.2 ± 0.9
Di-M-PGE_2 (n=5)	562 ± 144	4.6 ± 0.8
Adriamycin (n=5)	115 ± 20	1.0
Adriamycin plus Di-M-PGE_2	347 ± 27	3.0 ± 0.7

Table 9. The effect of splenectomy and Di-M-PGE$_2$ on B-16 tumor growth in vivo.

	Total viable cells $(\times 10^6)$	Tumor weight(g)	Diameters (mm)	Plating efficiency.
Control (n=13)	9.6±1.4	1.66±0.22	13.0±0.7	107.7± 4.6
Splenectomy (n=9)	16.1±3.1	2.41±0.32	14.6±1.0	117.0±14.4
Splenectomy plus Di-M+PGE$_2$ (n=13)	10.4±2.8	1.39±0.22	11.7±0.8	95.2± 7.6

In the second set of studies, splenectomy (performed 7 days prior to inoculation with tumor cells) was utilized to induce immunosuppression, which was manifested by the acceleration of the rate of B-16 tumor growth. In this group of experiments, Treatment of thymectomized animals with di-M-PGE$_2$ essentially normalized the rates of tumor growth (Table 9).

4. CONCLUSIONS

The data which initially seemed contradictory, are now totally consistent. Prostaglandins have antagonistic effect on normal animals (in which they are immunosuppressive) and in immunosuppressed mice (where they restored immunocompetence). The mechanism of these differentially effect are not known but are currently being worked out.

ACKNOWLEDGMENTS

This work was supported in part by Grant CH 103A from the American Cancer Society, by Grant 80.00451.04 from the C.N.R. in conjunction with the National Science Foundation U.S.A. - Italy Cooperative Program in Science, and the Foundation for Surgical Education and Investigation.

REFERENCES

Anderson, C.B., Newton, W.T., and Jaffe, B.M., 1975, Circulating Pro-
    staglandin E and Allograft Rejection, Transplantation, 19:527.
Anderson, C.B., Jaffe, B.M., and Graff, R.J., 1977, Prolongation of
    Murine Skin Allografts by Prostaglandin E1 , Transplantation,
    23:444.
Bonta, I.L., and de Vos, C.J., 1965, The Effect of Estradiol 16,17-
    Dihemisuccinate on Vascular Permeability as Evaluated in the Rat
    Paw oedema Test, Acta Endocrinol., 49:403.
Cunningham, A.J. and Szenberg, A., 1968, Further Improvements in
    the Plaque Technique for Detecting Single Antibody-Forming
    Cells, Immunol., 14:599.
Favalli, C., Garaci, E., Etheredge, E.E., Santoro, M.G., and Jaffe,
    B.M., 1980, Influence of PGE on the Immune Response in Melanoma-
    Bearing Mice, J. Immunol.,125:897.
Favalli, C., Garaci, E., Santoro, M.G., Santucci, L., and Jaffe, B.
    M., The Effect of PGA$_1$ on the Immune Response in B-16 Melanoma-
    Bearing Mice, Prostaglandins, 19:587.
Hofer, D., Dubitsky, A.M., and Jaffe, B.M., 1980, Prostaglandin Poten-
    tiation of the Effect of chemotherapy on B-16 Melanoma, Surg.
    Forum, 31:417.
Jaffe, B.M., Parker, C.W., Marshall, G.P., and Needleman, P., 1972,
    Renal Concentrations of Prostaglandins in Acute and Chronic Re-
    nal Ischemia, Biochem. Biophys. Res. Comm, 49:799.
Jaffe, B.M., Behrman, H.R., and Parker, C.W., 1973, Radioimmunoassay
    Measurement of Prostaglandins E, A, and F in Human Plasma, J.
    Clin. Invest, 52:398.
Jaffe, B.M., and Moore, T.C., 1974, Elevation in Prostaglandin E
    Activity of Rat Heart Allograft Coronary Sinus Venous Blood,
    IRCS Med. Sci, 2:1417.
Jaffe, B.M., Moore, T.C., and Vigran, T.S., 1975, Tissue levels of
    Prostaglandin E Following Heterotopic Rat Heart Allografting.,
    Surgery, 78:481.
Mittal, K.K., Mickey, M.R., Singal, D.P., and Terasaki, P.I., 1968,
    Serotyping for Homotransplantation. XVIII. Refinement of Micro-
    droplet Lymphocyte Cytotoxicity Test, Transplantation, 6:913.
Moore, T.C., and Jaffe, B.M., 1974, Prostaglandin E levels of Hetero-
    topic Rat Heart Allografts and Host lymphoid Tissues at Inter-
    vals Postgrafting, Transplantation, 18:383.
Ono, K., and Lindsey, E.S., 1969, Improved Technique of Heart Tran-
    splantation in Rats, J. Thoracic Cardiovasc. Surg, 57:225.
Santoro, M.G., Philpott, G.W., and Jaffe, B.M., 1976, Inhibition of

Tumor Growth "in vivo" and "in vitro" by Prostaglandin E_2, Nature, 263:777.

Santoro, M.G., Philpott, G.W., and Jaffe, B.M., 1977, Inhibition of B-16 Melanoma Growth "in vivo" by a Synthetic Analog of Prostaglandin E_2, Cancer Res., 37:3774.·

Santoro, M.G., Philpott, G.W., and Jaffe, B.M., 1977, Dose Dependent Inhibition B-16 Melanoma Growth "in vivo" by a synthetic Analogue of PGE_2 , Prostaglandins, 14:645.

Santoro, M.G., and Jaffe, B.M., 1979, Inhibition of Friend and Erythroleukaemia-Cell Tumors "in vivo" by a Synthetic Analogue of Prostaglandin E_2, Brit. J. Cancer, 319:408.

Sever, J.L., 1962, Application of Microtechnique to Viral Serologic Investigations, J. Immunol., 88:320.

BEHAVIORAL CONDITIONING AND IMMUNITY

Robert Ader

Department of Psychiatry, University of Rochester
School of Medicine and Dentistry
Rochester, New York 14642

1. INTRODUCTION

Modern investigators no longer think of a central nervous system and an endocrine system, but of an integrated neuro-endocrine system. In the same way, a growing body of experimental data suggests that one cannot think of an immune system that is independent of other biologic processes that function to maintain or restore homeostatic balance. While it has generally been assumed that (or, at least, immunologists have behaved as if) the immune system is an autonomous agency of defense, this is no longer a tenable assumption. Converging evidence, from immunology, neuroendocrinology, neurophysiology pharmacology and psychology indicate that the immune system, like any other system operating in the interests of homeostasis, is integrated with other physiological processes and is therefore subject to regulation or modulation by the brain (Ader, 1981a).

Much of the evidence for an integrated network of neuroendocrine-immune system interactions has been described in previous chapters dealing with anatomical and neurochemical and functional connections between the central nervous system, the endocrine system and the immune system. These studies suggest that considerable information is being transmitted in all possible directions. It is left for me, then, to point out and attempt to document the potential impact of behavioral factors in immuno-regulation. What follows is a brief overview of some relevant literature and illustrative studies of conditioning effects.

1.1. Behavioral Factors and Susceptibility to Disease

A part of the existing literature relevant to behavioral factors in immunoregulation describes the effects of psychosocial factors (or "stress") on the predisposition to or on the precipitation and/or perpetuation of disease processes that are thought to involve immunologic competence. To the extent that some cancers may have a viral etiology. I would refer you to an extensive review of studies in humans by Fox (1981) and reviews of the animal literature prepared by La Barba (1970) and Riley et al.(1981). Experientially, the manipulation of early life experiences (Ader and Friedman, 1965 a,b; La Barba et al., 1970 a,b; Levine and Cohen, 1959; Otis and Scholler, 1967), social factors (Ader and Friedman, 1964; Andervont, 1944; De Chambre and Gosse, 1973; Kaliss and Fuller, 1968; Lemonde, 1959; Sklar and Anisman, 1980) and noxious stimulations such as electric shock or conditioning procedures (Amkraut and Solomon, 1972; Kavetsy et al., 1966; Marsh et al., 1959; Newberry et al., 1972; Plaut et al., 1980; Rashkis, 1952) or, conversely, the minimization of environmental disturbances (Riley et al., 1981) can influence the development and/or the response to spontaneously developing or experimentally-induced neoplastic disease in animals. Also, the capacity to cope with (stressful) environmental circumstances can attenuate tumor growth and mortality (Sklar and Anisman, 1979).

Abundant clinical, mostly retrospective evidence documents a relationship between "life change" or "stress" and a variety of (immunologically mediated?) disease processes (Gunderson and Rahe, 1974; Plaut and Friedman, 1981). Both susceptibility to (Jacobs et al., 1970; Kasl et al., 1979; Meyer and Haggerty, 1962) and recovery from (Greenfield et al., 1959; Imboden et al., 1961) infectious diseases have been related to life stresses in humans. Similar data exists for allergic conditions (Engels and Wittkower, 1975) and for autoimmune disorders (Solomon, 1981). Again, most of the experimental data have been obtained from animals.

Stimulation that is usually referred to as "stressful" has been shown to increase susceptibility to herpes simplex (Rasmussen et al.,1957), Coxsackie B (Johnson et al.,1959), polyoma (Chang and Rasmussen, 1965), and vesicular stomatitis (Jensen and Ras-

mussen,   1963;   Yamada et al., 1964) viruses in mice. Paralleling a
clinical   paradigm   (Holmes   et   al.,   1951),   Friedman et al. (1965)
found   that neither stress nor an inoculation of Coxsackie B virus,
alone,   was   sufficient   to   induce disease in adult mice. However,
the   combination   of   stress   and inoculum could elicit symptoms of
disease.

With   respect   to   parasitic infection, fighting (Weinmann and
Rothman,   1967) and exposure to a predator (Hamilton, 1974) decreased   the resistance to H. nana in direct proportion to the frequency   of the stress experience. In contrast, resistance to P. berghei
is   increased   when   rats   are subjected to stressful environmental
regimens   (Friedman   et   al., 1973). Increased resistance to polio-
myelitis   has   been   found to follow avoidance conditioning in monkeys   (Marsh   et   al., 1963), and physical restraint (but not a cold
bath)   suppresses   development   of experimental allergic encephalomyelitis in rats (Levine et al., 1962).

This   diversity in findings is further illustrated in the case
of   autoimmune disease. Amkraut et al. (1971) found that "crowding"
increased   susceptibility to adjuvant-induced arthritis in the rat.
Using   a   collagen-induced arthritis, Rogers et al. (1980) observed
an   increased   resistance among rats exposed to a cat. In contrast,
they   also   found   that   auditory stress would exacerbate the incidence of this autoimmune disorder (Rogers et al., 1981).

It   seems clear from this illustrative survey that the variety
of   environmental   manipulations   and   the   variety   of   pathologic
processes   that   have   been studied yield a seemingly contradictory
pattern   of results that preclude definitive generalizations regarding   the   effects   of   "stress." In addition to the several, undoubtedly   different,   stimulus   conditions, that are labelled as being
"stressful,"   the   observed increases and/or decreases in the incidence   of   disease would appear to depend upon the pathogen and the
response measure chosen for analysis.

1.2. Stress and Immunologic Reactivity

Attention   has   also   been directed to the effects of "stress"
on   some   parameter of immunologic competence, per se. A variety of
genetically   and   experientially determined host factors, influence
immunologic   reactivity   as   measured   by   a variety of assays that

reflect different specific and non specific immune defense mechanisms. Age, for example, is a major factor determining immunologic
competence (Makinodan and Yunis, 1977; Yunis et al., 1976).
Nutritional factors, especially during early development (Gross
and Newberne, 1980), are also relevant for an analysis of stress
effects in terms of both undernutrition (Holm and Palmblad, 1976;
Palmblad, 1976; Palmblad et al., 1977a) and obesity (Palmblad et
al., 1977b). Sleep deprivation has also been used to assess the
effects of "stress" on immune responses (Palmblad, 1981).
The death of a spouse reflects a common and particularly stressful
experience. Bartrop et al. (1977) noted that bereavement was accompanied by a depression in lymphocyte function that was independent of the hormonal responses that were also measured. These
observations have been repeated by Schleifer et al.(1980). Recently, several other programs have been initiated to explore the
relationship between stressful life events and coping styles and
immunologic competence, i.e. lymphocyte cytotoxicity, natural killer cell activity (Dorian et al., 1981; Greene et al., 1978; Locke
et al., 1978; Roessler et al., 1979). Preliminary results suggest
that high "stress scale scores", combined with unsuccessful coping
skills, are correlated with depressed immunologic defenses.

Studies in animals (Monjan, 1981) have found increases as
well as decreases in immunologic reactivity following a variety of
"stressful" experiences. Repeated sampling procedures have uncovered a biphasic response: first a depression and then an increase
in the lymphocyte response to mitogenic stimulation (Folch and
Waksman, 1974; Monjan and Collector, 1976). Gisler et al. (1971)
found suppressed activity in splenic lymphocytes obtained from
mice subjected to acceleration or anesthetization, the effect
being a function of the animals' strain. These "in vitro" effects
could be mimicked by ACTH (Gisler and Schenkel-Hulliger, 1971),
but neither Gisler nor Solomon (Solomon et al., 1979) were able to
reproduce "in vivo" effects by ACTH treatment.

In response to a topically applied irritant, electric shock
has been reported to increase immunologic reactivity in guinea
pigs (Guy, 1952; Mettrop and Visser, 1969). By using mice, others
(Christian and Williamson, 1958; Funk and Jensen, 1967; Smith et
al., 1960) have reported that auditory stimulation reduces the
inflammatory response. Pitkin (1965) observed a reduced hypersensitivity response in mice exposed to high temperature, and
Wistar and Hildemann (1960) observed prolonged survival of a skin

allograft in mice subjected to an avoidance conditioning regimen. A depressed graft-vs-host response was also observed among animals subjected to a limited feeding schedule (Amkraut et al., 1973).

Avoidance conditioning reduces the severity of anaphylactic responses (Rasmussen et al., 1959). This result is usually attributed to stress-induced elevations in adrenocortical steroid levels. Contrary to their expectations, however, these authors found that, depending upon challenge dose, individually housed mice were more resistant to anaphylaxis than animals housed in groups (Treadwell and Rasmussen, 1961).

A variety of noxious stimuli and, again, social factors have been shown to increase or decrease primary and secondary humoral responses to different antigens in several species (Edwards et al., 1980 ; Glenn and Becker, 1969 ; Hill et al., 1967 ; Joasoo and McKenzie, 1976; Solomon, 1969; Vessey, 1964). Pavlidas and Chirigos (1980) have reported that macrophages from immobilized mice show a decreased non specific tumoricidal activity. In another recent study (Keller et al., 1981) rats were either kept in their home cages, placed into an experimental apparatus, or placed into the apparatus and subjected to low or high intensity electric shock. There was a progressively greater suppression of lymphocyte function corresponding to increases in the degree of stress. Early life experiences, which can chronically alter behavioral and physiologic reactivity, have also been shown to influence animals' subsequent immunologic reactivity (Michaut et al., 1981; Monjan and Mandell, 1980; Solomon et al., 1968).

Psycho-social or stressful environmental circumstances are evidently capable of affecting humoral and cell mediated immune responses "in vitro" and "in vivo". These environmentally-induced alterations in immunologic competence are presumably mediated by neuroendocrine changes or responses to "stressful" events. Like the data on disease susceptibility, there is little uniformity to the results obtained thus far. In general, the impact of psycho-social or stressful events on immune function is determined by several major factors including the quality and quantity of environmental stimulation, the quality and quantity of immunogenic stimulation, the myriad host factors (e.g., age, diet, circadian rhythmicity, etc.), upon which psycho-social events and immunogenic stimuli are superimposed, the temporal relationship between stress and immunogenic stimulation, procedural factors such as the nature of the dependent variable and sampling parameters, and the interaction among any or all such factors. Reviews of many of these aspects of the behavioral effects on the immune system can be found in Ader (1981a) and Solomon and Amkraut (1981).

1.3. Conditioning Studies

The use of behavioral conditioning techniques is probably the oldest experimental approach to the study of the relationship between the central nervous system and the immune system. The first such studies were conducted more than 50 years ago by Metal'nikov and Chorine (1926). Under normal conditions, for example, peritoneal exudate is comprised primarily of mononuclear leukocytes. The introduction of antigen results in a rapid increase in the number of polynucleated cells. Metal'nikov and Chorine attempted to condition this response. Guinea pigs were subjected to repeated pairings of intraperitoneal injections of foreign material and specific external (conditioned) stimuli. After a rest period to allow the peritoneal exudate to return to normal, the conditioned stimulus was presented without the injection of antigen. Within five hours of antigenic stimulation, 90% of the peritoneal exudate consisted of polynucleated cells. In response to the conditioned stimulus, this same animal showed an increase in polynucleated cells from 0.6 to 62% within five hours. Other guinea pigs showed similar responses.

These original observations on conditioned leukocyte reactions were confirmed by several other investigators (Benatato, 1955; Diacono, 1933; Nicolau and Antinescu-Dimitriu, 1929; Ostravskaya, 1930; Podkopaeff and Saatchian, 1929; Riha, 1955; Ul'yanov, 1953; Vygodchikov and Barykini, 1927). Other non-specific defense mechanisms such as phagocytosis (Golovkova, 1947; Hadnagy and Kovats, 1954; Pel'ts, 1955; Strutsovskaya, 1953), complement (Berezhnaya, 1956; Dolin et al., 1960), and lysozyme activity (Gasanov, 1953) were also shown to be influenced by conditioning.

Metal'nikov and Chorine (1928) were also the first to report that the repeated association of a presumably neutral conditioned stimulus with antigenic stimulation resulted in an increase in specific antibody titer when the neutral stimulus was subsequently presented alone. These observations have been confirmed under a variety of experimental circumstances, with a variety of antigens

(bacterial, cellular, viral, anatoxic), and in different species
(Luk'ianenko, 1961). A detailed review of this early Soviet
research has been provided elsewhere (Ader, 1981b).

2. THE CONDITIONING PARADIGM

The experimental protocol used in our studies of conditioned
immunopharmacologic effects is based on a simple, extremely effective paradigm referred to as taste aversion learning (Garcia et
al., 1974). In this passive avoidance situation, consumption of a
novel, distinctively flavored drinking solution may be followed by
the injection of a pharmacologic agent that induces a transient
gastrointestinal upset. Water deprived rats, for example, might be
offered a novel sodium saccharin drinking solution, the conditioned stimulus (CS), and injected with any of several drugs with
noxious gastrointestinal effects, the unconditioned stimulus (US).
After a single pairing of the CS and the US, animals will avoid
drinking that flavored solution when it is subsequently presented
alone or when the animal is given a choice between the flavoured
solution and plain water (a preference test). Moreover, avoidance
of the CS solution can be observed even if it is not offered to
the animal until three months after the conditioning trial. Since
the ability to form rapid associations between gustatory cues and
gastrointestinal consequences has obvious survival value for the
individual, it is not surprising that taste aversion learning is a
highly reproducible experimental phenomenon.

Another relevant feature of this experimental paradigm is
that learned preferences for distinctively flavored drinking solutions can be established on the basis of their association with
recovery from illness or with drugs that correct experimentally-
-induced deficiency states (Garcia et al., 1967; Soughers and
Etscorn, 1980; Spasrenborg et al., 1981; Zahorik et al., 1974).

The essential features of our experimental procedures are
outlined in Table 1. Individually caged rats or mice are first
adapted to drinking their total daily allotment of water during a
single 15- or 30-min. period, at the same time each day. On the
training day, animals are randomly divided into conditioned, non
conditioned, and placebo groups. Conditioned animals are provided
with a 0.1-0.15% solution of sodium saccharin in tap water (the
CS) instead of plain water and immediately thereafter they are

Table 1. Experimental protocol

Group	Adaptation	Conditioning Day (treatment)	Antigenic stimulation		Days after antigen .....+n
			Sub-group	treatment	
Conditioned	H_2O	SAC + CY	US	H_2O + CY	Samples
	(15-30 min)		CSo	H_2O -	Samples
			CS	SAC + SAL	Samples
Non-conditioned[a]	H_2O	H_2O + CY	NC	SAC -	Samples
	(15-30 min)				
Placebo	H_2O	H_2O or SAC + SAL	P	H_2O or SAC	Samples

[a]Non conditioned animals received saccharin drinking solution one day after CY injection.

injected i.p. with cyclophosphamide (CY). Non conditioned animals also receive a saccharin drinking solution and an i.p. injection of CY, but these stimuli are not paired; they are introduced on different days. Placebo animals receive plain water (or saccharin) and are injected with saline. Some time after conditioning (from 3 days to 7 weeks in different experiments), all animals are exposed to antigenic stimulation.

Coincidental with the injection of antigen (e.g., sheep erythrocytes), previously conditioned animals are randomly divided into three sub-groups. Group US is provided with plain water and again injected with CY in order to define the unconditioned immunosuppressive effects of the drug. Group CS is also provided with plain water to drink and is included to control for the effects of prior conditioning, per se. Group CS, the critical experimental group, is re-exposed to the conditioned stimulus on one or more occasions on or following the day of antigen treatment, i.e., is provided with the saccharin-flavored drinking solution and injected i.p. with saline. Non conditioned (NC) animals are provided with the saccharin drinking solution on whatever schedule applies to animals in Group CS. Placebo-treated

animals receive either plain water or saccharin during the regu-
larly scheduled drinking periods.

Immunologic reactivity is measured at one or more times following antigenic stimulation. All assays are performed according
to standard procedures and without knowledge of the group to which
an animal belongs.

3. CONDITIONED IMMUNOPHARMACOLOGIC RESPONSES

3.1. Conditioned Suppression of Humoral Response

The following pattern of results was predicted on the basis
of an hypothesized conditioning of immunosuppresion: Placebo-
-treated animals without prior CY treatment would show relatively
high hemagglutinating antibody titers in response to the injections of SRBC. In contrast, NC rats and those conditioned animals
that were not re-exposed to the saccharin drinking solution (Group
CSo) were expected to have relatively high antibody titers but,
because of the CY, injected on the training day, they were expected to show slightly lower titers than animals in Group P. Conditioned animals treated with CY at the same time that antigen was
injected (Group US) were expected to show a minimal antibody
response. The critical experimental group, conditioned animals
that were re-exposed to saccharin at the time of antigen stimulation (Group CS) were expected to show an attenuated antibody
response relative to NC and CSo animals.

Our initial findings (Ader and Cohen, 1975), based on
antibody titers measured six days after treatment with SRBC,
conformed precisely to the predicted relationship among the
several groups (Figure 1). Placebo-treated animals had the highest
antibody titers and CY, administered at the time of antigenic stimulation, suppressed antibody production. Non conditioned animals
and conditioned animals that were not re-exposed to the CS did not
differ; both groups had lower antibody titers than placebo-treated
animals. This difference presumably reflects the residual effects
of CY. Conditioned animals that were re-exposed to the CS on the
day of antigenic stimulation or three days later (Group CS1), or
re-exposed to the CS on both of these days (Group CS2), had
antibody titers that were significantly lower than the titers in
Groups NC and CSo. These results, then, were taken as evidence of

a conditioned immunosuppressive response. Published studies by
Rogers et al. (1976) and Wayner et al. (1978) have confirmed this
phenomenon (Figure 1).

In my own laboratory, the phenomenon of conditioned immunosuppression has been replicated under a variety of circumstances.
Changing the CS, for example, still results in a conditioned
response. Increasing the dose of CY from 50 to 75 mg/kg alters the
kinetics of antibody production, and a conditioned immunosuppressive effect is observed eight days rather than six days after
treatment with SRBC. An attenuated antibody response is observed
in conditioned animals that are re-exposed to the CS even when the
interval between conditioning and antigenic stimulation is increased (in order to reduce the residual immunosuppressive effects
of CY), or when a preference procedure rather than a forced exposure to the CS is used (in order to equate fluid consumption among
the experimental and control groups). The details of these experiments are described elsewhere (Ader and Cohen, 1981). Although
the magnitude of the effect is not large, conditioned immunosuppression is a highly consistent phenomenon.

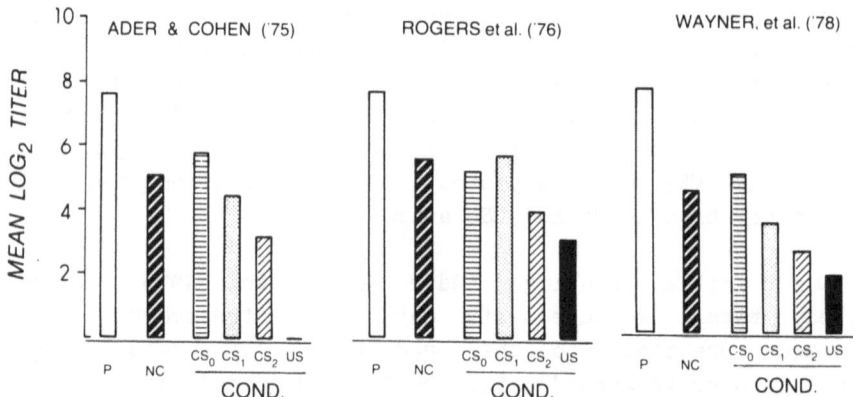

Fig. 1. Hemagglutinating antibody titers (mean + SEM) measured six
days after injection of SRBC. NC = non conditioned rats;
CSo = conditioned animals that were not re-exposed to the
CS after antigen treatment; CS1 = conditioned animals re-
-exposed to the CS on one occasion; CS2 = conditioned animals re-exposed to the CS on two occasions; US = conditioned rats treated with CY at the time of antigenic stimulation; P = placebo-treated animals. From Ader (1981c), reprinted by permission of Pergamon Press.

Wayner et al. (1978) were able to repeat our results using SRBC, but they did not observe a conditioned immunosuppressive response in rats exposed to Brucella abortus, a thymus independent antigen. Any one of several interacting procedural variables might account for the lack of an effect since we have been able to demonstrate the phenomenon using a T-cell independent system. In these experiments (Cohen et al., 1979), BDF1 mice were treated in much the same manner as the rats in previous experiments. Mice, however, received 200 or 300 mg/kg CY on the conditioning day and the interval between conditioning and antigenic stimulation was two weeks. All mice were injected with 50 μg of the hapten 2,4,6-trinitrophenol coupled to the thymus independent carrier lipopolysaccharide (TNP-LPS). The results of two experiments varied with the dose of CY and other procedural innovations, but conditioned mice that were re-exposed to the CS showed lower antibody titers than controls.

As a reflection of immunologic responsivity, antibody titer is the result of a complex chain of events which, at any of several levels, might be influenced by the neuroendocrine changes that accompany a conditioned response or that are the direct effect of conditioning (Ader, 1976). Under certain circumstances, high levels of adrenocortical steroids can be immunosuppressive. It was therefore hypothesized that the depressed antibody response observed in conditioned animals resulted from a conditioned elevation in corticosterone level. Studies designed to evaluate this possibility (Ader and Cohen, 1975; Ader et al., 1979), however, failed to confirm the hypothesis. Like CY, lithium chloride (LiCl) is an effective unconditioned stimulus for inducing a taste aversion and will unconditionally elicit an adrenocortical response. LiCl is not immunosuppressive, however, and animals conditioned with LiCl instead of CY do not show an immunosuppressive response to SRBC. In experiments conducted to examine the possibility that an elevation in steroid level, superimposed upon the residual immunosuppressive effects of CY, might be responsible for the conditioning effect, additional groups of conditioned rats were injected with LiCl or corticosteroids instead of being re-exposed to the CS previously paired with CY. Neither of these circumstances attenuated antibody titer relative to NC or CSo groups, whereas conditioned animals, that were re--exposed to the CS again, showed an attenuated antibody response. These results, therefore, provide no support for the hypothesis that the conditioned immunosuppressive response is mediated by an experimentally-induced differential elevation of corticosterone.

3.2. Conditioned Suppression of a Graft-vs-Host Response

The generality of conditioned immunosuppression is further extended by our observations that the phenomenon applies to a cell-mediated as well as humoral responses (Bovbjerg et al., 1982). To accomplish this, we capitalized upon a report by Whitehouse et al. (1973), that multiple low doses of CY could suppress a popliteal graft-vs-host (GvH) response if the drug was injected on the day of and the two days following injection of splenic lymphocytes. In a preliminary experiment we repeated the results of Whitehouse et al. and established that a single low dose injection of CY was only moderately immunosuppressive and was not sufficient to approximate the effects of three low dose injections. Our conditioning study, then, was predicated on the possibility that a single low dose of CY in conjunction with repeated re-exposure to a CS, previously paired with CY , would suppress a GvH response to a greater extent than a single injection of CY alone.

In this study, rats were conditioned by pairing saccharin consumption with 50 mg/kg CY 48 days before grafting. Recipient Lewis x Brown Norwegian hybrid females were initially divided into conditioned, non conditioned, and placebo groups. On the test day (Day 0), all rats were injected into a hind footpad with a suspension of splenic leukocytes obtained from female Lewis donors. The critical group of conditioned animals (Group CSr) was treated as follows: On Day 0 they were re-exposed to the CS (in a preference testing procedure) and injected ip with saline; on Day 1 they were re-exposed to the CS and injected ip with 10 mg/kg CY; on Day 2 they were re-exposed to the CS and injected with saline. As in previous studies, there was another conditioned group that was not re-exposed to the CS, but these animals did receive the single injection of 10 mg/kg CY on Day 1. Also, a US group was injected with CY on Days 0, 1, and 2, to define the unconditioned response to the immunosuppressive treatment. Non conditioned animals were, as in previous studies, exposed to saccharin and CY according to the schedule that applied to the experimental group.

The data are shown in Figure 2. Injections of 10 mg/kg CY on

Days 0, 1, and 2 (Group US) suppressed the GvH response relative to placebo-treated animals, replicating, again, the results of Whitehouse et al. (1973). A single low dose injection of CY caused only a slight attenuation of the response; that is, non-conditioned animals did not differ from the placebo group but Group CSo did show a lower node weight response that Group P. The control groups that received a single low dose injection of CY did not differ and showed a greater GvH response than animals that received three injections of CY (Group US). In contrast, animals that received a single low dose injection of CY and re-exposure to the saccharin drinking solution previously paired with CY showed a suppressed GvH response. Stimulated lymph nodes, harvested from Group CSr, weighed significantly less than those from NC and CSo

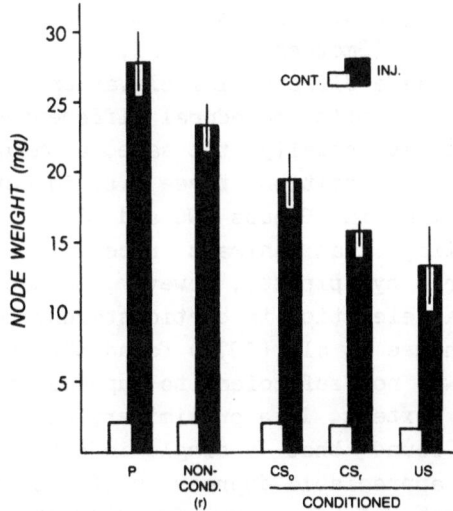

Fig. 2. Popliteal lymph node weights determined five days after inoculation with splenic leukocytes. Values for injected and contralateral footpads are given for placebo-treated rats; for non conditioned (NCr) animals exposed to a single low dose of CY administered one day after the cellular graft, and for conditioned animals given a single low dose of CY and provided with plain water (CSo), conditioned animals given a single low dose of CY and re-exposed to the CS on Days 0, 1, and 2 after the cellular graft (CSr), and conditioned animals given three low dose injections of CY (on Days 0, 1, and 2) and provided with plain water. From Ader and Cohen (1981), reprinted by permission of Academic Press.

animals. There was no significant difference in lymph node weight between Group CSr and the animals that received three injections of CY.

The physiological mechanisms underlying the conditioned suppression of a GvH response have yet to be determined. Elevated adrenocortical steroid levels would not seem to be involved in the conditioned suppression of humoral responses, but that possibility can not be completely excluded in the case of a GvH response. Conditioning may have involved effects on host cells, donor cells, or both, and although the initiating donor cells are resistant to changes in the level of circulating corticosterone, it has been shown (Cohen and Claman, 1971) that the treatment of recipients with hydrocortisone reduces splenomegaly. Steroid levels were not measured in our experiment, but it has been reported that the use of a preference testing procedure does not differentially influence corticosterone level (Smotherman et al., 1976). Also, it is not likely that there was a differential elevation in steroid levels attributable to non specific procedural differences. The handling of all animals was essentially the same, although experimental animals did receive, in addition, three i.p. injections (compared to one i.p. injection in Groups NC and CSo). This stimulation added to the handling that animals received in administering saccharin (or water) by pipette, however, is not likely to have caused a differential elevation in corticosterone level (Cohen and Crnic, 1982). Whitehouse et al. (1973) found that three injections of 1 or 3 mg/kg CY was not sufficient to suppress the GvH response to any appreciable extent. In a preliminary experiment (Bovbjerg et al., 1982) we found that a single injection of 10 mg/kg CY would not cause an appreciable depression of the GvH response and that three injections of 5 mg/kg CY did not suppress the GvH response any more than a single injection of 10 mg/kg CY. It is unlikely, therefore, that, in the absence of conditioning, additional ip injections of saline would suppress the GvH response.

3.3. Conditioned Suppression in the Chemotherapy
    of Systemic Lupus Erythematosus

We have recently initiated studies to assess the impact of conditioned immunosuppressive responses in New Zealand mice (Ader and Cohen, 1982). These studies are aimed at determining the effect of conditioning within a biological model and in determi-

ning the applicability of conditioning procedures to the regulation and control of immunologic disorders. The female NZBxNZW F1
mouse has become a standard experimental model for systemic lupus
erythematosus (Steinberg et al., 1981; Talal, 1976; Theofilopoulos
and Dixon, 1981). These animals develop a lethal glomerulonephritis between approximately 8 and 14 months of age. Weekly treatment
with cyclophosphamide, however, delays the onset of proteinuria
and prolongs survival (Casey, 1968; Hahn et al., 1975; Lehman et
al., 1976; Morris et al., 1976; Russell and Hicks, 1968; Steinberg
et al., 1975). Based on the above studies indicating that immune
responses could be suppressed by conditioning procedures, it was
hypothesized that the substitution of conditioned stimuli for
immunosuppressive drug, might delay the development of systemic
lupus erythematosus (SLE) in conditioned animals relative to non
conditioned animals that were treated with the same amount of
drugs.

When NZBxNZW F1 females were four months old, an 8-week
chemotherapeutic regimen was begun. On one day of each week all
animals were given a 0.15% solution of sodium saccharin in tap
water by pipette (up to a maximum of 1.0 ml). Cyclophosphamide (30
mg/kg) treatment was administered according to the following
schedule:

Group C100 was treated on a traditional chemotherapeutic
regimen. That is, CY was injected once each week immediately after
the mice drank a saccharin solution. This occurred at the same
time and on the same day of each week. As expected, this dosage of
CY and this duration of chemotherapy was effective in prolonging
survival but was not sufficient to prevent the ultimate development of autoimmune disease in these mice.

Group C50 also received saccharin administered at the same
time and on the same day of each week. For these conditioned
animals, however, CY injections followed exposure to saccharin
only half the time; on 2 of every 4 weeks, these animals received
an i.p. injection of saline instead of CY. In effect, these
conditioned mice were treated under a partial reinforcement
schedule; saccharin consumption was pharmacologically reinforced
on only 50% of the occasions when saccharin was administered.

Group NC50 was a non conditioned group that received the same
weekly exposures to saccharin and the same number of CY and saline

injections as Group C50. For these animals, however, the CY (or saline) injections were not paired with comsumption of saccharin; the taste stimulus and pharmacologic stimulus were presented on different days of the same week.

A control group received no CY. These animals did, however, receive weekly exposure to saccharin and saline injections on a non contingent basis.

Non conditioned animals that received only half the total amount of CY administered under the traditional therapeutic schedule were expected to show symptoms of disease and die sooner than animals treated weekly and somewhat later than animals that were not treated at all. Animals in Group C50 were also treated with half the amount of drug given to animals in Group C100. If, however, the pairing of saccharin and CY is capable of eliciting a conditioned immunosuppressive response, one would predict that Group C50 would develop SLE at a slower rate than non conditioned

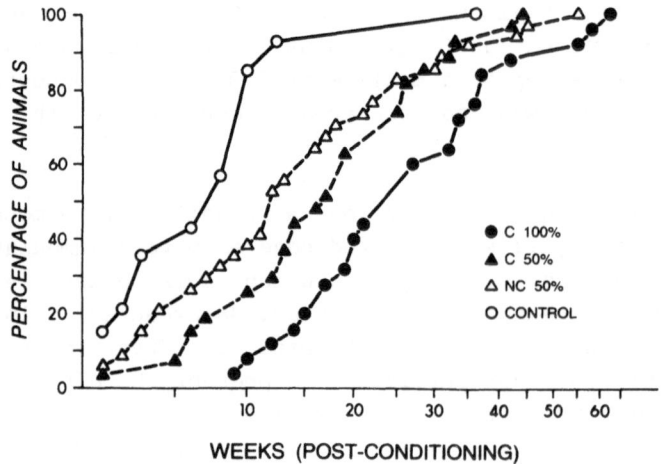

Fig. 3. Rate of development of an unremitting proteinuria in NZBxNZW F1 female mice under different chemotherapeutic regimens. Group C100 (N = 25) received weekly presentations of saccharin followed by ip injection of 30 mg/kg CY; Group C50 (N = 27) received weekly presentations of saccharin with injection of CY following saccharin on 2 of every 4 weeks; Group NC50 (N = 34) received weekly presentations of saccharin and unpaired injections of CY on 2 of every 4 weeks; Control mice (N = 14) received weekly presentations of saccharin but no CY. From Ader and Cohen (1982), reprinted by permission of Science.

mice treated with exactly the same number and distribution of CY injections. This is precisely what happened.

Weekly treatment with CY delayed the onset of proteinuria and prolonged survival in these NZBxNZW mice. Considering the entire population of animals that developed autoimmune disease (Figure 3), there was a significant difference in the development of an unremitting proteinura. When all animals can be expected to develop disease and die, the longer one follows the progression of disease, the less likely it is to discriminate statistically among differentially treated groups. As can be seen in Figure 4, differences among these groups are especially dramatic when one considers the development of SLE using as a point of reference the rate of development of proteinuria in the initial 50% of the animals to develop disease. Group C100 developed proteinuria later than the groups treated with half the amount of drugs or no drug. Group NC50 did not differ significantly from untreated control animals. Group C50, however, developed proteinuria significantly later than untreated controls and non conditioned animals treated with the same amount of CY.

Essentially the same results were observed with respect to mortality. While there was an overall difference among the total population of animals (Figure 5), the differences are especially

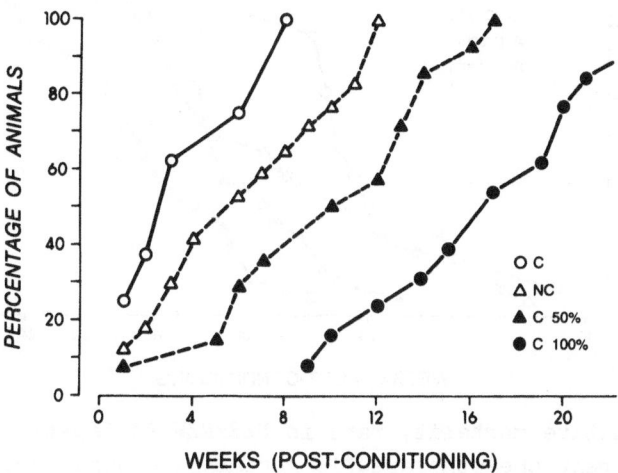

Fig. 4. Time required for 50% of differentially treated NZBxNZW F1 female mice to develop an unremitting proteinuria. Group designations are the same as in Fig. 3.

apparent when one considers the rate at which the first half of
each group died (Figure 6). In this case, animals treated with CY
weekly differed significantly from untreated controls and from
Group NC50. Group NC50 did not differ significantly from untreated
animals, but conditioned animals that received the same amount of
drug survived significantly longer than untreated controls and non
conditioned animals. The difference between Groups C50 and C100
was not statistically significant.

The results of this study were precisely based on the
hypothesis that the pairing of saccharin consumption and CY
injection would enable saccharin, acting as a CS, to suppress
immunologic reactivity and thereby delay the onset of SLE under a
chemotherapeutic regimen that was not, in itself, sufficient to
influence the development of autoimmune disease. As such, these
observations constitute further elaboration of conditioned immunopharmacologic effects and document the biologic impact of conditioned immunosuppressive responses.

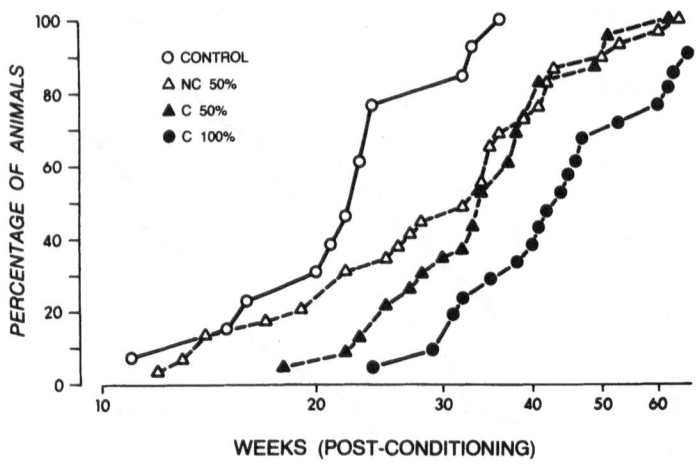

Fig. 5. Cumulative mortality rate in NZBxNZW F1 female mice following
different chemotherapeutic regimens. Groups C100 (N = 21),
C50 (N = 23), NC50 (N = 29), and Control (N = 13) are defined as in Fig. 3. From Ader and Cohen (198), reprinted by
permission of Science.

4. DISCUSSION

It was hypothesized that the pairing of a neutral, gustatory stimulus with the immunosuppressive effects of a pharmacologic agent would enable the neutral or conditioned stimulus to suppress the immune response to antigenic stimulation i.e., immunopharmacologic responses could be conditioned. Using a one-trial passive avoidance conditioning paradigm, consumption of a novel, distinctively flavored drinking solution, saccharin, was paired with an injection of an immunosuppressive drug, cyclophosphamide. When rats or mice were subsequently treated with SRBC, a T-cell dependent antigen, or TNP-LPS, a T-cell independent antigen, conditioned animals that were re-exposed to the saccharin drinking solution showed attenuated antibody responses relative to conditioned animals, that were not reexposed to the conditioned stimulus and non conditioned animals that were exposed to saccharin. These observations of conditioned immunosuppression have been repeated in our laboratory under a variety of experimental conditions (Ader and Cohen, 1981) and by others (Rogers et al., 1976; Wayner et al., 1978).

The generality of these findings is further illustrated in

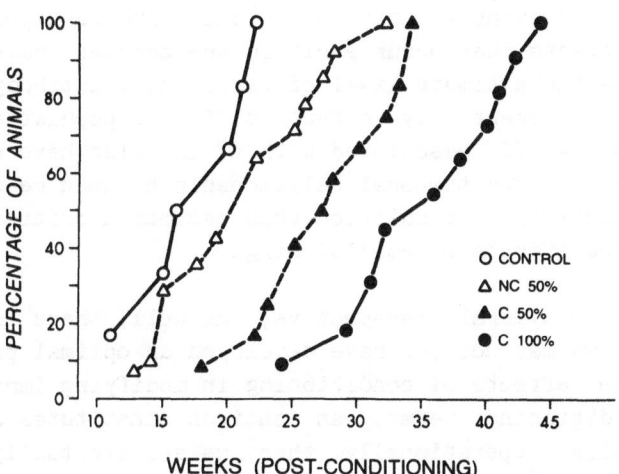

Fig. 6. Rate at which a 50% mortality is reached in differentially treated NZBxNZW F1, female mice. Group designations are the same as in Fig. 3.

the conditioned suppression of a cell-mediated immune response. Forty-eight days after pairing saccharin consumption with an injection of CY, re-exposure of conditioned animals to the CS effected a significant reduction of a GvH response.
By extending the impact of conditioned immuno-pharmacologic responses from the humoral responses previously demonstrated to a cell-mediated reaction, these results significantly expand upon the potential of the brain to regulate or modulate immunologic reactivity.

It would appear, then, that conditioned immunosuppression is a highly reproducible phenomenon and, although the effects of conditioning on antibody responses are relatively small, the biologic effects are clearly demonstrable.
Incorporating conditioning techniques (and, presumably, conditioned immunosuppressive responses) within an immuno-pharmacotherapeutic regimen for the treatment of systemic lupus erythematosus in New Zealand mice, a delay in the onset of proteinuria and mortality was accomplished using an amount of drug that would normally be minimally effective in modifying the development of autoimmune disease.

From an immunological perspective, hemagglutinating antibody titers measured several days after antigenic stimulation may not be the most sensitive index of the effects of conditioning. It may be presumed, for example, that conditioning and re-exposure to the CS exerts effects that occur early in the complex chain of events that determine the ultimate level of circulating antibody.
Besides, CY differentially affects different populations of lymphocytes and a CS associated with CY may also have such differential effects. The temporal relationship between re-exposure(s) to a CS and antigenic stimulation thus becomes a critical issue in determining the effects of conditioning.

From a behavioral perspective, as well, there is reason to believe that we may not yet have developed an optimal paradigm for assessing the effects of conditioning in modifying immune responses. In conditioning terms, an antigen constitutes an unconditioned stimulus. Operationally, then, we are eventually pairing a conditioned stimulus for suppression of antibody production with an unconditioned stimulus for initiation of that very same response.

This descriptive analysis of our current paradigm is consistent with the data thus far available and is discussed in greater detail elsewhere (Ader and Cohen, 1981). It should be noted here, though, that this analysis suggests that a potentiation of immunologic reactivity might constitute a more sensitive model in which to explore conditioned immunopharmacologic effects.

As indicated above, the physiological mechanisms mediating conditioned humoral or cell-mediated responses remain to be determined. At this point, we assume that the effects of conditioning are mediated by neuroendocrine changes influencing afferent, central, and/or efferent immune processes.

The direct and indirect evidence for anatomical and neurochemical innervetion of lymphoid organs, receptors for hormones and neurotransmitters on lymphocytes, endocrine involvement in immune responses and autoimmune disorders (and vice versa), and the myriad host factors (age, sex, nutritional state, circadian rhythmicity, etc.) that influence immunologic reactivity provide compelling evidence for a "dynamic flow of information" among the central nervous system, the endocrine system, and the immune system. Based on these data (described by Goldstein, Talal, Sorkin, Besedovsky, Spector and others elsewhere in this volume), there would appear to be multiple neuroendocrine pathways that might profitably be explored in analyzing the documented effects of behavioral factors in immunoregulation.

ACKNOWLEDGEMENTS

The research described in this chapter was supported by a USPHS Research Scientist Award (K05-MH-06318) from the National Institute of Mental Health (RA) and a Research Career Development Award (K04-AI-70736) from the National Institute of Allergic and Infectious Diseases (to N.C.) and by research grants from the W.T. Grant Foundation, the National Institute of Child Health and Human Development (HD-09977), the National Institute of Neurological and Communicative Disorders and Stroke (NS-15071)and the Kroc Foundation.

Cyclophosphamide was generously supplied by the Mead Johnson Research Center, Evansville, Indiana, U.S.A.

REFERENCES

Ader, R., 1976, Conditioned adrenocortical steroid elevations in the
    rat, J. Comp. physiol. Psychol, 90:1156.
Ader, R. Ed., 1981a, "Psychoneuroimmunology," Academic Press, New
    York.
Ader, R., 1981b, An historical account of conditioned immunobiologic
    responses, in: "Psychoneuroimmunology," R. Ader, ed., Academic
    Press, New York, p. 321.
Ader, R., 1981c, The central nervous system and immune responses:
    Conditioned immunopharmacologic effects, in: "Advances in Immu-
    nopharmacology," J. Hadden, L. Chedid, P. Mullen, and F. Sprea-
    fico, eds., Pergamon Press, Oxford, p. 427.
Ader, R., and Cohen, N., 1975, Behaviorally conditioned immuno-sup-
    pression, Psychosom. Med., 37:333.
Ader, R., and Cohen, N., 1981, Conditioned immunopharmacologic re-
    sponses, in: "Psychoneuroimmunology," R. Ader, ed., Academic
    Press, New York, p. 281.
Ader, R., and Cohen, N., 1982, Behaviorally conditioned immunosup-
    pression and murine systemic lupus erythematosus, Science, Vol.
    215, p. 1534-1536.
Ader, R., Cohen, N., and Grota, L.J., 1979, Adrenal involvement in
    conditioned immunosuppression, Int. J. Immunopharmac., 1:141.
Ader, R., and Friedman, S.B., 1964, Social factors affecting emotio-
    nality and resistance to disease in animals: IV. Differential
    housing, emotionality, and Walker 256 carcinosarcoma in the rat,
    Psychol. Rep., 15:535.
Ader, R., and Friedman, S.B., 1965a, Differential early experiences
    and susceptibility to transplanted tumor in the rat, J. Comp.
    Physiol. Psychol., 59:361.
Ader, R., and Friedman, S.B., 1965b, Social factors affecting emotio-
    nality and resistance to disease in animals: V. Early separa-
    tion from the mother and response to a transplanted tumor in the
    rat, Psychosom. Med., 27:119.
Amkraut, A.N., and Solomon, G.F., 1972, Stress and murine sarcoma
    virus (Moloney)-induced tumors, Cancer Res., 32:1428.
Amkraut, A.N., Solomon, G.F., Kasper, P., and Purdue, P., 1973,
    Stress and hormonal intervention in the graft-versus-host re-
    sponse, in: "Microenvironmental Aspects of Immunity," B.D. Jan-
    kovic and K. Isakovic, eds., Plenum, New York, p. 667.
Amkraut, A.N., Solomon, G.F., and Kraemer, H.C., 1971, Stress, early
    experience and adjuvant-induced arthritis in the rat, Psychosom.
    Med., 33:203.

Andervont, H.B., 1944, Influence of environment on mammary cancer
    in mice, J. Nat. Cancer Inst., 4:579.
Bartrop, R.W., Lazarus, L., Luckhurst, E., Kiloh, L.G., and Penny,
    R., 1977, Depressed lymphocytes function after bereavement,
    Lancet., i:834.
Benetato, G.R., 1955, Le mechanisme nerveux central de la reaction
    leucocytaire et phagocytaire, J. Physiologie, 47:391.
Bereznykh, D.V., 1955, On the question of conditioned reflex resto-
    ration of immunogenesis, Bull. Exp. Biol. Med., 40:49.
Bovbjerg, D., Ader, R., and Cohen, N., 1982, Behaviorally conditio-
    ned immunosuppression of a graft-vs-host response, Proc. Natl.
    Acad. Sci., in press.
Casey, T.P., 1968, Immunosuppression by cyclophosphamide in NZB/NZW
    mice with lupus nephritis, Blood, 32:436.
Chang, S., and Rasmussen, A.F. Jr., 1965, Stress-induced suppression
    in interferon production in virus-infected mice, Nature,
    205:623.
Christian, J.J., and Williamson, H.O., 1958, Effect of crowding on
    experimental granuloma formation in mice, Proc. Soc. Exp. Biol.
    Med., 99:385.
Cohen, J.J., and Claman, H.N., 1971, Hydrocortisone resistance of
    activated initiator cells on graft-versus-host reactions, Natu-
    re, 229:274.
Cohen, J.J., and Crnic, L.S., 1982, Glucocorticoids, stress and the
    immune response, in: "Immunopharmacology," D.R. Webb, Jr., ed.,
    Marcel Dekker, New york, in press.
Cohen, N., Ader, R., Green, N., and Bovbjerg, D., 1979, Conditioned
    suppression of a thymus-independent antibody response, Psycho-
    som. Med., 41:487.
DeChambre, R.P., and Gosse, C., 1973, Individual versus group caging
    of mice with grafted tumors, Cancer Res., 33:1401.
Diacono, H., 1933, Le phenomene hemolytique: Contribution a l'etude
    de l'hemolyse: XI. Reflexes conditionnels et hemolyse, Arch.
    Inst. Pasteur, Tunis, 22:376.
Dolin, A.O., Krylov, V.N., Luk'ianenko, V.I., and Flerov, B.A., 1960,
    New experimental data on the conditioned reflex reproduction
    and suppression of immune and allergic reactions, Zh. vyssh,
    nerv. Deyatel., 10:832.
Dorian, B.J., Keystone, E., Garfinkel, P.E., and Brown, G.M., 1981,
    Immune mechanisms in acute psychological stress, Psychosom.
    Med., 43:84.
Edwards, E.A., Rahe, R.H., Stephens, P.Mand Henry, J.P., 1980, Anti-
    body response to bovine serum albumin in mice: The effects of

psychosocial environmental change, <u>Proc. Soc. Exp. Biol. Med.</u>, 164:478.

Engels, W.D., and Wittkower, E.D., 1975, Psychophysiological allergic and skin disorders, <u>in</u>: "Comprehensive Textbook of Psychiatry, II," A.M. Freedman, H.J. Kaplan and B.J. Sadock, eds., Williams and Wilkins, Baltmore, p. 1685.

Folch, H., and Waksman, B.H., 1974, The splenic suppressor cell: Activity of thymus dependent adherent cells: Changes with age and stress, <u>J. Immunol.</u>, 113:127.

Fox, B.H., 1981, Psychosocial factors and the immune system in human cancer, <u>in</u>: "Psychoneuroimmunology," R. Ader, ed., Academic Press, New york, p. 103.

Friedman, S.B., Ader, R., and Glasgow, L.A., 1965, Effects of psychological stress in adult mice inoculated with Coxsackie B viruses, <u>Psychosom. Med.</u>, 27:361.

Friedman, S.B., Ader, R., and Grota, L.J., 1973, Protective effect of noxious stimulation in mice infected with rodent maleria, <u>Psychosom. Med.</u>, 35:535.

Funk, G.A., and Jensen, M.M., 1967, Influence of stress on granuloma formation, <u>Proc. Soc. Exp. Biol. Med.</u>, 124:653.

Garcia, J., Ervin, F.R., Yorke, C.H., and Koelling, R.A., 1967, Conditioning with delayed vitamine injections, <u>Science</u>, 155:716.

Garcia, J., Hankina, W.G., and Rusiniak, K.W., 1974, Behavioral regulation of the milieu interne in man and rat, <u>Science</u>, 185:824.

Gasonov, G.T., 1953, Experimental data on the study of the effect and excretion of lysozyme, unpublished dissertation.

Gisler, R.H., Bussard, A.E., Mazie, J.C., and Hess, R., 1971, Hormonal regulation of the immune response: I. Induction of an immune response in vitro with lymphoid cells from mice exposed to acute systemic stress, <u>Cell. Immunol.</u>, 2:634.

Gisler, R.H., and Schenkel-Hulliger, L., 1971, Hormonal regulation of the immune response: II. Influence of pituitary and adrenal activity on immune responsiveness in vitro, <u>Cell. Immunol.</u>, 2:646.

Glenn, W.G., and Becker, R.E., 1969, Individual versus group housing in mice: Immunological response to time-phased injections, <u>Physiol. Zool.</u>, 42:411.

Golovkova, I.N., 1947, The influence of nociceptive and conditioned reflex stimulation on phagocytic capability or leukocytes in the organism, <u>Bull. Eksp. Biol. Med.</u>, 24:268.

Greene, W.A., Betts, R.F., Ochitill, H., Niker, H.P., and Douglas, R.G., 1978, Psychosocial factors and immunity: Preliminary report, Psychosom. Med., 40.

Greenfield, N.S., Roessler, R., and Crosley, A.P., 1959, Ego strength and length or recovery from infectious mononucleosis, J. Nerv. Ment. Dis., 128:125.

Gross, R.L., and Newberne, P.M., 1980, Role of nutrition in immunologic function, Physiol., Rev., 60:188.

Gunderson, E.K., and Rahe, R.H., 1974, "Life Stress and Illness", Thomas, Springfield, Illinois.

Guy, W.B., 1952, Neurogenic factors in contact dermatitis, Arch. Dermatol. Syphil., 66:1.

Hadnagy, C.S., and Kovts, I., 1954, Die rolle der hirnrinde bei den veranderungen der fahigkeit des serums zur stimulation der phagozytose, Acta. Physiol. Acad. Hung., 5:325.

Hahn, B.H., Knotts, L., Ng, M., and Hamilton, T.R., 1975, Influence of cyclophosphamide and other immuno-suppressive drugs on immune disorders and neoplasia in NZB/NZW mice, Arthr. Rheum., 18:145.

Hamilton, D.R., 1974, Immunosuppressive effects of predator induced stress in mice with acquired immunity to Hymenolepsis nana, Psychosom. Med., 18:143.

Hill, C.W., Greer, W.E., and Felsenfeld, O., 1967, Psychological stress, early response to foreign protein, and blood cortisol in vervets, Psychosom. Med., 29:279.

Holm, G., and Palmblad, J., 1976, Acute energy deprivation in man: Effect on cell-mediated immunological reactions, Clin. Exp. Immunol., 25:207.

Holmes, T.H., Treuting, T., and Wolff, H.G., 1951, Life situations, emotions and nasal disease: Evidence on summative effects exhibited in patients with "hay fever," Psychosom. Med., 13:71.

Imboden, J.B., Canter, A., and Cluff, L.E., 1961, Convalescence from influenza: A study of the psychological and clinical determinants, Arch. Int. Med., 108:393.

Jacobs, M.A., Spilken, A.Z., Norman, M.M., and Anderson, L.S., 1970, Life stress and respiratory illness, Psychosom. Med., 32:233.

Jensen, M.M., and Rasmussen, A.F., Jr., 1963, Stress and susceptibility to viral infection. I. Response of adrenals, liver, thymus, spleen and peripheral lymphocyte counts to sound stress, J. Immunol., 90:17.

Jensen, M.M., and Rasmussen, A.F., Jr., 1963, Stress and susceptibility to viral infections: II. Sound stress and susceptibility to vesicular stomatitis virus, J. Immunol., 90:21.

Joasoo, A., and McKenzie, J.M., 1976, Stress and the immune response in rats, Int. Arch. Allergy., 50:659.

Johnson, T., Lavender, J.F., and Marsh, J.T., 1959, The influence of avoidance learning stress on resistance to Coxsackie virus in mice, Fed. Proc., 18:575.

Kaliss, N., and Fuller, J.L., 1968, Incidence of lymphatic leukemia and methylcholanthrene-induced cancer in laboratory mice subjected to stress, J. Nat. Cancer Inst., 41:967.

Kasl, S.V., Evans, A.S., and Neiderman, J.C., 1979, Psychosocial risk factors in the development of infectious mononucleosis, Psychosom. Med., 41:445.

Kavetsky, R.E., Turkevitch, N.M., and Balitsky, K.P., 1966, On the psychophysiological mechanism of the organism's resistance to tumor growth, Ann N.Y. Acad. Sci., 125:933.

Keller, S.E., Weiss, J., Schleifer, S.J., Miller, N.E., and Stein, M.,1981, Suppression of immunity by stress: Effect of a graded series of stressors on lymphocyte stimulation in the rat, Psychosom. Med., 43:91.

La Barba, R.C., 1970, Experimental and environmental factors in cancer, Psychosom. Med., 32:259.

La Barba, R.C., Klein, M.L., White, J.L., and Lazar, J., 1970a, Effects of early cold stress and handling on the growth of Ehrlich carcinoma in BALB/C mice, Develop. Psychol., 2:312.

La Barba, R.C., White, J.L., Lazar, J., and Klein, M., 1970b, Early maternal separation and the response to Ehrlich carcinoma in BALB/C mice, Develop. Psychol., 3:78.

Lehman, D.H., Wilson, C.B., and Dion, F.J., 1976, Increased survival times of New Zealand hybrid mice immunosuppressed by graft-versus-host reactions, Clin. Exp. Immunol., 25:297.

Le Monde, P., 1959, Influence of fighting on leukemia in mice, Proc. Soc. Exp. Biol., Med., 102:292.

Levine, S., and Cohen, C., 1959, Differential survival to leukemia as a function of infantile stimulation in DBA/2 mice, Proc. Soc. Exp. Biol. Med., 102:53.

Levine, S., Strebel, R., Wenk, E.J., and Harman, P.J., 1962, Suppression of experimental allergic encephalomyelitis by stress, Proc. Soc. Exp. Biol. Med., 109:294.

Locke, S.E., Hurst, M.W., Heisel, J., and Williams, R.M., 1978, The influence of stress on the immune response, Paper presented at the annual meetings of the American Psychosomatic Society.

Luk'ianenko, V.I., 1961, The problem of conditioned reflex regulation of immunobiologic reactions, Usp. Sovrem. Biol., 51:170.

Mkinosi, T., and Yunia, E., 1977, "Immunology and Aging," Plenum, New York.

Marsh, J.T., Lavender, J.F., Chang, S., and Ramussen, A.F., Jr.,
    1963, Poliomyelitisin monkeys: Decreased susceptibility after
    avoidance stress, Science, 140:1415.
Marsh, J.T., Miller, B.E., and Lamson, B.G., 1959, Effect of repea-
    ted brief stress on growth of Erhlich carcinoma in the mouse,
    J. Natl. Cancer Inst., 22:961.
Metal'nikov, S., and Chorine, V., 1926, Role des reflexes condition-
    nels dans la formation des anticorps, Comp. Rendu Soc. Biol.,
    99:142.
Mettrop, P.J.G., and Visser, P., 1969, Exteroceptive stimulation as
    a contingent factor in the induction and elicitation of delayed-
    type hypersensitivity reactions to 1-chloro-, 2-4, dinitrobenze-
    ne in guinea pigs, Psychophysiol., 5:385.
Meyer, R.J., and Haggerty, R.J., 1962, Streptococcal infections in
    families: Factors altering individual susceptibility, J. Pediat.,
    29:339.
Michaut, R.J., De Chambre, R.P., Doumerc, S., Lesourd, B., Deville-
    chabrolle, A., and Moulias, R., 1981, Incluence of early mater-
    nal deprivation on adult humoral immune response in mice,
    Physiol. Behav., 26:189.
Monjan, A.A., 1981, Stress and immunologic competence: Studies in
    animals, in: "Psychoneuroimmunology," R. Ader, ed., Academic
    Press, New york, p. 185.
Monjan, A.A., and Mandell, W., 1980, Fetal alcohol and immunity: De-
    pression of mitogen-induced lymphocyte blastogenesis, Neurobe-
    hav. Toxicol., 2:213.
Morris, A.D., Esterly, J., Chase, G., and Sharp, G.C., 1976, Vycol-
    phosphamide protection in NZB/NZW disease, Arthritis. Rheum.,
    19:49.
Newberry, B.H., Frnkie, G., Beatty, P.A., Maloney, B.D., and Gilch-
    rist, J.C., 1972, Shock stress and DMBA-induced tumors, Psycho-
    som. Med., 34:295.
Nicolau, I., and Antinescu-Dimitriu, O., 1929, L'influence des refle-
    xes conditionnels sur l'exsudat peritoneal, Comp. Rendu Soc.
    Biol., 102:144.(b)
Ostravskaya, O.A., 1930, Le reflex conditionnel et les reactions de
    l'immunite, Ann. Inst. Pasteur, 44:340.
Otis, L.S., and Scholler, J., 1967, Effects of stress during infancy
    on tumor development and tumor growth, Psychol. Rep., 20:167.
Palmblad, J., 1976, Fasting in man: Effect on PMN granulocyte func-
    tion, plasma iron and serum transferrin, Scand. J. Haematol.,
    17:217.
Palmblad, J., 1981, Stress and immunologic competence: Studies in

man, in: "Psychoneuroimmunology," R. Ader, ed., Academic Press,
    New York, p. 229.
Palmblad, J., Cantell, K., Holm, G., Norberg, R., Stander, H., and
    Sundblad, L., 1977a, Acute energy deprivation in man: Effect of
    serum immunoglobulin, antibody response, complement factors
    3 and 4, acute phase reactants and interferon producing capacity
    of blood lymphocytes, Clin. Exp. Immunol., 30:50.
Palmblad, J., Hallberg, D., and Rossner, S., 1977b, Obesity, plasma
    lipids and polymorphonuclear (PMN) granulocyte functions, Scand.
    J. Haematol, 19:292.
Pavlidas, N., and Chirigos, M., 1980, Stress-induced impairment of
    macrophage tumoricidal function, Psychosom. Med., 42:47.
Pel'ts, D.G., 1955, The role of the cerebral cortex in the modifica-
    tions of phagocytic activity of blood leukocytes of animals from
    the application of electrocutaneous stimuli, Bull. Exp. Biol.
    Med., 40:55.
Pitkin, D.H., 1965, Effect of physiological stress on the delayed hy-
    persensitivity reaction, Proc. Soc. Exp. Biol. Med., 120:350.
Plaut, S.M., Esterhay, R.J., Sutherland, J.C., Wareheim, L.E., Fried-
    man, S.B., Schnaper, N., and Wiernik, P.H., 1980, Psychological
    effects on resistance to spontaneous AKR leukemia in mice, Psy-
    chosom. Med., 42:72.
Plaut, S.M., and Friedman, S.B., 1981, Psychosocial factors in infec-
    tious disease, in: "Psychoneuroimmunology," R. Ader, ed., Aca-
    demic Press, New York, p.3.
Podkopaeff, N.A., and Saatchian, R.L., 1929, Conditioned reflexes
    for immunity: I. Conditioned reflexes in rabbits for cellular
    reaction of peritoneal fluid, Bull. Battle Creek Sanit. Hosp.
    Clinic, 24:375.
Rashkis, H.A., 1952, Systemic stress as an inhibitor of experimental
    tumors in Swiss mice, Science, 116:169.
Rasmussen, A.F., Jr., Marsh, J.T., and Brill, N.C., 1957, Increased
    susceptibility to herpes simplex in mice subjected to avoidance-
    learning stress or restraint, Proc. Soc. Exp. Biol. Med., 96:183.
Rasmussen, A.F. Jr., Spencer, E.S., and Marsh, J.T., 1959, Decrease
    in susceptibility of mice to passive anaphylaxis following avoi-
    dance-learning stress, Proc. Soc. Exp. Biol. Med., 100:878.
Riha, I., 1955, A contribution to the question of conditioned reflex
    formation of antibodies, Folia Biol., 1:139.
Riley, V., Fitzmaurice, M.A., and Spackman, D.H., 1981, Psychoneuro-
    immunologic factors in neoplasia: Studies in animal, in: "Psy-
    choneuroimmunology," R. Ader, ed., Academic Press, New York,
    p. 31.

Roessler, R., Cate, T.R., Lester, J.W., and Couch, R.B., 1979, Ego strength, life events, and antibody titers, Paper presented at the annual meetings of the American Psychosomatic Society.

Rogers, M.P., Reich, P., Strom, T.B., and Carpenter, C.B., 1976, Behaviorally conditioned immunosuppression: Replication of a recent study, Psychosom. Med., 38:447.

Rogers, M.P., Treatham, D.E., McCune, W.J., Ginsberg, B.I., Rennke, H.G., Reich, P., and David, J.R., 1980, Effect of psychological stress on the induction of arthritis in rats, Arthritis. Rheum., 23:1337.

Rogers, M.P., Treatham, D.E., and Reicn, P., 1981, Modulation of collagen-induced arthritis by different stress protocols, Psychosom. Med., 42:72.

Russel, P.J., and Hicks, J.D., 1968, Cyclophosphamide treatment of renal disease in (NZBxNZW) F1 hybrid mice, Lancet, i:440.

Schleifer, S.J., Keller, S.E., McKegney, F.P., and Stein, M., 1980, Bereavement and lymphocyte function, Paper presented at the meeting of the American Psychiatric Association.

Sklar, L.S., and Anisman, H., 1979, Stress and coping factors influence tumor growth, Science, 205:513.

Sklar, L.S., and Anisman, H., 1980, Social stress and tumor growth, Psychosom. Med., 42:347.

Smith, L.W., Molomut, N., and Gottfried, B., 1960, Effect of subconvulsive audiogenic stress in mice on turpentine induced inflammation, Proc. Soc. Exp. Biol. Med., 103:370.

Smotherman, W.P., Hennessy, J.W., and Levine, S., 1976, Plasma corticosterone levels during recovery from LiCl produced taste aversions, Behav. Biol.,16:401.

Solomon, G.F., 1969, Stress and antibody response in rats, Int. Arch. Allergy, 35:97.

Solomon, G.F., 1981, Emotional and personality factors in the onset and course of autoimmune disease, particularly rheumatoid arthritis, in: "Psychoneuroimmunology," R. Ader, ed., Academic Press, New York, p. 159.

Solomon, G.F., and Amkraut, A.A., 1981, Psychoneuroendocrinological effects on the immune response, Ann. Rev. Microbiol., 35:155.

Solomon, G.F., Amkraut, A.A., and Rubin, R.T., 1979, Stress and psychoimmunological response, in:"Mind and Cancer Prognosis," B.A. Stoll, ed., Wiley, New York, p.73.

Solomon, G.F., Levine, S;, and Kraft, J.K., 1968, Early experience and immunity, Nature, 220:821.

Soughers, T.K., and Etscorn, F., 1980, A learned preference in the mouse using potassium deficiency as the induced need state,

Bull. Psychon. Soc., 16:62.

Sparenborg, S.P., Buskist, W.F., Miller, H.L., Jr., Fleming, D.E., and Duncan, P.C., 1981, Attenuation of taste-aversion conditioning in rats recovered from thiamine deficiency: Atropine vs. lithium toxicosis, Bull. Psycho. Soc., 17:237.

Steinberg, A.D., Gelfand, M.C., Gardin, J.A., and Lowenthl, D.T., 1975, Therapeutic studies in NZB/W mice: III. Relationship between renal status and efficiancy of immunosuppressive drug therapy, Arthritis. Rheum., 18:9.

Steinberg, A.D., Huston, D.P., Taurog, J.D., Cowdery, J.S., and Raveche, E.S., 1981, The cellular and genetic basis of murine lupus, Immunol. Rev., 55:121.

Strutsovkaya, A.L., 1953, An experiment on the formation of conditioned phagocytic reactions in children, Zh. Vyssh. Nerv. Deyatel., 3:238.

Talal, N., 1976, Disordered immunologic regulation and autoimmunity, Transplant. Rev., 31:240.

Theofilopoulos, A.N., and Dixon, F.J., 1981, Etiopathogenesis of murine SLE, Immunol. Rev., 55:179.

Treadwell, P.E., and Rasmussen, A.F., Jr., 1961, Role of the adrenals in stress-induced resistance to anaphylactic shock, J. Immunol. 87:492.

Ul'yanov, M.I., 1953, On the question of cortical regulation of the leukocyte composition of peripheral blood, Klin. Med., 31:52.

Vygodchikov, G.V., and Barykini, O., 1927, The conditioned reflex and protective cell reactions, J. Biol. Med. Exp. (Moscow), 6:538.

Wayner, E.A., Flannery, G.R., and Singer, G., 1978, Effects of taste aversion conditioning on the primary antibody response to sheep red blood cells and Brucella abortus in the albino rat, J. Comp. Physiol. Psychol., 21:995.

Weinmann, C.J., and Rothman, A.H., 1967, Effects of stress upon acquired immunity to the dwarf tapeworms Hymenolepsis nana, Exp. Parasitol., 21:61.

Whitehouse, M.W., Levy, L., nad Beck, F.J., 1973, Effect of cyclophosphamide on a local graft-versus-host reaction in the rat, Influence of sex, disease and different dosage regimens, Agents Actions, 3:53.

Wistar, R., Jr., and Hildemann, W.H., 1960, Effect of stress on skin transplantation immunity in mice, Science, 131:159.

Yamada, A., Jensen, M.M., and Rasmussen, A.F. Jr., 1964, Stress and susceptibility to viral infections: III. Antibody response and viral retention during avoidance learning stress, Proc. Soc.

Exp. Biol. Med., 116:677.

Yunis, E.I., Fernandes, G., and Greenberg, L.J., 1976, Tumor immunology, autoimmunity and aging, J. Amer. Geriat. Soc., 24:253.

Zahorik, D.M., Maier, S.F., And Pies, R.W., 1974, Preferences for
tastes paired with recovery from thiamine deficiency in rats:
Appetitive conditioning or learned satiety? J. Comp. Physiol.
Psychol., 87:1083.

NEUROENDOCRINE IMMUNOREGULATION

Hugo O. Besedovsky, Adriana del Rey and Ernst Sorkin

Swiss Research Institute, Medical Department
CH-7270 Davos, Switzerland

1. INTRODUCTION

Considerable advances have been made in understanding the cellular elements of the immune system, antibody structure, and the generation of antibody diversity at the genetic and somatic level. How immunological cells, antibodies and other cell products interact and how these interactions are regulated have now become major issues. In view of the enormous complexity of the immune system, it is hardly surprising that different levels of regulation exist such as antibody feedback, idiotypic-anti-idiotypic responses, suppressor and helper T-cells, lymphokine signals and genetic requirements. The common feature of these control mechanisms is that they are based on interactions involving elements of the immune system itself.

This characteristic attests to the autonomy of the immune system but leaves open the question of the limit of such autonomy. The most obvious limit is determined by the metabolic requirements of immunological cells, which as for all types of cells, are under control of hormones and neurotransmitters. In our view, however, control of metabolism is by no means the only influence of these agents upon immune cells. Therefore, we propose, that the CNS and the endocrine system impose another, more integrative level of regulation for the immune system.

Indeed, our findings support the hypothesis of the existence of immune-neuroendocrine circuits which are based on a dynamic

315

flow of information between the immune system and the endocrine and nervous systems.

As we shall show, signals emitted by activated immunological cells reach central structures resulting in neuroendocrine changes capable of affecting the course of the immune response.

2. MINIMAL REQUIREMENTS FOR NEUROENDOCRINE
CONTROL OF THE IMMUNE RESPONSE

There is no question that hormones and neurotransmitters are present within the micro- and macro-environment in which the immune response takes place. However, it is a pertinent question whether immunologic cells can "see" these agents and be influenced by them.

2.1. Lymphocytes and Accessory Cells Express Receptors for
Hormones and Neurotransmitters

An essential requirement for neuroendocrine control of the immune system is the presence of receptors for hormones and neurotransmitters on immunologic cells. In fact, receptors for corticosteroids (Cake and Litwack, 1975; Werb et al.,1978) insulin (Hollenberg and Cuatrecasas, 1974; Helderman and Strom, 1978), growth hormone (Arrenbrecht, 1975), oestradiol (Gilette and Gilette, 1979), testosterone (Abraham and Bug, 1976), β-adrenergic agents (Hollenberg and Cuatrecasas, 1974; Singh et al., 1979), and acetylcholine (Strom et al., 1974a; Richman and Arnason, 1979) have been demonstrated in lymphoid and accessory cells.

It seems a reasonable assumption that most of the effects of hormones and neurotransmitters at the cellular and subcellular levels are exerted via such receptors. β-adrenergic receptors and insulin receptors were found to appear in higher numbers in lymphocyte membranes only after their activation (Hollenberg and Cuatrecasas, 1974). This event helps to increase the sensitivity of lymphocytes towards these hormones when compared with unstimulated cells and may thereby modulate the magnitude of a given response. It will be important to eventually study the kinetics of appearance or modulation of hormonal receptors in the various subsets of lymphocytes.

2.2. Hormones and Neurotransmitters Interfer with Processes
      Essential for the Immune Response

There is agreement that several hormones and neurotransmitters influence a variety of cellular and subcellular processes
which are essential for the immune response, e.g. metabolism,
transport of substances and allosteric changes in membranes, lymphoid cell proliferation and transformation, lymphokine synthesis
(for refs. see Besedovsky and Sorkin, 1977a).

2.3. Common Immune-neuroendocrine Pathways Control Immunological
     Activation

Hormones and neurotransmitters can modulate, in lymphocytes
and accessory cells, the levels of intracellular nucleotide (cAMP,
cGMP), i.e. of messengers which are supposed to participate in the
process of lymphocyte activation. This subject is discussed in
detail by Hadden in this volume and by Hadden et al. (1975).

Such data attest to the existence of intracellular pathways
common to hormones and neurotransmitters on the one hand and antigens and signals intrinsic to the immune system on the other hand.

2.4. Interference with Neuroendocrine Functions Influences the
     Immune Response

Investigations on the participation of hormones in the immune
response have generally involved either the parenteral administration of hormones or the ablation or blockade of endocrine
glands. Numerous reports agree that hormone administration can
lead to depressed or stimulated immune responses depending on the
kind and dose of hormones and the timing of their administration.
In general, glucocorticoids, androgens, oestrogens, and progesterone depress the immune response "in vivo", whereas growth
hormone, thyroxine, and insulin increase the response.
It is beyond the scope of this presentation to review the vast literature on this subject. The reader may find the following papers
to be especially helpful (Billingham et al., 1951; Dougherty et
al., 1964; Wolstenhome and Knight, 1970; Claman, 1975; Fabris, 1977;
Besedovsky and Sorkin, 1977b). Work on thymic hormones is discussed
by A. Goldstein in this volume.

Data on the effects of mediators of the autonomic nervous system on the immune system are contradictory, but in the main they indicate that neurotransmitters can influence the immune response, both "in vitro" and "in vivo". Some of the previously obtained data on catecholamines have been discussed elsewhere (see Besedovsky et al., 1979a). Examples of manipulation of the sympathetic nervous system and its suppressive action on the immune system are described below.

Parasympathetic agents have been reported to increase antibody formation (Marat, 1974) and cytotoxicity (Strom et al., 1972, 1974b). In addition, direct manipulation of the brain can affect the immune response. Thus, electrolytic lesions or stimulation of different parts of the brain yielded results which were interpreted to influence the immune response either directly or by alterations of hormonal controls (Jankovic and Isakovic, 1973; Stein et al., 1976). Also, studies on effects of stress and conditioning showed that environmental stimuli can interfere with the immune response (see Ader, 1981 and this volume; Riley, 1981).

2.5. Immune-neuroendocrine Interactions Exist under Physiological and Pathological Conditions

Sex differences in the immune response are well documented and such differences are important in autoimmune diseases (Talal, 1977 and this volume). There are also well established examples of immune-endocrine interactions during ontogeny (for ref. see Besedovsky and Sorkin, 1977b). Disruption of these interactions at either the immunological or endocrine level produces simultaneous changes in both.
a) Absence of external antigenic challenge in germfree animals leads to alterations in immunological and endocrine development.
b) Endocrine deficiency, e.g. in hypopituitary dwarf mice leads to deficient cell-mediated immunity.
c) The thymus and bursa of Fabricius which control immune development are also involved in the maturation of several endocrine functions.

2.6. Do Neuroendocrine Influences Imply Immunoregulation?

The previously described facts show important neuroendocrine effects on immunity but in our view are not sufficient proof for immunoregulation.

Manipulations of neuroendocrine structures such as organ extirpation, denervation, administration of hormones or neuro-transmitters, brain lesions or stimulation are necessary to iden-tify neuroendocrine influences on the immune response which may or not be operative under physiological conditions. However, such procedures often represent extreme situations (e.g. injection of pharmacological doses of hormones) and may lead to definitive alterations in the host (e.g. endocrine gland extirpation).

Also the mentioned examples of immune-neuroendocrine inter-actions which occur over a protracted period of time, cannot be used as valid argument for intervention of hormones and neuro-transmitters in regulation of a phasic phenomenon such as the immune response.

Regulation requires a dynamic flow of signals between the parameters to be regulated and the regulatory agencies. Thus the signals are integrated in circuits which guide the system under regulation towards a given program. Attempts to analyse external immunoregulation must be based on knowledge of the circuitry between the immune system to be regulated and the neuroendocrine structures.

A physiological approach to analyse such links is to trigger the immune response by antigen and study changes in those para-meters which are thought to exert regulatory effects. After establishing such changes, the next step should be the characte-rization of the signals causing them. Such knowledge would orient us towards possible targets at the level of the neuroendocrine system or immune system at which regulation occurs.

3. IMMUNE-NEUROENDOCRINE CIRCUITS

3.1. Evidence for a Glucocorticoid Associated Immunoregulatory
     Circuit. Increased Blood Glucocorticosteroid Levels during
     the Immune response.

We have shown that during the primary immune response of rats to a particulate antigen, sheep red cells (SRBC), or to soluble

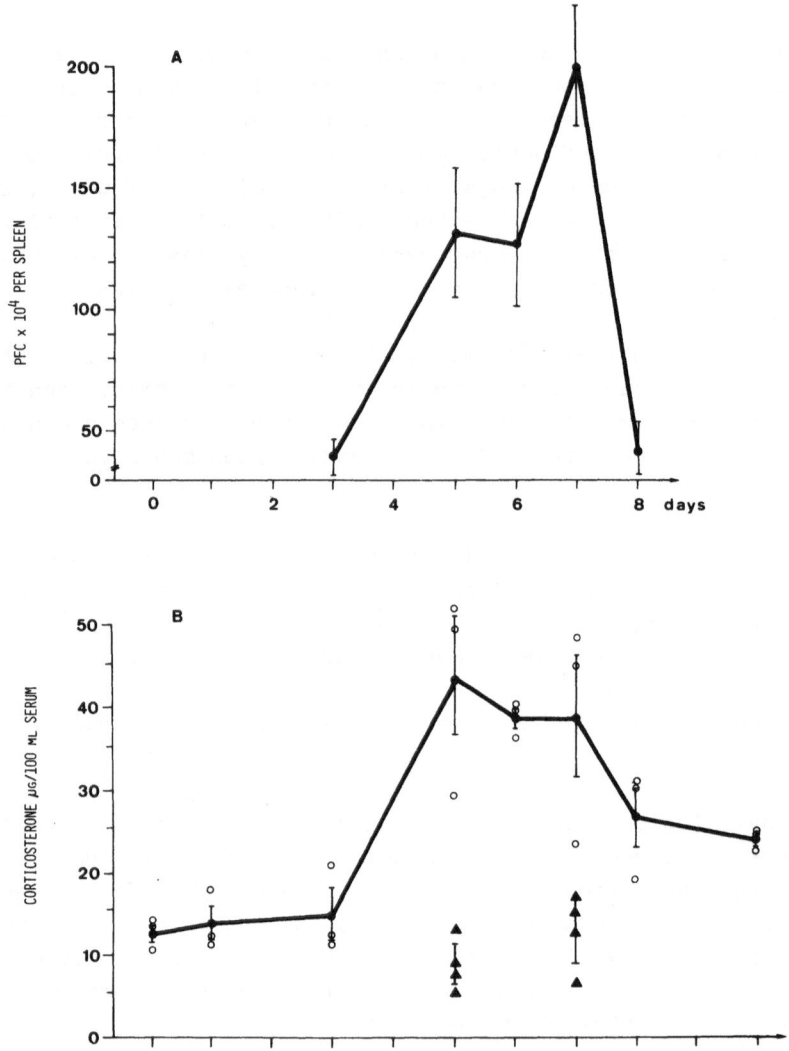

Fig. 1. Changes in serum corticosterone levels during the immune
response to sheep red cells (SRBC) in rats. (A) Plaque forming cells (PFC)x10^4 per spleen. (B) Corticosterone levels
in serum: animals immunized with SRBC:O, controls injected with rat red blood cells (RRBC):▲. Besedovsky, H.O.
et al., 1975. Reprinted by permission from Academy Press.

antigen, Trinitrophenyl-haemocyanin (TNP-Hae), and of mice to
TNP-horse red blood cells (TNP-HRBC), corticosterone levels
increased several fold.

Fig. 1 shows a two- to three-fold increase in serum corticosterone levels above normal at 5, 6, 7 or 8 days after injection
of 4×10^9 SRBC into female rats. No significant changes in the
serum corticosterone level occurred on days 1 and 3 after
immunization or at any time after injection of homologous red
cells, implying that the animals were not stressed by handling or
the injection of the cells.

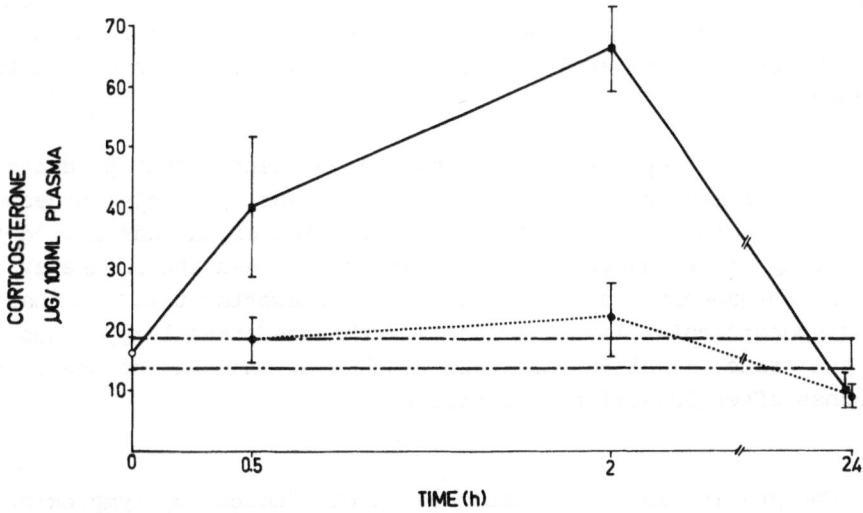

Fig. 2. Lymphokine containing supernatants from Con A-stimulated
rat spleen cells increase corticosterone blood levels in
rats. Female Holtzman rats received an i.p. injection of 1
ml of one of the following supernatants: ■ , supernatants
from Lewis rat spleen cells, stimulated with Con A.● , control supernatant: Con A was added only after the collection
of the supernatants. Plasma were obtained 0,5 hr, 2 h, or
24 hr after the injection of supernatants and corticosterone levels determined by RIA. Each point in the curve represents the mean ± SEM of plasma corticosterone values from 7
individual animals. O, mean of all controls. Besedovsky, et
al., 1981, reprinted by permission from J. Immunology.

3.2. Lymphokines Increase Glucocorticoid Blood Levels

The above experiments suggest that during the immune response
there is a flow of information from the immune system to
neuroendocrine structures. The nature of these messages remains
unknown but lymphokines (LK) released upon activation of immunocytes are likely candidates, particulary since some are present in
blood (Neta and Salvin, 1981). We found that administration of
lymphokine-containing supernatants from human peripheral blood
leukocytes or rat spleen cells, both stimulated with concanavalin
A (Con A) evoked in rats within 30 min to 2 hr a several-fold increase in corticosterone blood levels (Besedovsky et al., 1981)
(Fig. 2)The supernatants applied were tested for a variety of biological activites and shown to contain MIF, TCGF (IL2), mitogenic
activity and LAF (IL1). No change in blood pressure or body temperature was noted in lymphokine-injected animals. Our results with
lymphokines were recently confirmed in humans by Dumonde (see this
volume).

Our data represent the primary evidence that products of
activated lymphoid cells (lymphokines) and possibly accessory
cells (monokines) can affect the function of the adrenal cortex
reflecting interchange of information between the immune system
and neuroendocrine structures. It is noteworthy that the changes
in glucocorticoid levels induced by the preformed lymphokines are
of the same magnitude as those reached at the peak of the immune
response after injection of antigens.

3.3. Changes in Glucocorticosteroid Levels Induced by Lymphokines
     are Centrally Mediated

The site of lymphokine action responsible for increasing
corticosteroid blood levels was analysed. Lymphokines (LK) could
act either directly at the level of the adrenal cortex or
centrally via the pituitary-adrenal axis. That the increase of
blood corticosterone levels by LK is mediated centrally is
supported by the following:
a. After administration of LK containing supernatants, ACTH in
blood increased several fold, e.g. after 2 hrs control: $118,00^{\pm}$
$10,73$ pg/ml, LK injected: $314,75$ $^{\pm}39,61$ pg/ml.
b. In hypophysectomized (Hx) or dexamethasone treated rats the
effect of LK was abolished.

These results show that lymphokines operate through the pituitary gland, most likely via increased corticotrophin releasing factor (CRF) output from the hypothalamus. Whatever the nature of the lymphoid cell products involved, there appears to exist a flow of afferent signals to central structures.

3.4. Increased Glucocorticoid Levels During the Immune Response are Immunosuppressive

The question arises whether the observed increase of glucocorticoid blood level affects the immune response. We studied this problem using antigenic competition where two non-cross reactive, non-toxic antigens (horse and sheep red cells) are injected sequentially (Besedovsky et al., 1979b). We administered the second antigen when the glucocorticoid blood level had increased several fold in response to challenge with the first antigen.

When the increase in corticosterone levels is impeded by prior adrenalectomy, antigenic competition can be overcome in a large proportion of the animals. We take this as a strong indication that the increase in glucocorticoid can reach immunosuppressive levels during the immune response. Also other studies show that the described increase in corticosteroid blood levels can inhibit the immune response (Gisler and Schenkel-Hulliger, 1971).

Summarizing results thus far, we have shown that following immunization, glucocorticoid concentrations in blood can reach immunosuppressive levels. Lymphokines preformed "in vitro", upon administration to normal animals, also provoke an equivalent increase of corticosterone. The effect of LK is observed in hours whereas during the immune response increase in glucocorticoid is maximal after several days. These observations favour LK as afferent signals to endocrine structures. The data obtained with dexamethasone treated or hypophysectomized animals show that the endocrine response is mediated primarily through the pituitary--adrenal-axis and most likely integrated at the hypothalamic level. The observed increase in glucocorticosteroid in turn may affect production of LAF (IL1) by macrophages, different sets of T-lymphocytes, and growth factor production (e.g. TCGF-IL2) by T-lymphocytes (Gillis et al., 1979 a,b).

4. IMMUNE-NEUROENDOCRINE CIRCUITS: EVIDENCE FOR SYMPATHETIC
   IMMUNOREGULATORY CIRCUIT

It is known that lymphoid organs are innervated by sympathetic nerves. More recently the distribution of sympathetic
fibers in lymphoid tissue has been investigated (Reilly et al.,
1976). Fluorescent microscopy of spleen and thymus in rodents has
revealed varicose noradrenaline (NA) fibers in both organs.
Furthermore, perivascular plexuses within the splenic white
pulp send single NA fibers between the surrounding lymphocytes
(Williams and Felten, 1981). This distribution pattern of noradrenergic fibers in spleen corresponds to the site where T
lymphocytes are found and where the first antibody forming cells
migrate after immunization (Fitch et al., 1969). These morphological data make it likely that an interaction between these nerve
elements and lymphoid cells exists, but do not provide sufficient
evidence for an immunomodulatory role for this innervation.

4.1. Disruption of Sympathetic Innervation increases Immune
     Response

In order to evaluate the significance of sympathetic innervation for the immune response, we have performed both local
surgical denervation of the spleen as well as chemical sympathectomy by 6-hydroxydopamine (6-OH-DA) followed by adrenalectomy
(Besedovsky et al., 1979a). In both experimental models, immunization increased the number of antibody forming cells as compared
to controls. Table 1 shows the enhancing effect on the immune
response following neonatal chemical sympathectomy combined with
adrenalectomy in adult life.

4.2. Effect of Alpha-adrenergic Agonists on Immune Response

In view of the above results, administration of sympathetic
neurotransmitter catecholamines (CA) and agonist drugs influence
immune functions. Indeed, numerous studies have been reported and
the collective "in vivo" and "in vitro" data support the notion
that sympathetic agonists influence immune processes (Besedovsky
et al.,1979a; Hadden et al., 1975). For example, we observed that
the "in vitro" induced primary immune response to sheep red blood
cells (SRBC) is decreased by the alpha-agonist drugs methoxamine

Table 1. Chemical sympathectomy combined with adrenalectomy enhances
the immune response

Treatment	Solv. & Sham Group 1	6-OH-DA & Sham Group 2	Solv. & Ax Group 3	6-OH-DA & Ax Group 4
$PFCx10^3/$ spleen	904 ± 204	1.225 ± 205	771 ± 196	1.690 ± 237
n	10	10	13	14

Group 1: rats injected i.p. with $2 \mu l \ g^{-1}$ body weight of solvent
(solv. H_2O) daily the first 5 days of life and sham operated at 2
months. Group 2: as group 1 but injected with 150 mg kg^{-1} 6-OH-DA
(6-hydroxydopamine) and sham operated. Group 3: as group 1 but adrenalectomized (Ax). Group 4: as group 1, but injected with 6-OH-DA
and adrenalectomized. All animals were injected with antigen (SRBC)
5 days after the operation and number of plaque forming cells (PFC)
determined 5 days later. Adrenalectomy alone (Group 3) did not significantly change the magnitude of the immune response, whereas
combined treatment of 6-OH-DA with adrenalectomy (Group 4) resulted
in an increase in number of PFC in the spleen ($p \leqslant 0.01$). Group 4
differed also significantly from Group 1 ($p \leqslant 0.01$).

and clonidine, over a wide range of concentrations (Besedovsky et
al., 1979a). Furthermore, methoxamine "in vivo" was found to be
highly immunosuppressive in rats when the drug was injected
together with the antigen (SRBC).

The mechanism of this suppression is unknown, but the fact
that methoxamine has little or no central effects and acts also
"in vitro", indicate that these alpha-agonists exert a direct
effect on lymphocytes or accessory cells.

4.3. Immune Response Induces Phasic Sympathetic Changes in
Lymphoid Organs

The above described data on innervation and denervation of
lymphoid organs as well as the effects of sympathetic neuro-

transmitters point to a symphathetic modulation of the immune response. In view of the complexity of such a response, it is unclear whether such effects reflect the existence of sympathetic immunoregulatory circuits or are merely effects upon the basal conditions of the immune system. The first possibility requires an active exchange of signals between the immune system and the sympathetic nervous system.

Our approach to the problem was to measure NA levels in lymphoid tissue following antigenic stimulation (Besedovsky et al., 1979a) because under physiological conditions, NA levels in tissue reflect the activity of sympathetic nerves. Rats were immunized with SRBC and the levels of NA in spleen determined by radioenzymatic assay during the immune response.

We found a slight decrease in NA content in the spleen on day 2 after antigen challenge, followed by a marked decrease on day 3 and day 4 compared with the controls (P < 0.001). By day 8, when few direct plaque forming cells were detectable, the NA content had returned to normal. In several similar experiments the reduc-

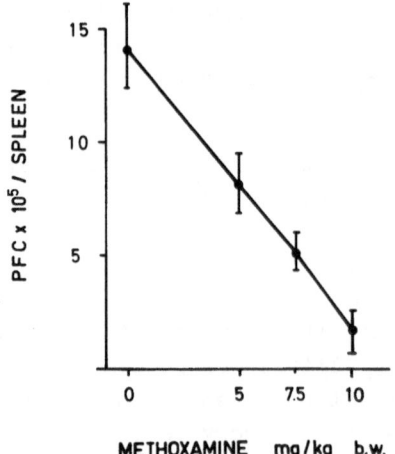

Fig. 3. Methoxamine suppresses immune response in vivo. Rats received one i.p. injection of methoxamine 15 min prior to the i.p. administration of 3×10^9 sheep red blood cells. The immune response was determined 5 days later by counting the number of plaque forming cells in the spleen. Each point corresponds to at least 10 animals.

tion in NA content ranged from 40 to 70%. When the results were
expressed as total splenic NA content, a similar reduction was
noted. The NA content of a nonlymphoid organ, the heart, was also
determined and no changes in its level were discerned at various
intervals after immunization. The data reported above were obtained in the main in immunologic high responder animals. Further
analysis of these and other experiments showed that the degree and
the persistance of splenic NA decrease is inversely related to the
magnitude of the response (del Rey et al., 1981).

These findings constitute the first definitive evidence that
a physiologically meaningful change in the splenic content of NA
occurs in the environment of antibody forming cells. By analogy to

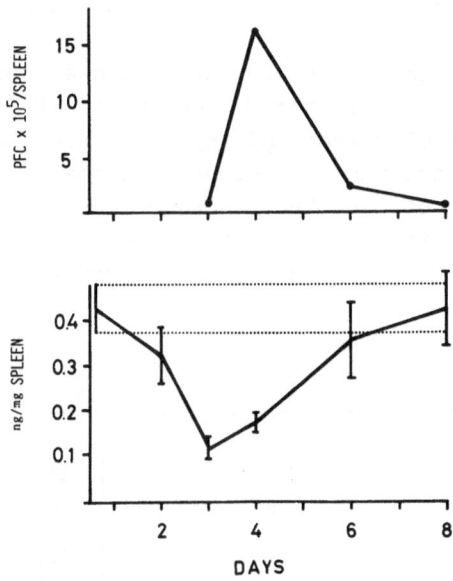

Fig. 4. Decreasing noradrenaline levels in the spleen during the
immune response. Rats were injected with 5×10^9 SRBC or physiological saline and the number of PFC and the NA content
determined on days 2, 3, 4, 6, and 8. Saline injected controls showed no significant changes in splenic NA content
and were used to define the normal control range (16 animals). Each point of the NA curve represents the mean value $\pm$ SEM obtained from determinations in spleen of 4 animals. Upper curve: plaque forming cells (PFC). Lower curve: splenic NA content.

the described data on denervation and effects of alpha-agonists,
this decrease in NA can be expected to affect the performance of
immunological cells.

4.4. Noradrenaline Levels in Lymphoid Tisue are Influenced by the
     Degrees of Antigenic Exposure

     The decrease of NA levels in animals challenged with antigen
under conventional conditions led us to investigate the basal
levels of NA in animals under germ-free (GF) conditions (del Rey
et al., 1981). Since environmental antigenic stimuli and consequently immune responses are reduced to minimum levels in this
state, we anticipated that the basal levels of NA in lymphoid
organs should be higher in germ-free (GF) rats than in specific
pathogen-free (SPF) animals. Fig. 5 shows the results.

     The lymphoid tissues of SPF rats, such as spleen, thymus and
lymphnodes had about half the NA content of GF animals. Also the
total content of NA of spleen and thymus is significantly lower in
SPF rats. In contrast the NA content of stomach and intestine was
similar regardless of whether the rats were kept in SPF or in GF
conditions. We explain these results by postulating that antigenic
exposure of conventional or SPF animals over their whole lifespan

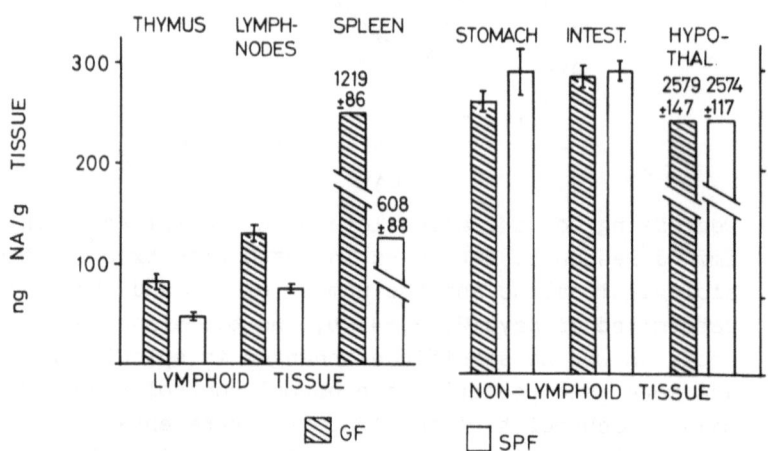

Fig. 5. SPF rats have lower NA content in lymphoid tissues than
        germ-free rats.

contributes to or even causes the described lower NA content in
the lymphoid organs. In order to evaluate the function of the
adrenal medulla, adrenalin (A) and NA contents of the adrenal
gland were simultaneously determined. GF animals had larger adrenals than SPF animals and, as shown in Fig. 6, the total adrenal
NA and A content was significantly higher in GF animals. The fact
that adrenal catecholamine content is lower in SPF than in GF
animals indicates that products of activated lymphoid cells reach
central structures which directly or indirectly control adrenal
medulla function.

The above data suggest that the sympathetic nervous system
participates in immunoregulation. In particular, the decrease of
NA levels during the immune response in the spleen but not in
non-lymphoid organs can be interpreted as a physiological mechanism for releasing the immunologically responding cells from
sympathetic inhibitory influences. The decrease in splenic NA
content is inversely related to the magnitude of the immune
response. This evidence favours a relevant role for sympathetic
signals in immunoregulation. In addition to direct effects on
immunological cells, changes in sympathetic activity could also
influence lymphoid cell traffic by affecting the blood flow in
lymphoid organs. The mechanisms underlying the NA decrease, the
nature of the afferent signals and the type of immunological cells
affected by sympathetic signals need to be elucidated.

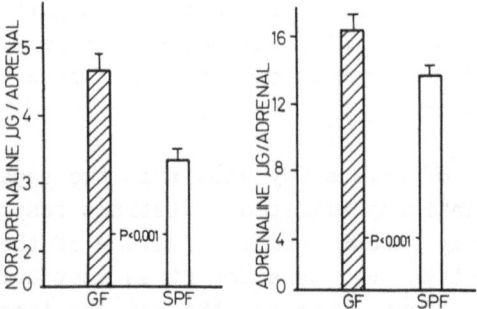

Fig. 6. Adrenal glands of SPF rats contain less catecholamines
        than those of GF animals.

5. IMMUNE-NEUROENDOCRINE CIRCUIT: EVIDENCE FOR CENTRAL
   INTEGRATION OF IMMUNE-NEUROENDOCRINE CIRCUITS

The described peripheral hormonal and sympathetic changes
make it very likely that they are integrated at central levels,
such as the hypothalamus. For proving the existence of such
integration it is mandatory to demonstrate electrophysiological
and biochemical changes in this organ during the immune response.
We have approached the problem by studying the rate of firing of
hypothalamic neurons and the catecholamine turnover in the hypothalamus.

5.1. Increase in Firing Rate of Hypothalamic Neurons During Immune
     Response

We have studied both the immune response and the rate of
firing of individual hypothalamic neurons at various intervals
after injection of SRBC or TNP-haemocyanin (TNP hae) (Besedovsky
et al., 1977a). Typical data for animals stimulated with SRBC are
summarized in Figure 7.

On day 1, no plaque forming cells were evident and no changes
in firing frequency were demonstrable compared with controls. On
day 5, PFC in spleen were maximal and there was more than a
twofold increase in the firing rate of the ventromedial neurons.
In several rats which were immunologically non responders, no
increase in firing rates occurred. Furthermore, no changes in
firing rates were observed in the anterior hypothalamic nucleus.

Hypothalamic responses to TNP-hae were also studied in rats
on days 1 through 5 after injection. A significant increase in
frequency of neuronal firing was noted on days 1, 2, 4 and 5; the
highest activation occurred on day 2, a time that precedes the
peak of the direct PFC.

The results of this study show that two separate, non toxic,
non infectious antigens elicited a distinct response in the hypothalamus. The only known common feature of these two agents is
their immunogenicity. We consider it as most unlikely that these
physiologic alterations involve the antigen itself. In fact, the
highest concentration of antigen is available upon injection when
no hypothalamic changes occurred. Therefore, it is concluded that

the hypothalamic events are linked to the immune response rather than to the antigen itself.

5.2. Decreased Rate of Noradrenaline Synthesis in the Hypothalamus During the Immune Response

It is well known that NA releasing neurons exert control over several types of hypothalamic neurons. In order to study whether noradrenergic pathways in the brain are affected by the immune response, we analysed in collaboration with Prof. Da Prada, Basel, the catecholamine turnover in the hypothalamus. SRBC injected rats showed a marked decrease in hypothalamic NA turnover as compared with controls on day 4 after antigen injection. The NA turnover rate was 377,05 $\pm$ 69,9 ng/g/h in controls and 154,33 $\pm$ 51,15 ng/g/h in immunized animals. The dopamine turnover was unchanged.

We interpret these results as evidence that the immune re-

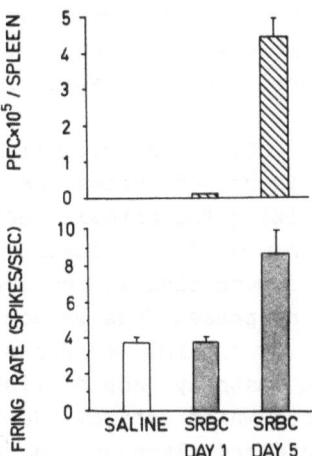

Fig. 7. Immune response changes hypothalamic neuronal activity. Increase in firing rates of neurons of ventromedial nuclei in the rat hypothalamus after antigenic stimulation. (A) Antibody-producing PFC in rats spleen; (B) firing rates. Rats were injected i.p. with 5×10^5 SRBC. From "Hypothalamic changes during the immune response" by Besedovsky, H.O., et al., 1977c. Reprinted by permission from Verlag Chemie GmbH, Heidelberg.

sponse can alter the rate of NA synthesis. It is unknown if the
increased firing rates and the decreased NA turnover in the
hypothalamus elicited by the immune response are causally related.
However, NA exerts an inhibitory effect on firing rates in neurons
of different parts of the brain, including the ventromedial
nucleus of the hypothalamus (Nishino, 1976). Thus, the decrease in
NA synthesis during the immune response may release from inhibition of hypothalamic neurons causing the observed increase in
firing.

6. DISCUSSION

The present paper has provided definitive evidence that
antigen elicits an immune response which triggers neuroendocrine
changes. Further, a flow of information occurs from the stimulated
immune system to central integrative structures e.g. the hypothalamus. As a result of these events, such structures respond by
inducing endocrine and autonomic changes which in turn influence
the course of the immune-neuroendocrine interactions (Besedovsky
and Sorkin, 1977b). The bidirectional flow of information with
reciprocal influences between the immune and the neuroendocrine
system, in our view, closely approaches the fulfilment of the
requirements for neuroendocrine participation in immunoregulation.

We will concentrate now on the mechanisms by which corticosteroid blood levels are increased during the immune response. The
antigens used for immunizing the animals were of quite different
nature, non-toxic and non-self replicating. Furthermore, the
changes in hormone levels were clearly temporally correlated with
the course of the immune response. Thus we concluded that hormonal
changes were brought about by the immune response itself.
Accordingly, an afferent pathway should exist from immunological
cells to those structures which control adrenocortical function.
Amongst others, we considered lymphokines and monokines as the
most likely candidates. Indeed, supernatants from activated lymphocytes and accessory cells, containing a variety of preformed
lymphokines and monokines, mimicked this increase in corticosterone levels and as expected this increase occurred rapidly
after their administration.

The effect of the lymphokines does not occur at the level of
the adrenals but is centrally integrated. This conclusion derives

from the fact that lymphokines increased ACTH levels and this event was absent in hypophysectomized or dexamethasone blocked animals.

One way by which the immune response via lymphokines may affect hypothalamic function is by decreasing NA synthesis in this organ. It is well documented (Ganong, 1974a,b,) that corticotrophin-releasing factor (CRF) production is inhibited by NA. Thus, the immune response, by decreasing NA turnover in the hypothalamus, may induce an increase in CRF and thereby increase the ACTH and corticosterone output.

The physiologically raised glucocorticosteroid levels may affect the performance of immunological cells by several mechanisms. For instance, glucocorticoids block production of lymphokines which may be essential for clonal expansion of T- and possibly B-cells. Thus, release of T-cell growth factor (IL2) from T-cells is suppressed by glucocorticoids whereas TCGF responder

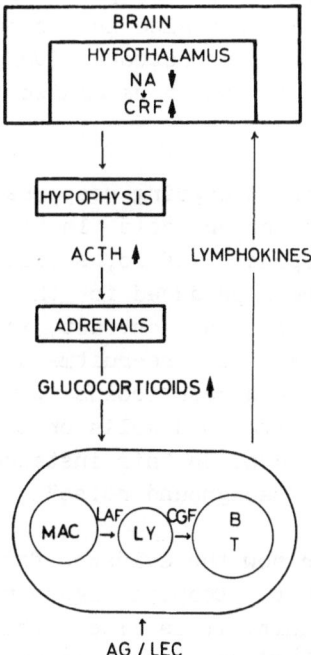

Fig. 8. Centrally mediated glucocorticoid-associated immunoregulatory circuit.

cells are not affected (Smith, 1981). However, the primary site of action of glucocorticoid hormones seems to be production of IL1 by macrophages.

In addition, it was shown that the synthesis of other lymphokines, such as MIF, MAF and chemotactic factors (Weston et al., 1973; Wahl et al., 1975) can be inhibited by glucocorticoids.

The overview concept of the glucocorticoid-associated immunoregulatory circuit is depicted in the following schematic diagram (Fig. 8).

A major conceptual difficulty to consider hormones and neurotransmitters in immunoregulation is how these non-specific agents exert control over a system involving specific effector cells and products. The same difficulty holds for nonspecific lymphokines and monokines. Burnet's early concept of the immune system as being totally compartmentalized into individual clones of cells with different specificities has undergone radical modification.
The discovery that distinctive cellular products, presumably lymphokines with polyclonal effects, participate in different stages of the immune response has revealed interclonal influences.
In addition, the idiotypic network (Jerne, 1974) also involves clones other than those which recognize and respond to a particular external antigen.

It is likely that an ongoing response may proceed relatively undisturbed because glucocorticoid levels increase late in the developing immune response. If so, sufficient cell growth factor would already have been produced for the clonal expansion of the antigen committed cells. In contrast, increasing glucocorticoid levels would suppress excessive recruitment of noncommitted cells. Thus, the effect of glucocorticoids would be to inhibit clonal expansion of unrelated lymphoid cells or cells with only low affinity for a given antigen. In this instance, specificity would be controlled by reducing "background noise".

We will consider now the evidence for a possible sympathetic immunoregulatory circuit. Despite ignorance about many steps of such a proposed circuit, it is likely that central participation elicits the peripheral NA decrease encountered in the course of an immune response. A purely local phenomenon such as NA consumption by spleen cells or other local factors is unlikely to cause the decrease of NA. The main reason for assuming a minor contribution of local mechanisms is the relative constancy of NA content in organs during varying conditions which is based on a feedback mechanisms operating with a high degree of precision. Free NA influences NA synthesis at the rate-limiting step of tyrosine--hydroxylase activity (Euler, 1972). Consequently, unless it is assumed that activated lymphocytes release a specific enzymatic inhibitor, locally induced NA changes will be rapidly compensated for via the aforementioned mechanisms. The fact that the thymus, an organ with only marginal direct involvement in immune respon-ses, has a lower NA content in SPF animals, favours the interpre-tation that factor(s) released locally by immunologically respon-ding cells are not directly inhibiting the sympathetic nerve acti-vity of lymphoid organs. Furthermore, adrenal catecholamine con-tent is lower in SPF than in GF animals indicating that products of activated lymphoid cells may reach central structures which directly or indirectly control adrenal medulla function.

Accordingly, it is proposed that changes in NA content in lymphoid organs during the immune response represent the efferent limb of a reflex mechanism triggered by antigen-stimulated cells. In view of the previously described evidence that sympathetic innervation and neurotransmitters exert inhibitory effects on immune mechanisms we assume that changes in tissue NA content represent immunoregulatory signals.

The links between the sympathetic peripheral changes and those in the hypothalamus need further clarification. Neverthless, the fact that both the peripheral and central sympathetic mecha-nisms are inhibited during the immune response, indicates that peripheral and central noradrenergic neurons may respond in a similar way to stimuli from activated immunological cells.

The experimental findings reported here, present persuasive evidence for physiological external immunoregulation. However, since hormonal and also autonomic mechanisms normally act in a highly integrated fashion (Houssay, 1957), it is a reasonable prediction that still other immune-neuroendocrine circuits will be operative. External immunoregulation can be viewed as being super--imposed on autoregulation which thereby becomes subject to and is integrated with a complex system of hormonal feed-backs and neural signals. Since the central nervous system coordinates multiple external and internal signals, it can be visualized that several

central inputs can affect the basal operation of the neuroendocrine control of the immune response. Numerous questions
remain concerning the nature of the afferent and efferent signals,
their kinetics and cellular targets and how they are to be
synchronized with autoregulatory mechanisms within the immune
system. However, it is hoped that as this kind of exploration
continues, we will come to understand better how immunological
cells operate in their physiological environment.

ACKNOWLEDGEMENTS

We thank Prof. S. Normann for careful readings of the manuscript and constructive criticism. We also thank Ms. Marianne
Furlenmeier for typing of the manuscript. This work was supported
by the Swiss National Science Foundation, Grant No. 3.603.80.

REFERENCES

Abraham, A.D., and Bug, G., ^{3}H-testosterone distribution and binding
in rat thymus cells in vivo, Molecular and Cellular Biochemistry, 13:157.

Ader, R., 1981, "Psychoneuroimmunology", Acad. Press, New York.

Arrenbrecht, S., 1974, Specific binding of growth hormone to thymo-
sytes, Nature, 252:255.

Besedovsky, H.O., and Sorkin, E., 1977a, Hormonal control of immune
processes, in: "Endocrinology," Vol. 2, V.H.T. James, ed.,
Exerpta Medica, Amsterdam, Oxford, p. 504.

Besedovsky, H.O. and Sorkin, E., 1977b, Network of immune-neuroendocrine interactions, Clin. Exp. Immunol., 27:1.

Besedovsky, H.O., Sorkin, E., da Prada, M. and Keller, H.H., 1979,
Immunoregulation mediated by the sympathetic nervous system,
Cell. Immunol., 48:346.

Besedovsky, H.O., Sorkin, E., Keller, M. and Muller, J., 1975, Changes in blood hormone levels during the immune response, Proc.
Soc. Exp. Biol. Med., 150:466.

Besedovsky, H.O., del Rey, A. and Sorkin E., 1979, Antigenic competition between horse and sheep red blood cells as a hormone-depen-
dent phenomenon, Clin. exp. Immunol., 37:106.

Besedovsky, H.O., del Rey, A. and Sorkin E., 1981, Lymphokine containing supernatants from Con A stimulated cells increase corticosterone blood levels, J. Immunol., 126:385.

Besedovsky, H.O., Sorkin, E., Felix, D. and Haas, H., 1977c, Hypothalamic changes during the immune response., Europ. J. Immunol., 7:323.

Billingham, R.E., Krohn, P.L., and Medawar, P.B., 1951, The effect of cortisone on the survival of skin homografts in the rabbit, Brit. Med. J., 2:1049.

Cake, M.H., and Litwack, G., 1975, The glucocorticoid receptors, in: "Biochemical actions of hormones," Vol. 3, G. Litwack, ed., Academic Press, New York, San Francisco, London, p. 317.

Claman, H.N., 1975, How corticosteroids work, J. Allergy Clin. Immunol., 55:145.

Dougherty, T.F., Berliner, M.L., Schneebeli, G.L., and Berliner, D.L., 1964, Hormonal control of lymphatic structure and function, Ann. N. Y. Acad. Sci., 113:825.

Euler, U.S., 1972, Synthesis, uptake and storage of catecholamines in adrenergic nerves. The effect of drugs, in: "Handbook of experimental pharmacology," Vol. 33, O. Eichler, A. Rarah, H. Herken and A.D. Welch, eds., Springer, Berlin, Heidelberg, New York, p. 186.

Fabris, N., 1977, Hormones and aging,in: "Immunology and aging," T. Makinodan and E. Yunis, eds., Plenum Medical Book Co., New York, p. 73.

Fitch, F.W., Stejskal, R., and Rowley, D.A., 1969, Histologic localization of hemolysin-containing cells, in: "Advances in experimental medicine and biology," L. Fiore-Donati and M.G., Hanna jr., eds., Plenum Press, New York, vol. 5, p. 223.

Gilette, S. and Gilette, R., 1979, Changes in thymic estrogen receptor expression following orchidectomy, Cell. Immunol., 42:194.

Gillis, S., Crabtree, G.R., and Smith, K., 1979a, Glucocorticoid-induced inhibition of T cell growth factor production. I. The effect on mitogen-induced lymphocyte proliferation, J. Immunol., 123:1624.

Gillis, S., Crabtree, G.R., and Smith, K.A., 1979b, Glucocorticoid-induced inhibition of T cell growth factor production. II. The effect on the in vitro generation of cyctolytic T cells, J. Immunol., 123:1632.

Gisler, R.H., and Schenkel-Hulliger, L., 1971, Hormonal regulation of the immune response. II. Influence of pituitary and adrenal activity on immune responsiveness in vitro, Cell. Immunol., 2:646.

Ganong, W.F., 1974a, Brain mechanisms regulating the secretion of the pituitary gland, in: "The neurosciences," Third study program, F.O. Schmitt, F.G., Worden, eds., Cambridge MIT Press,

p. 549.

Ganong, W.F., 1974b, The role of catecholamines and acetylcholine in the regulation of endocrine function, Life Sci., 15:1401.

Hadden, J.W., Johnson, E.M., Hadden, E.M., Coffey, R.G., and Johnson, L.D., 1975, Cyclic GMP and lymphocyte activation, in: "Immune recognition," A.S. Rosenthal, ed., Academic Press, New York, San Francisco, London, p. 359.

Helderman, J.H., and Strom, T., 1978, Specific insulin binding site on T and B lymphocytes as a marker of cell activation, Nature, 274:62.

Hollenberg, M.D., and Cuatrecasas, P., 1974, Hormone receptors and membrane glycoproteins during in vitro transformation of lymphocytes, in: "Control of proliferation of animal cells," B. Clarkson and R. Baserga, eds., Cold Spring Harbour Lab., p.423.

Houssay, B.C., 1957, Comments, in: "Hormonal regulation of energy metabolism," Springfield, p. 111.

Jankovic, B.D., and Isakovic, K., 1973, Neuro-endocrine correlates of immune response. I. Effects of brain lesions on antibody production, Arthus reactivity and delayed hypersensitivity in the rat, Int. Arch. Allergy, 45:360.

Jerne, N.K., 1974, Towards a network theory of the immune system, Ann. Immunol. Inst. Pasteur., 125C:373.

Marat, B.A., 1974, Effect of central cholinolytics on the primary immune response in rabbits, Bull. Exp. Biol. Med., 76/8:971.

Neta, R., and Salvin, S.B., 1981, Production of lymphokines in vivo, in: "Lymphokines," E. Pick, ed., Acad. Press, New York., vol. 2, p. 295.

Nishino, H., 1976, Suprachiasmatic nuclei and circadian rhythms, Role of suprachiasmatic nuclei in rhythmic activity of neurons in the lateral hypothalamic area, ventromedian nuclei and pineal gland, Folia Pharmacol. Jap., 72:941.

Reilly, F.D., McCuskey, R.S., and Meineke, H.A., 1976, Studies on the hemopoietic microenvironment. VIII. Adrenergic and cholinergic innervation of the murine spleen, The Anatomical Record, 185:109.

Del Rey, A., Besedovsky, H.O., Sorkin, E., Da Prada, M., and Bondiolotti, G.P., 1981, Immunoregulation mediated by the sympathetic nervous system, Difference between immunological high and low responder animals, Am. J. Physiol., in press.

Del Rey, A., Besedovsky, H.O., Sorkin, E., Da Prada, M., and Arrenbrecht, S., 1981, Immunoregulation mediated by the sympathetic nervous system, Cell. Immunol., in press.

Richman, D.P., and Arnason, B.G., 1979, Nicotinic acetylcholine re-

ceptor: Evidence for a functionally distinct receptor on human
    lymphocytes, Proc. Natl. Acad. Sci., USA, 76:4632.

Riley, V., 1981, Psychoneuroendocrine influences on immunocompetence
    and neoplasia, Science, 212:1100.

Sinch, U., Millson, D.S., Smith, P.A., and Owen, J.J.T., 1979, Iden-
    tification of -adrenoceptors during thymocyte ontogeny in mice,
    Eur. J. Immunol., 9:31.

Smith, K.A., 1981, T-cell growth factor: Present status and future
    implications, in: "Lymphokines," E.Pick, ed., Academic Press,
    New York, vol. 2, p. 21.

Stein, M., Schiavi, P.C., and Camerino,M., 1976, Influence of brain
    and behavior on the immune system, Science, 191:435.

Strom, T.B., and Sytkowski, A.J., 1974a, Cholinergic augmentation of
    lymphocyte-mediated cytotoxicity, A study of the cholinergic
    receptor of cytotoxic T lymphocytes, Proc. Natl. Acad. Sci.
    USA, 71:1330.

Strom, T.B., Deisseroth, A., Morganroth, J., Carpenter, Ch.B., and
    Merill, J.P., 1972, Alteration of the cytotoxic action of sen-
    sitized lymphocytes by cholinergic agents and activators of
    adenylate cyclase, Proc. Natl. Acad. Sci., USA, 69:2995.

Strom, T.B., Sytkowski, A.J., Carpenter, C.B., and Merill, J.P.,
    1974b, The cholinergic receptor of cytotoxic T-lymphocytes,
    in: "Lymphocyte recognition and effector mechanism. Procee-
    dings of the 8th Leucocyte Culture conference," K., Lindahl-
    -Kiessling and D., Osoba, eds., Academic. Press, New York,
    London, p. 509.

Talal, N., 1979, Autoimmunity and lymphoid malignancy: Manifestation
    of immunoregulatory disequilibrium, in: "Autoimmunity," N.
    Talal, ed., Academic. Press, New York, p. 194.

Wahl, S.M., Altmen, L.C., and Rosenstreich, D.L., 1975, Inhibition
    of in vitro lymphokine synthesis by glucocorticosteroids, J.
    Immunol., 115:476.

Werb, Z., Foley, R., and Munck, A., 1978, Interaction of glucocorti-
    coids with macrophages, Indentification of glucocorticoid recep-
    tors in monocytes and macrophages, J. Exp. Med., 147:1684.

Weston, W.L., Claman, H.N., and Krueger, G.G., 1973, Site of action
    of cortisol in cellular immunity, J. Immunol., 110:880.

Williams, J.M. and Felten, D.L., 1981, Sympathetic innervation of
    murine thymus and spleen: A comparative histofluorescence study.
    The Anatomical Record, 199:531

Wolstenholme, G.E.W. and Knight, J.(eds)1970, Hormones and the immune
    response. Ciba Foundation Study Group No. 36., J. and A.
    Churchill, London.

THYMUS-NEUROENDOCRINE NETWORK

N. Fabris, E. Mocchegiani, M. Muzzioli and R. Imberti*

Immunological Centre, Gerontological Research Dept.
I.N.R.C.A., Ancona, and *Rehanimation Unit
University of Pavia, Italy

1. INTRODUCTION

The idea that the thymus might be considered as an endocrine gland integrated in the complex hormonal network regulating the growth and the internal homeostasis of high organisms was first suggested by the observations that this organ seemed to be functionally active only before puberty, when the majority of endocrine glands are involved in body development and that alterations of its growth pattern was frequently accompanied by modifications of the growth rate of whole organism (Chiodi, 1939).

The trials to give an experimental support to these observations, although they were quite numerous at that time, failed however to support the main hypothesis. Neither experiments correlating the thymus to sexual maturation (Andersen, 1932) or to developmental growth (Szent-Gyorgyi et al., 1962) nor those trying to involve the thymus in basic metabolic processes, such as glucose metabolism (Gudernatsch, 1937), offered substantial evidence to the hypothesis.

The discovery, in the early 1960's, of the immunological role of thymus, (Miller, 1961; Good et al., 1962) brougth forth the idea that the thymus and its cellular products were a kind of "task force" against external noxae, totally autonomous and independent from the physiological alterations of the "internal milieu" (Miller and Osoba, 1967).

A number of observations in recent years, have, however
demostrated that, although the thymus-dependent immunity has an
highly sophisticated autoregulatory mechanism, much of its efficiency is influenced by extra-immunological regulatory circuits
(Fabris, 1981a). Central and autonomic nervous system, endocrine
balance and metabolic turnover have been shown to play a role in
the development and maintanance of the immune system (Fabris,
1981a), thus representing a kind of second regulation of level
superimposed on the intrinsic mechanism of self-regulation of the
immune system.

The comprehensive picture of these integrative mechanisms
still waits, however, for a systematic experimental approach,
which should take into consideration not only the fact that the
majority of homeostatic regulation mechanisms are interdigitated
with each other, but also of the discovery of a consistent endocrine activity of the thymus (Goldstein et al., 1972).

This point is of striking biological importance, since it
introduces new humoral factor(s), which, although specifically
acting upon the immune system, cannot be considered as depleted of
physiological relevance for the whole neuroendocrine system.

From an experimental point of view the existence of a
fuctional relationship between the thymus and the neuroendocrine
system has been suggested by a number of observations dealing
either with possible neurohormonal alterations following the removal of the thymus or with the modifications wich may be induced
within the thymus itself by different endocrine manipulations.

Different experimental animal models have been used in such a
research; congenital mutants, ectomized animals and physiologically aged animals, these last, on the assumption that they suffer
from alterations of both neuroendocrine and immune system (for
review see Fabris, 1981a, and Fabris and Piantanelli 1982).
Much less has been done in humans, although neuroendocrine-immune
interactions have been observed in selected human endocrine pathology (MacCuish et al., 1974; Sympson et al., 1975). Also in
some genetic abnormalities, such as Down's syndrome, Duchenne's
muscular dystrophy, ataxia-teleangectasia and athopic asthma, the
alterations observed at thymic level might, to some extent, depend on neurological and/or endocrinological modifications, which
are frequently associated whit those diseases.

Aim of this work is to summarize the findings which, at present, support the functional relationship between the thymus (and particularly its endocrine activity) and the neuroendocrine system.

2. INLUENCE OF NEUROENDOCRINE SYSTEM ON THYMUS ACTIVITY

The idea that the thymus is under the influence of the neuroendocrine system stemmed from the observation that alterations at the level of the nervous system or of the endocrine balance might alter the growth pattern of the thymus and, consequently, the efficiency of the thymus-dependent immunity.

2.1. Endocrine Glands

The surgical removal of the adeno-hypophysis in rats (Duquesnoy et al., 1979) or congenital hypopituitarism, as it occurs in dw/dw mice (Fabris et al., 1971a), causes hypotrophy of the thymus and decreased peripheral T-cell function, both of which can be restored to normal by treatment with developmental hormones and particulary with growth hormone and thyroxine (Fabris et al., 1971b). In humans, no clear-cut pictures have been described.
In anencephalic foetuses, hypertrophy of the thymus has been recorded, and interpreted as being due to hypofunction of adrenals (Bearn, 1966). With regard to thymus-dependent immunity, while, according to some authors (Amman et al., 1970), no deficiences are observable in hypopituitary humans, other authors have reported a clear-cut reduction in T mitogen response, which are corrected to normal by treatment with growth hormone preparations (Bianchi et al., 1980).

Also the thyroid has great influence on the growth rate of the thymus: hypo- and hyperfunction of the gland cause respectively reduced or increased size of the thymus both in rodents (Fabris, 1973) and in man (Sympson et al., 1975). The administration of exogenous thyroxine to otherwise normal animals results in enlargement of both central and peripheral lymphoid organs; in particular, the outflow of lymphocytes from the thymus increases during treatment with thyroxine (Ernstrom and Larsson, 1966) and peripheral immune efficiency is found augmented (Oaki et al., 1976; Basso et al., 1981). The effect of thyroxine on thymus-de-

pendent immunity is even more evident in old mice: the age-associated reduction of PHA response and of PHA:ConA ratio is significantly recovered by short-term treatment with L-thyroxine
(Fabris et al., 1982).

The influence of the endocrine pancreas on thymus growth is
still a debated problem. While there seem to be a general
agreement on the existence of modulatory actions of insulin on the
performance of peripheral mature lymphocytes (see Hadden, this
volume), contradictory findings have been reported on the thymus
function. Decreased cellularity of this organs has been observed
in rats (Fabris and Piantanelli, 1977) and can be restored to
normal by treatment with insulin. However, according to other
authors the effect might depend on the hyperglicemic state rather
than on the hypoinsulinemia (Fernandes et al., 1978).

The effect of adrenals on thymus growth has been extensively
studied in rodents; both in mice and rats overproliferation of
lymphatic tissues, including the thymus, and cellular depletion
have been recorded after adrenalectomy or corticosteroid treatment, respectively (Gunn et al., 1970). Also the physiological
variations of blood corticosteroid level, due to cyrcadian rythmi-
city seem to significantly modify not only the number and function
of peripheral mature cells (Abo et al., 1980), but also the rate
of cellular proliferation within the thymus itself (Pauly et al.,
1976). In this context, it has to be noted, however, that, in
addition to the effect of adrenal cortex hormones, also pituitary
corticotropin may act on the thymus: increased adenine uptake by
the thymus of adrenalectomized rats under corticotropin injection
(Brick-Johnson and Dougherty, 1965) and increased thymidine uptake
in cultures of thymic epithelial cells after "in vitro" administration of corticotropin would support the idea that it is the
ACTH-adrenal axis which may modulate thymic activity, rather than
a single component of it (Deschaux, 1977).

With regard to sexual glands, enlargement of the thymus following gonadectomy and hypotrophy after treatment with steroid
hormones are well known phenomena (Castro, 1974). As for adrenals,
however, it is difficult, at present, to dissociate the effects
exerted on the thymus by sexual gland hormones "per se" (Szemberg,
1970; Waltman et al., 1971; Barnes et al., 1974) from those due to
pituitary gonadotropins (Addock et al., 1973; Fabris et al.,
1977). The interrelationship between pituitary and target gland

hormones suggest that in some peculiar endocrinological situations, such as menstrual cycle or pregnancy, it is the day by day
readjustement of hormonal balance, that determines the level of
thymic function. That one of the targets of sexual hormones is the
thymus is further supported either by the observation that in
hamster, post-thymectomy wasting disease effects males, but not
females (Sherman and Dameshek, 1963), or by the finding that
impressive modifications can be induced by sex hormones treatment
on the epithelial component of the thymus (Cherry et al., 1968)
which is responsible for the production of thymic hormones
(Dardenne et al., 1974).

2.2. Central and Autonomous Nervous System

The experimental evidences for a neural control on the thymus
function are still quite few and frequently controversial. It is
out of doubt that the thymus possesses a rather complex innerva-
tions (see Spector, this volume) which does not seem to be involved only in the modulation of blood vessel tone. But it is also
true that the nervous system may act on different organs also
through the modulation of the secretion of hormones and neurotransmitters, which can reach the target organ without requiring
innervation. A clear-cut dissection of this multifaced functional
patterns is therefore quite difficult. Among the experimental
models which can support the idea that the nervous system acts on
the thymus function, there may be listed the following.

Electrolytic lesions of selected brain areas, particularly in
the hypothalamic region result in hypotrophy of thymus, whereas
lesions of other areas do not have significant effects on thymus
function (Stein et al., 1976).

Lethargic mice (Lh/Lh) suffer from a neurological abnormality
which develops at preweaning time, lasts 30 to 60 days and than
progressively disappears. The neurological disease is associated
with thymic atrophy which is reversed to normal as soon as the
neural disturbances disappear (Dung, 1977). Quite similar thymic
pictures have been reported in pathological alterations of the
neuromuscular function, such as miotonic dystrophy in mice,
chicken and humans (see Horrobin, this volume).

Table 1. Modification of FTS circulating level in different congenital or experimental disendocrinopaties.

Exp. animals	Time after gland removal (days)	FTS titre ($1/\text{Log}_2$)	P[y]
DwJ normal	–	5.50 ± 0.17	–
DwJ dwarf	congenital	2.88 ± 0.30	A
sham-operation	15	5.30 ± 0.20	–
thyroidectomy[a]	5	3.80 ± 0.57	NS
"	15	1.00 ± 0.37	A
exp. diabetes[b]	5[c]	3.32 ± 0.82	B
	15	1.82 ± 0.32	A
castration[a] (prepuberal)	5	4.52 ± 0.20	NS
	15	5.07 ± 0.45	NS
castration[a] (post-puberal)	5	4.32 ± 0.32	NS
	15	4.65 ± 0.33	NS
adrenalectomy[a]	5	4.52 ± 0.20	NS
	15	4.32 ± 0.41	NS

[a] Ectomy has been performed at 60 days of age in Balb/c mice.
[b] Diabetic condition has been induced in Balb/c mice by i.p. injection of alloxan (200 mg/kg b.w.).
[c] Time has been recorded from the beginning of glucosuria.
[y] P was evaluated by comparing ectomized animals with sham-operated
controls. A = P< 0.01, B = P< 0.05.

Treatment of newborn mice with beta-blocking agents, such as
propanolol, arrests the development of the thymus and, consequently, of thymus dependent function (Goldstein G. et al., 1976).
Also during maturity, administration of propanolol prevents the
enlargement of the thymus, usually associated with hyperthyroid
conditions (Sympson et al., 1975).

On the other hand "in vitro" administration of cathecolamines
to thymic explants may affect subsequent growth and differentiation of thymus dependent lymphocytes (Upendra and Owen, 1976).

All these observations clearly support the existence of relationships between both the central and the autonomic nervous system and thymic function.

With regard to the mechanisms by which hormones and neuro-transmitters may affect thymic function, two alternatives can be taken into consideration. Firstly, the action of these factors may be directly exerted on thymocytes. Such a possibility is suppor-ted by the existence on the cellular membrane of thymocytes, or at cytoplasmic level, of receptor sites for different hormones and neurotransmitters (Gavin III, 1977). Further more both prolifera-tion and differentiation of thymocytes might also be influenced by hormone dependent alterations of metabolic turnover (Pandian and Talwar, 1971).

An alternative possibility is that hormones and neurotrans-mitters act on thymocyte turnover by modulating the synthesis and/or the release of thymic humoral factors (Golstein A. et al., 1972; Bach et al., 1973). In order to investigate this point we have measured the circulating level of thymic factor (FTS) (Bach et al., 1972) in different experimental and human disendocrino-paties.

3. INFLUENCE OF NEURO-ENDOCRINE SYSTEM ON THE SYNTHESIS AND/OR SECRETION OF FTS

3.1. Effect of Experimental Disendocrinopaties

Table 1 shows the circulating level of FTS, as measured by the Azathioprine rosette inibition test (Bach et al., 1972), in animals deprived of different endocrine glands, either because of congenital absence, or because of surgical removal or chemical blockade. Congenital hypopituitarism, experimental hypothyroidsm and diabetes, all cause a reduction of plasma level of FTS, whe-reas removal of the gonads or of adrenals do not induce any significant modification.

Reconstitution experiments by means of substitutive hormonal therapy have demonstrated (Table 2) that the circulating level of FTS returns to normal already few days after the beginning of the hormonal treatment (Fabris and Mocchegiani, submitted).

Table 2. Recovery of FTS level in thyroidectomized or diabetic mi-
         ce by substitutive therapy.

Exp. Group	Treatment	Time of treatment (days)[a]	FTS titre (1/Log$_2$)	P[y]
sham-operated	-	-	5.82 ± 0.50	-
thyroidectomized	-	-	1.00 ± 0.0	-
"	L-thyroxine	2	4.32 ± 0.36	A
"	"	4	6.02 ± 0.75	A
diabetic	-	-	1.82 ± 0.58	-
"	Insulin	7	6.36 ± 0.49	A
"	"	14	5.72 ± 0.55	A

[a]Hormonal treatment begun in thyroidectomized animals at 15 days
after operation, in diabetic mice 15 days after the appearance
of glucosuria.
[x]Geometric mean ± standard error.
[y]P was calculated by comparing treated with untreated ectomized
animals. A = P ≤ 0.01.

3.2. Findings in Human Disendocrinopaties

The FTS level in human hypo- and hyperthyroidism has been
measured in sera of patients of different ages, suffering either
from hypothyroidism following surgical thyroidectomy or from
hyperthyroidism due to diffuse nodular goitre (Table 3). Since the
physiological level of FTS declines with advancing age, data have
to be compared with age-matched controls. Hypopituitarism in young
age (under 30) is associated with consistent reduction of FTS
level; the extent of this decrease is not evaluable in patients
over 40, since at this age also the physiological level of FTS is
low (Bach et al., 1972). By contrast, hyperthyroidism, occurring
in patients over 40 years of age, is associated with high levels
of FTS, sometimes even higher than those detected in young age,
when FTS level is at its maximal values.

These data clearly confirm the findings in mice, i.e. that
modifications of the turnover of thyroid hormones may influence

Table 3. Circulating plasma levels of FTS in primary hypo- and hyperthyroidism.

	No. of cases	Age range (years)	FTS titre $(1/\text{Log}_2)$	P[y]
Normal	10	20 - 30	4.25 ± 0.25[a]	-
Hypothyroid	8	20 - 30	1.50 ± 0.29	A
Normal	10	40 - 60	1.57 ± 0.30	-
Hyperthyroid	7	40 - 60	4.86 ± 0.26	A

[a]Geometric mean $\pm$ standard error.
[y]P was calculated by comparing thyroid patients which age-matched
normal individuals. A = $P < 0.01$.

the synthesis and/or the secretion of FTS.
Moreover, the functional relationship between thyroid and thymus
is not evident only in such extreme situations as removal of the
thyroid or of clear-cut hyperfunctional state. Also in less
critical situations affecting the turnover of thyroid hormones,
such as the low T_3 syndromes associated with prematurity or trauma
(Hesch, 1981), a correlation between the blood level of thriiodo-
thyronin (T_3) and the level of FTS is observable (Fabris, 1981b).

At birth the level of FTS is usually quite low, but already
by the fifth day of life it reaches the physiological level of
young age. In premature infants the time required in order to
reach normal value is much longer, from 40 to 60 days (see also
Chandrá, 1979). Prematurity is also associated with low levels of
T_3, likely due to impaired T_3 to T_4 peripheral conversion, and
there exists a strict correlation between the values of FTS and
those of T_3.

Quite similar findings have been obtained in the low T_3
syndrome following traumatic lesions. Patients suffering from
traumatic car accidents show low levels of T_3 and concomittantly
low FTS levels. In both premature infants and traumatic patients
the recovery of thyroid hormone turnover is followed by normalization of FTS level.

Table 4. Recovery of FTS plasma level and spleen PHA response in old Balb/c mice after 15 days treatment with L-thyroxine.

Exp. Group	FTS titre ($1/\text{Log}_2$)	PHA response (cpm/culture/$\text{x}10^3$)
Young	5.82 ± 0.50^a	55.2 ± 3.6^a
Old	1.00 ± 0.0	16.6 ± 3.0
Old + thyroxine	4.80 ± 0.37	40.7 ± 5.6

[a]Geometric mean $\pm$ standard error.

3.3. Effect of Age-associated Endocrinological Disturbances

In mice with advancing age there occur a progressive alteration of thyroid hormone turnover: both T_3 and T_4 serum levels
decline with age (Fabris et al., 1982). Old mice treated with
L-thyroxine regain the capacity to produce FTS (Table 4).

The recovery of FTS secretion in old mice is not a sterile
event since it induces an increased functionality of the peripheral immune system as assessed by the reconstitution of the
number of T-lymphocytes and of their responsiveness to mitogen
stimulation, which are abnormally low in old mice (Fabris et al.,
1982).

It is of interest to note that, in addition to the recovery
of FTS level and of peripheral immune efficiency in old mice,
thyroxine seems to rejuvenate the thymus, so that when such a
thymus is transplanted into young thymectomized recipient, its
behaviour rensembles more that of a young thymus, than that of an
old one. These findings, while on one hand clearly confirm the
influence of the endocrine system on the thymic humoral activity,
on the other hand strongly support the idea that the functional
decline of thymic factor production is to a large extent a
reversible phenomenon. From preliminary experiments it seems,
however, that such a reversibility disappears in very old age.
Thyroxine treatment does not seem to be equally active in very old

Table 5. Low circulating level of FTS in genetic syndromes (adapted from Franceschi et al., 1981).

	No. of cases[a]	FTS titre ($1/Log_2$)	FTS titre (range)
Normal	23	4.96 ± 0.12	1/16 - 1/64
Down	15	2.53 ± 0.26	1/2 - 1/16
Duchenne	12	1.55 ± 0.20	1/2 - 1/4

[a]All cases were young subjects (age range: 5-20 years).
[b]Geometric mean $\pm$ standard error.

(over 26 months) mice. This fact does not exclude, however, the possibility that by neuroendocrinological manipulations other than thyroxine treatment, a recovery of thymic factor production in old mice may still be achieved.

3.4. Findings in Congenital Genetic Diseases

In the course of the study on the factors which may influence the production of FTS in humans, we have measured FTS level in different congenital genetic diseases, such as Down's syndrome and Duchenne muscular dystrophy.

In the majority of these cases a reduced circulating level of FTS has been observed (Franceschi et al., 1981) (Table 5). Down's syndrome is characterized by a number of immunological disturbances, quite similar to those observed in physiological aging (see Walford, this volume). The interpretation of these findings in the view of neuroendocrine-immune interaction is quite difficult at present. It is out of doubt that Down's subjects are suffering from many different disturbances, including alterations of the neuroendocrine homeostasis, as supported by the frequency of hormonal and dismetabolic diseases. Further work is needed, however, in order to assess the eventual neuroendocrinological component in the FTS alteration recorded in these patients.

A more easy interpretation may be offered to the findings on Duchenne syndrome, according at least to the hypothesis of Horrobin (see this volume). The concomittancy of neuromuscular disorders and immune disturbances is frequently recurrent in both animals and man, including ataxia-teleangectasia (see Gatti, this volume). More integrative studies are however needed in order to understand these apparently anomalous connections.

4. THYMUS VS NEUROENDOCRINE SYSTEM INTERACTIONS

The idea that the thymus may act, particularly during early stages of life, on the physiologic development of non-immunologic functions has already been proposed (Comsa, 1977; Pierpaoli and Sorkin, 1972a; Fabris et al., 1972), and supported by the original observation that post-thymectomy wasting disease, in addition to the obvious immunological disturbances, is characterized by pathological signs, which can hardly be linked to the direct effect of immune deficiency itself (McIntire et al., 1964).

Mice thymectomized at birth, show in fact a progressive impairement of body growth with reduced lenght of ears and tail, microsplancnia, microsomia, thinness of the skin and lack of subcutaneous fat, osseal alterations, particularly evident in the vertebrae with consequent hunched posture, and hypotrophy of various tissues including submaxillary gland, hair follicles and bone marrow (McIntire et al., 1964).

The majority of pathological signs observed in thymectomized animals are present also in nude mutations (Gershwin et al., 1975; Vos et al., 1980); however, some of them, including altered age/weight ratio, do not seem to appear when animals are maintained in germ-free conditions.

More focused investigation on the morphological and functional aspects of the neuroendocrine system in both thymectomized and nude animals, have confirmed that these animals display a profoundly disturbed neuroendocrine balance.

4.1. Effect of Thymus Hypofunctioning on Neuroendocrine Homeostasis

At hypophyseal level, progressive degranulation of growth hormone and prolactin producing cells has been observed in both thymectomized and thymusless nude mice (Pierpaoli et al., 1971; Comsa et al ., 1977).

Determinations of blood levels of pituitary hormones have demonstrated a reduction of plasma level of prolactin and an increased level of luteotropic hormone (LH) in thymectomized mice (Pierpaoli et al., 1976). In neonatally thymectomized rats transitory decrements of ACTH levels and increased blood concentrations of LH were observed (Deschaux et al., 1979).

By contrast, no alterations in the morphology of the pituitary gland have been observed in the nude mutation of rats (Vos et al., 1980). Hormonal determinations in these animals have not been done thus far.

Transitory signs of thyroid stimulation have been observed in thymectomized guinea pigs and ascribed to pituitary involvement (Comsa, 1971). In nude mice (Pierpaoli and Sorkin, 1972b; Pierpaoli and Besedovsky, 1975; Vos et al., 1980) but not in nude rats features of hypotrophy of the gland with reduced plasma levels of T_3 and T_4 have been reported.

In old normal mice, which are characterized by an involuted thymus and by low levels of T_3 the implantation of a neonatal syngeneic thymus under the kidney capsule induces a significant increment of plasma T_3 levels (Piantanelli et al ., 1978).

Both neonatally thymectomized and nude mice have been reported to show an abnormal histological picture of adrenals (Pierpaoli and Sorkin, 1972b), accompained by a transient increase of plasma levels of corticosterone (Pierpaoli and Besedovsky, 1975). Similar pictures of adrenal stimulation have been observed in neonatally thymectomized guinea pigs (Comsa,1971) and rats (Fachet et al., 1962).

According to other authors, neonatal thymectomy in rats induces on the contrary reduction of corticosterone plasma levels, which, in the presence of the concomittant low levels of ACTH,

would suggest an action of the thymus on the adrenals via the
hypophysis (Deschaux et al., 1979).

Gonadal function in thymus-deprived animals has been deeply
investigated, since it was demonstrated that neonatal thymectomy
in hamster had quite different effects according to sex (males
undergo wasting diseases, females do not) (Sherman and Dameshek,
1963). In mice, thymectomy causes sterility in females, but not in
males (Nishizuka and Sakakura, 1969; Deschaux et al., 1979).

Further investigations in both thymectomized and athymic nude
mice, have shown that both thymus-deprived conditions are characterized by a delayed vaginal opening time, with deeper sexual
underdevelopment in nude mice than in thymectomized animals
(Besedovsky and Sorkin, 1974).

In the intricate picture derived from such contradictory
results, only one finding seems certainly well observable in all
animal models, including the nude rat: the sexual dimorphysm which
characterizes submaxillary glands is absent in thymus-deprived
animals (Wortis, 1975; Vos et al, 1980).

With regard to the endocrine pancreas very little is presently
known. Preliminary experiments in nude mice have shown, that while
there are not differences in the basal levels of plasma insulin
between nude and normal littermates the insulin-dependent esokinase
pattern in the liver is strongly altered in nude animals (Fabris
and Piantanelli, 1979). Moreover in old normal mice, the abnormally
high plasma level of insulin is restored to young values by trans-
planting a syngeneic neonatal thymus (Piantanelli et al., 1978).

Finally, some physiological reactions induced by the stimulation of beta-adrenergic receptors, such as the increased rate of
DNA synthesis in submandibular glands or the increment of total
water intake shortly after the injection of isoproterenol are reduced in nude, in thymectomized and in old normal mice and can be
restored by a syngeneic neonatal thymus transplant (Piantanelli
et al., 1978; Fabris and Piantanelli, 1979). Preliminary experiments suggest, furthermore, that such an action of the thymus on
the beta-adrenergic receptor-adenyl cyclase-cAMP system is exerted
through modification of the beta-adrenergic receptor density on
the surface of target cells (Piantanelli et al., 1980).

4.2. Effect of Thymus Hypofunctioning on Parameters of Aging

To the above reported list of thymus vs neuroendocrine system interactions there should be added also some observations on the influence of the thymus on other extra-immunological parameters, which are strongly dependent on the neuroendocrine balance. Among there phenomena these are to be quoted the alterations of collagen, the osteoporosis, the osseal malformations (for ref. see Pierpaoli and Sorkin, 1972a; and Piantanelli and Fabris, 1978) and the increased ploydity of liver cells recorded in thymus-deprived animals (Giuli et al., 1980).

To note that these alterations appear also as a consequence of aging (for review see Piantanelli and Fabris, 1978; Fabris and Piantanelli, 1982) and, furthermore, the majority of them can be corrected by a neonatal thymus transplant performed even in old age (Piantanelli et al., 1978; Pieri et al., 1980).

These findings, taken together, on one hand give further support to the idea that the thymus exerts a wide-spread influence on the neuroendocrine system, on the other hand strongly suggest that such an influence is operating throughout the whole span of life and that its deterioration may represent an important component of the aging process.

With regard to the mechanism, by which the thymus may influence the neuroendocrine system very little is known. A candidate may certainly be the cellular product of the thymus, i.e. T-derived cells, since humoral secretion of them, such as lymphokines, seem to act on the neuroendocrine balance (see Sorkin, this volume). Since lymphokines are produced as a consequence of antigenic stimuli, this interpretation would necessarily suppose that either the degree of antigenic stimulation or the degree of lymphokine response are modified in the different animal models, the aging animal included.
It is to be noted, however that some of the extra-immunological parameter tested are strictly age-dependent, i.e. the function under study starts to decline (or to increase) very early in life and the modification with age follows a quasi-linear pattern. This kind of profile is not, however, that one followed by the majority of immunological functions, which reach the maximal efficiency in middle-aged animals (Walford, 1976) and decline only thereafter. Based on these consideration it seems to us unlikely that the

mediation of lymphokines might fully explain our findings, although it can not be excluded a their role in very old age.

By contrast, the profile of the age-dependent decline of the endocrine function of the thymus, as measured by bioassays (Bach et al., 1972; Lewis et al., 1978) or by RIA (see Hall and Goldstein, this volume) parallels that one of the aging parameters, taken into consideration in our studies (Piantanelli et al., 1978).
We favour, therefore, the interpretation, according which it is the endocrine function of the thymus, which mediates thymus-neuroendocrine interactions (Fabris, 1981; Piantanelli and Fabris, 1982). The recent observation that thymus may modify the rate of secretion of pituitary luteotropic hormone (Hall and Goldstein, this volume) gives the first experimental support to this hypothesis. Further work on this line will certainly elucidate, in the future, the role played by thymic humoral factor(s) in the thymus-neuroendocrine system interactions.

5. CONCLUSION

The existence of bidirectional interactions between the neuroendocrine system and thymic function is supported by the following observations:
a. Changes of the neuroendocrine balance, induced by experimental manipulation or physiologically occurring, such as those related to aging, modify the growth pattern of the thymus and greatly influence the synthesis and/or the secretion of thymic hormones, as measured in the circulation by bioassay.
b. Thymus absence, as in thymectomized and in athymic nude mice, or thymus hypofunctioning, as it occurs in aging, causes modifications in different components of the neuroendocrine network; most of these alterations are recovered by neonatal thymus transplant.

A key role in this thymus-neuroendocrine network is played by the endocrine function of the thymus, which on one hand is under the modulating action of the neuroendocrine balance, and on the other hand it seems to regulate some neuroendocrine function, in addition to the more obvious effect on the perypheral immune system.

The widespread action of the thymus, which seems to directly and indirectly influence such basic physiological mechanisms as hormonal turnover and beta-adrenoceptor-adenylate-cyclase complex, and its relevance during the whole span of life of the organism may not be enough to assign to the thymus the primary role in aging processes, but it may certainly justify reconsidering, at least at a speculative level, its possible role as a biological clock for physiological functions as important as immune and neuro-endocrine homeostasis.

ACKNOWLEDGEMENT

This work was in part supported by Grant no. CT81.00196.04 from Consiglio Nazionale delle Ricerche, Italy.

REFERENCES

Abo, T., Kawate, T., Hinuma, S., Iton, K. Abo, W., Sato, J. and Kumagai, K., 1980, The circadian periodicities of lymphocyte sub--populations and the role of corticosteroid in human beings and mice, in: "Recent advances in the chronobiology of allergy and immunology", Smolenzky, M.H., Reinberg, A., and MacGovern, J.P., eds., Pergamon Press, Oxford.

Addock, E.W., III, Teasdale, F., Agust, C.S., Cox, S., Meschia, G., Battaglia, F. C., and Naughton, M.A., 1973, Human chorionic gonadotrophin: its possible role in maternal lymphocytes suppression, Science, 181:835.

Amman, A.J., Duquesnoy, R.J., and Good, R.A., 1970, Endocrinological studies in ataxia telangiectasia and other immunological deficiency diseases, Clin. Exp. Immunol., 6:587.

Andersen, D.H., 1932, The relationship between the thymus and reproduction, Physiol. Rev., 12:1.

Bach, J.f., and Dardenne, M., 1973, Studies on thymus products. II. Demonstration and characterization of a circulating thymic hormone, Immunology, 25:353.

Bach, J.F., Dardenne, M., Papiernik, M., Barvis, A., Levasseur, P. and Lebrand, H., 1972, Evidence for a serum-factor secreted by the human thymus, Lancet, 2:1056.

Basso, A., Mocchegiani, E., and Fabris, N., 1981, Increased immunological efficiency in young mice by short-term treatment with L-thyroxine, J. Endocrinol. Invest., 4:431.

Bearn, J.G., 1966, Influence of the pituitary-adrenal axis on deve-
    loment of the rat foetal thymus, Proc. Soc. Exp. Biol. Med.,
    122:273.
Besedovsky, H.O., and Sorkin, E., 1974, Thymus involvement in female
    sexual maturation, Nature (London), 249:356.
Bianchi, E., Colombo, A., Salvatoni, A., Petrone, M., Gasperi, A.,
    Nespoli, L., and Severi, F., 1980, Isolated anterior pituitary
    aplasia in a newborn, in "Problems in Pediatric Endocrinology",
    C. La Cauza and A.W. Root, eds., Academic Press, London.
Barnes, E.W., Loudon, N.B., MacCuish, A.C., Jordan, J., and Irvine,
    W.J., 1974, Phytoemagglutinin-induced lymphocyte transformation
    and circulating autoantibodies in women taking oral contracep-
    tives, Lancet, i:898.
Brinck-Johnson, T., and Dougherty, T.F.,1965, Effect of cortisol and
    corticotropin on incorporation of adenine in the lymphatic
    tissue nucleic acids, Acta Endocrinol. (Copenhagen), 49:471.
Castro, J.E., 1974, Hormone mechanism of immunopotentiation in mice
    after castration, J. Endocrinol., 62:311.
Chandra, R.K., 1979, Serum thymic hormone activity in protein-energy
    malnutrition, Clin. Exp. Immunol., 38:338.
Cherry, C.I., Einstein, R. and Glucksmann, A., 1968, Epithelial
    cords and tubules of rat thymus: effects of age, sex, castra-
    tion, thyroid and other hormones on their incidence and secre-
    tory activity, Brit. J. of Exp. Pathol., 48:90.
Chiodi, H., 1939, Influence de la thymectomie sur la croissance et
    le development des rats blancs, Seances de la Soc. de Biologie,
    130:298.
Comsa, J., 1971, Thymic hormones, Hormones, 2:226.
Comsa, J., Leonhardt, H. and Ozminski, K., 1979, Hormonal influences
    on the secretion of the thymus, Thymus, 1:81.
Comsa, J., Philipp, E.M., and Leonhardt, H. 1977, Effects of thy-
    mectomy on the endocrines of the rat, Isr. J. Med. Sci., 13:354.
Dardenne, M., Papiernik, M., Bach, J.F. and Stutman, O., 1974, Studies
    on thymus products. III. Epithelial origin of the serum thymic
    factor, Clin. Exp. Immunol., 27:299.
Deschaux, P., 1977, Etude in vivo et in vitro des interactions du
    thymus avec certaines glandes endocrines, Lyon, Thesis.
Deschaux, P., Binimbi Massengo and Fontanges, R., 1979, Endocrine
    interaction of the thymus with the hypophysis, adrenals and
    testies: Effect of two thymic extracts, Thymus, 1:95.
Dung, H.C., 1977, Deficiency in the thymus-dependent immunity in
    "lethargic" mutant mice, Transplantation, 23:39.
Duquesnoy, R.J., Mariani, T., and Good, R.A., 1969, Effect of hypo-

physectomy on the immunological recovery from X-irradiation, Proc.Soc. Exp. Biol. Med., 132:1176.

Ernstrom, U., and Larsson, B., 1966, Thymic and thoracic duct contribution to blood lymphocytes in normal and thyroxin-treated guinea-pig, Acta Physiol. Scand., 66:189.

Fabris, N., 1973, Immunodepression in thyroid-deprived animals, Clin. Exp. Immunol., 15:601.

Fabris, N., 1981a, Body homeostasis mechanisms and immunological aging, in:" Immunology of Aging", Makinodan, T., and Kay, M.M.B., eds, CRC Press, Palm Beach.

Fabris, N., 1981b, Influence of thyroid hormones on the immune system,in: "The low T_3 syndrome", R.D. Hesch, ed., Academic Press, London and New York.

Fabris, N., 1981c, Ontogenic and phylogenetic aspects of neuro-endocrine-immune network, Develop. Comparat. Immunology, 5(1):46.

Fabris, N., and Mocchegiani, E, Endocrine control of thymic serum factor production in young-adult and old mice, submitted.

Fabris, N., Muzzioli, M., and Mocchegiani. E., 1982, Recovery of age-dependent immunological deterioration in Balb/c mice by short-term treatment with L-thyroxine, Mech. Age. Develop., 18:237.

Fabris, N., and Piantanelli, L., 1977, Differential effect of pancreatectomy on humoral and cell-mediated immune responses, Clin. Exp. Immunol., 28:315.

Fabris, N., and Piantanelli, L., 1979, Thymus, homeostatic regulation and aging, Proc. XI Int. Cong. Gerontology, Excerpta Medica, p. 451.

Fabris, N., and Piantanelli, L., 1982, Thymus-neuroendocrine interactions during development and aging, in: "Hormones and Aging", Adelman R., and J. Roth, eds., CRC Press, Palm Beach.

Fabris, N., Piantanelli, L., and Muzzioli, M., 1977, Differential effect of pregnancy or gestagens on humoral and cell-mediated immunity, Clin. Exp. Immunol., 28:306.

Fabris, N., Pierpaoli, W., and Sorkin, E., 1971a, Hormones and the immunological capacity. III. The immunodeficiency diseases of the hypopituitary Snell-Bagg dwarf mouse, Clin. Exp. Immunol., 9:209.

Fabris, N., Pierpaoli, W., and Sorkin, E., 1971b, Hormones and the immunological capacity. VI. Restorative effects of developmental hormones or of lymphocytes on the immunodeficiency syndrome of the dwarf mouse, Clin. Exp. Immunol., 9:227.

Fabris, N., Pierpaoli, W., and Sorkin, E., 1972, Lymphocytes, hormones and ageing, Nature, (London), 240:557.

Fachet, J., Stand, E., Vallent, K., and Paltkovits, M., 1962, Func-
    tional interaction between thymus and adrenal cortex, Acta Med.
    Acad. Hung., 18:461.

Fernandes, G., Handwerger, B.S., Yunis, E.J., and Brown, D.M., 1978,
    Immune response in the mutant diabetic C57BL/Ks-db+ mouse, J.
    Clin. Invest., 61:243.

Franceschi, C., Licastro, F., Chiricolo, M., Bonetti, F., Zanotti,
    M., Fabris, N., Mocchegiani, E., Fantini, M.P., Paolucci, P.,
    and Masi, M., 1981, Deficiency of autologous mixed lymphocytes
    reactions and serum thymic factor level in Down Syndrome, J.
    Immunol.,126:2161.

Gavin, J.R. III, 1977, Polipeptide hormone receptor on lymphoid
    cells, in:"Immunopharmacology", Hadden, J.W., Coffey, R.G. and
    Spreafico, F., eds., Plenum Press, New York, p.357.

Gershwin, M.E., Merchant, B., Gelfand, M.C., Vickers, J., Steinberg,
    A.D., and Hansen, C.T., 1975, The natural history and immuno-
    pathology of outbred athymic (nude) mice, Clin. Immunol.
    Immunopathol., 4:324.

Giuli, C., Pieri, C., Piantanelli, L., and Fabris, N., 1980, Electron
    microscopic morphometric analysis of mouse liver. I. Experimen-
    tal studies on the morphogenetic significance of the thymus
    in nude and normal mice, Mech. Age. Develop., 13:265.

Goldstein, A.L., Guba, A., Zats, M.M., Hardy, M.A., and While, A.,
    1972, Purification and biological activity of thymosin, a
    hormone of the thymus gland, Proc. Nat. Acad. Sci., 69:1800.

Goldstein, G., Scheid, M., Hammertring, U., Bose, E.A., Schlesinger,
    D.H., and Niall, H.D., 1976, Isolation of a polypeptide that
    as lymphocytes-differentiating properties and is probably
    represented universally in living cells, Proc. Nat. Acad. Sci.,
    U.S.A., 72:11.

Good, R.A., Dalmasso, A.P., Martinez, C., Archer, O.K., Pierce, J.C.,
    and Papermaster, B.W., 1962, The role of the thymus in develop-
    ment of immunologic capacity in rabbits and mice, J. Exp. Med.
    116:773.

Gudernatsch, F., 1937, The present status of the thymus problem,
    Med. Rec., 146:101.

Gunn, A., Lance, E.M., Medawar, P.B., and Nehlsen, S.L., 1970,
    Synergism between cortisol and antilimphocitic serum, in:
    "Hormones and the immune response", Ciba Study Group No. 36,
    Wolstenholme, G.E.W. and J. Knight, eds., Churcill, London.

Hesch, R.D., 1981, "The Low T3 Syndrome", Academic Press, London
    and New York.

Lewis, V.M., Twomey, J.J., Bealmear, P., Goldstein, G., and Good,

R.A., 1978, Age, thymic involution, and circulating thymic hormone activity, J. Clin. Endocrinol. Metab., 47:145.

MacCuish, A., Urbaniak, S.J., Campbell, C.J., Duncan, L.J.P., and Irvine, W.J., 1974, Phytohemagglutinin trasformation and circulating lymphocyte subpopulations in insulin-dependent diabetes, Diabetes, 23:708.

McIntire, K.R., Sell, S., and Miller, J.F.A.P., 1964, Pathogenesis of the post-neonatal thymectomy wasting syndrome, Nature, 204:151.

Miller, J.F.A.P., 1961, Immunological function of the thymus, Lancet, 2:748.

Miller, J.F.A.P., and Osoba, D., 1967, Current concepts on the immunological function of the thymus, Physiol. Rev., 47:437.

Nishizuka, J. and Sakakura, T., 1969, Thymus and reproduction: sex-linked dysgenesia of the gonad after neonatal thymectomy in mice, Science, 166:753.

Oaki, N., Wakisaka, G., and Nagata, I., 1976, Effects of thyroxine on T-cell counts and tumour cell rejection in mice., Acta Endocrinol., 81:104.

Pandian, M.R., and Talwar, G.P., 1971, Effect of growth hormone on the metabolism of thymus and on the immune response against sheep erythrocytes, J. Exp. Med., 134:1095.

Pauly, J.E., Lawrence, E., Scheving, E., Burnes, R., and Tien-Hu Tsai., 1976, Circadian rhythm in DNA synthesis in mouse thymus: Effect of altered lighting regimens, restricted feeding and presence of Ehrlich ascites tumor, Anat. Rec., 184(3):284.

Piantanelli, L., Basso, A., Muzzioli, M., and Fabris, N., 1978, Thymus-dependent reversibility of physiological and isoproterenol-evoked age-related parameters in athymic (nude) and old normal mice, Mech. Age. Develop., 7:171.

Piantanelli, L., and Fabris, N., 1978, Hypopituitary dwarf and athymic nude mice and the study of the relationships among thymus, hormones and aging, in: "Genetic effects on Aging", Harrison, D.E. and Bergsma, D., eds., Sinauer Ass., Suderland, Mass, p.315.

Piantanelli, L., Fattoretti, P., and Viticchi, C., 1980, Beta-adrenoceptor changes in submandibular glands of old mice., Mech. Age. Dev., 14:155.

Pieri, C., Giuli, C., Del Moro, M., and Piantanelli, L., 1980, Electron microscopic morphometric analysis of mouse liver. II. Effect of ageing and thymus transplantation in old animals, Mech. Age. Develop., 13:275.

Pierpaoli, W., and Besedovsky, N.O., 1975, Role of the thymus in programming of neuroendocrine function, Clin. Exp. Immunol.,

20:325.

Pierpaoli, W., Bianchi, H., and Sorkin, E., 1971, Modification of
    the growth-hormone producing cells in the hypophysis of neona-
    tally thymectomized mice, Clin. Exp. Immunol., 9:889.

Pierpaoli, W., Kopp, H.G., and Bianchi, E., 1976, Interdipendence
    of thymic and neuroendocrine functions in ontogeny, Clin.
    Exp. Immunol., 24:501.

Pierpaoli, W., and Sorkin, E., 1972a, Hormones, thymus and lympho-
    cyte functions. Experientia 28:1385.

Pierpaoli, W., and Sorkin, E., 1972a, Alterations of adrenal cortex
    and thyroid in mice with congenital absence of the thymus,
    Nature New Biol., 238:282.

Sherman, J.D., and Dameshek, W., 1963, "Wasting disease" following
    thymectomy in the hamster, Nature, Lond., 197:469.

Sympson, J.G., Gray, S.E., Michie, W., and Swanson Beck, J., 1975,
    The influence of preoperative drug treatment on the extent of
    hyperplasia of the thymus in primary thyrotoxicosis, Clin.
    Exp. Immunol., 22:249.

Stein, M., Schiavi, R.C., and Camerino, M., 1976, Influence of brain
    and behaviour on the immune system, Science, 191:435.

Szemberg, A., 1970, Influence of testosterone on the primary lymphoid
    organs of the chicken, in: "Hormones and Immune Responses",
    Ciba, Study Group No. 36, G.E.W. Wolstenholme and J. Knight,
    eds., Churchill, London, p.45.

Szent-Gyorgyi, A., Hegyeli, A., and Mc Laughlin, J.A., 1962, Consti-
    tuents of the thymus gland and their relation to growth, ferti-
    lity, muscle and cancer, Proc. Nat. Acad. Sci., 48:1439.

Upendra, S., and Owen, J.J.T., 1976, Studies on the maturation of
    thymus stem cells: the effects of catecholamines, histamine
    and peptide hormones on the expression of T cell alloantigens,
    Eur. J. Immunol., 6:59.

Vos, J.G., Berkvens, J.M., and Kruijt, B.C., 1980, The athymic nude
    rat, Clin. Immunol. Immunopathol., 15:213.

Walford, R.L., 1976, When is a mouse "old"? J. Immunol., 177:342.

Waltman, S.R., Burde, R.M., and Berrios, J., 1971, Prevention of
    corneal homograft rejection by estrogens, Transplantation,
    11:194.

Wortis, H.H., 1975, Pleiotropic effects of the nude mutation, in
    "Immunodeficiency in man and animals", Bergsma, D., ed. Birth
    Defects Series, Sinauer Ass. Mass., p.528.

MYASTHENIA GRAVIS: THYMIC AND PERIPHERAL BLOOD CELL

INTERACTIONS IN SPECIFIC ANTIBODY PRODUCTION

John Newsom-Davis

Department of Neurological Science
Royal Free Hospital School of Medicine
Pond Street, London NW3 2QG, England

1. INTRODUCTION

Myasthenia gravis is a disorder of neuromuscular transmission in which antibody is produced to the skeletal muscle receptor for the neurotransmitter acetylcholine. It is thus one of a group of autoimmune disorders predicted by Lennon and Carnegie (1971) and now increasingly being recognised, in which cell surface receptors to peptide hormones or neurotransmitters become the target for autoantibodies. Other examples of diseases which show this feature are thyrotoxicosis and some forms of diabetes.

A further feature of myasthenia is the evidence for involvement of the thymus, which is of special interest in the light of recent work suggesting that developing T-cells may learn to recognise self-antigens there. Thus, the study of myasthenia, and in particular of the role of the thymus in the disease, may throw some light on the defects in immune regulation that lead to disorders of this kind.

2. IMMUNOLOGICAL MECHANISMS

The illness is characterized clinically by fatiguable muscle weakness that can be life-threatening. Neuromuscular transmission depends on the reaction between acetylcholine, released in packets (quanta) from the nerve terminal, and the acetylcholine receptor (AChR) which is an integral membrane protein located on the peaks of the postsynaptic folds of the muscle fibres. The reaction causes receptor in channels to open briefly, allowing the influx of small cations that depolarises the muscle cell and leads to muscle contraction. The use of an iodinated snake toxin, ^{125}I--alpha bungarotoxin (α-butx), that binds specifically and with high affinity to the acetylcholine reaction site on the AChR, demonstrated that the number of functional AChRs was greatly reduced in myasthenia (Fambrough et al., 1973), and this reduction adequately accounted for the physiological abnormalities (Ito et al., 1978).

Anti-AChR antibody is implicated in the loss of receptor. This antibody is specific for myasthenia and is detectable in 90% of those with generalised disease (Lindstrom et al., 1977; Compston et al., 1980). It is a heterogeneous IgG antibody binding to more than one determinant on the receptor. It is usually assayed by an immuno-precipitation method, in which ^{125}I-α-Butx--labelled human AChR, detergent extracted from amputated calf muscle, is incubated with the test serum. Receptor-antibody complexes are then precipitated with anti-human IgG antiserum. The titre is expressed as moles of toxin-binding sites precipitated per litre of serum. Anti-AChR antibody leads to loss of AChR apparently by more than one mechanism. Cross-linking of AChRs by the divalent antibody increases the rate at which AChR is internalised into the muscle cell and there degraded by lysosomal enzymes (Drachman et al., 1978). Secondly, immunohistological techniques have demonstrated IgG and complement components C3 and C9 coating segments of the postsynaptic membrane and degraded products of the membrane shed into the synaptic cleft (Engel et al., 1977; Sahashi et al., 1980).

These changes are consistent with complement-dependent lysis of the postsynaptic membrane, and would account for the simplified appearance of the membrane in long-standing cases of myasthenia. There is at present no reliable evidence that antibody can produce direct immunopharmacological block of the acetylcholine reaction site on the receptor.

3. CLINICAL EVIDENCE FOR INVOLVEMENT OF THYMUS

The first report indicating that the thymus might be involved in the disease was that by Weigert (1901) who described a thymus tumour in a myasthenic patient. Over the next 40 years, occasional cases of thymic tumour (thymoma) associated with myasthenia were treated by thymectomy with apparent benefit, which led to this operation becoming the treatment of choice in the disease whether or not a thymic tumour was present. At this stage it became apparent that in non-thymomatous cases the thymus showed a distinctive pathology. In younger patients, whose age at disease onset was usually less than 40 years, the thymic medulla often contained numerous lymphoid follicles with active germinal centres, which clearly differed from controls of similar age in whom the thymus was typically atrophic. These changes were regarded by Sloan (1943), who first described them, as hyperplasia of the thymus, secondary to some unknown stimulus. Older myasthenic patients, in contrast, typically show involution of the thymus.

The appearance of thymic hyperplasia was not wholly confined to those with myasthenia gravis, and germinal centres have been reported in autoimmune disease in the absence of myasthenia such as thyrotoxicosis and systemic lupus erythematosus (Barnes and Irvine, 1973), raising the possibility that the thymus could be in some way implicated in these diseases too. Thymoma, which is present in 10% of myasthenics, also occurs in association with other immunological disorders including polymyositis, systemic lupus erythematosus and rheumatoid arthritis (Souadjian et al., 1974). In this context, the fact that myasthenia itself shows an increased association with other autoimmune diseases may possibly be relevant to the role of the thymus in these disorders.

The clinical response to thymectomy in myasthenia has provided further grounds for implicating the gland in the aetiology of the disease, but has also been a continuing source of controversy. Initial doubts about its value were largely settled when it was recognised that thymic pathology had to be taken into account when assessing the outcome (Simpson, 1958). Patients with thymic hyperplasia appeared to respond much better to thymectomy than those with thymoma. Many large series have since confirmed that in the former group about 25% can expect to enter remission following surgery, and a further 50% will improve. A problem with most of these studies has been the lack of satisfactory controls, but

their conclusions have been supported by the retrospective controlled study by Buckingham et al. (1976). 80 patients treated by
thymectomy were compared to controls, computer-matched for the important variables of age, sex, severity and duration of disease,
who were treated "medically" (but not with immunosuppressive
drugs). Thymectomy was shown to be significantly beneficial.

Analysis of the immune and HLA characteristics of myasthenic
patients according to the pathology of the thymus and the age of
onset of the disease also suggests that the thymus influences the
disease process (Compston et al., 1980). We distinguished three
main groups of patients, namely: 1) thymoma, 2) non-thymoma with
the age of onset less than 40 years (in whom the thymus typically
shows hyperphasia) and 3) non-thymoma with the age of onset
greater than 40 years (in whom the thymus when examined shows
involution). Females predominated in group 2 and males in group 3,
while the sex incidence was equal in group 1. Anti-AChR antibody
titres showed significant differences between the three groups
and, perhaps even more strikingly, serum anti-striated muscle
antibody is virtually always detectable in thymoma patients but
much less commonly so in non-thymoma cases. Frequencies of HLA
antigens A1, B8 and DRW3 were also significantly increased in
patients with thymic hyperplasia, and A3, B7 and DRW2 in the
non-thymoma older cases. No HLA association has yet convincingly
been shown with thymoma but a particular Gm haplotype occurs with
increased frequency in Japanese (Nakao et al.,1980).

4. THYMUS CELL POPULATIONS

Thymus germinal centres in myasthenia contain cells bearing B
cell markers (Staber et al., 1975). Anti-AChR antibody was
detected in thymic extracts from myasthenic patients with thymic
hyperplasia by Mittag et al. (1976), suggesting the possibility of
its production there. Lisak et al. (1978) have enumerated thymic B
cells in myasthenic and control thymuses. The population of B
cells was increased, while that of T cells was reduced in thymic
hyperplasia compared to control thymus, and to those with thymoma
who did not significantly differ from controls. Piantelli et al.
(1980) also showed that E-rosetting cells were decreased in
myasthenic thymus compared to normal. In addition, B cells were
very infrequent in normal thymus and in myasthenic thymuses that
showed few or absent germinal centres, but were numerous in those

with many germinal centres. The percentage of T-cells, i.e. cells bearing receptors for the Fc portion of IgM, in the myasthenic thymus, was not different from that in control thymus.

Thymic cells from cases of thymic hyperplasia also appeared able to stimulate autologous blood lymphocytes, as assessed by thymidine incorporation (Abdou et al., 1974). This effect is apparently mediated by the E-rosette negative population of thymic cells (B-cell enriched) (Opelz et al., 1978). Thymocytes from thymoma cases did not significantly stimulate.

5. THYMUS AND ACETYLCHOLINE RECEPTOR

Several groups have shown that the normal thymus contains acetylcholine receptor or AChR-like material. Lindstrom et al. (1976) were able to precipitate an α-Butx-binding protein from rat thymus, and Engel et al. (1977) reported binding of peroxidase-labelled α-Butx to epithelial cells in myasthenic thymus and also in a thymus from a patient with dermatomyositis.
Muscle-like "myoid" cells grown out from thymus could also be labelled autoradiographically with iodinated α-Butx (Kao and Drachman, 1977), indicating that they express acetylcholine receptor on their surface. Recently, it has been shown that mouse thymic lymphocytes bear a surface AChR-like antigen, as judged by their ability to bind antibody to torpedo nicotinic acetylcholine receptor (Fuchs et al., 1980).

6. THYMUS AND ANTI-AChR ANTIBODY PRODUCTION

The presence of germinal centres in the myasthenic thymus and the relatively high number of thymus B cells in these cases points to the thymus as a site of antibody production. We have now studied anti-AChR antibody production by cultured thymic lymphocytes obtained from over 50 patients undergoing thymectomy (Vincent et al., 1978; Scadding et al., 1981; Newsom-Davis et al., 1981).
Cells are cultured for 8-12 days and the supernatant assayed for anti-AChR antibody production. This was detected in about 60% of cases in whom the thymus showed hyperplasia. Those in this group in whom antibody production was not detected usually, had low levels of serum anti-AChR. In neither group did pokeweed mitogen significantly increase anti-AChR production.

The rate of antibody production, which reached over 40 fmols/10^6 cells/24 hours in one patient, did not correlate with the degree of thymic hyperplasia which was assessed without knowledge of the culture results (Scadding et al., 1981). Cells from involuted thymuses, or from those containing thymoma, produced little or no anti-AChR culture.

In cases with thymic hyerplasia, the duration of the illness at the time of thymectomy correlated positively with the rate of antibody production. But even in those with long-standing disease and high rates of antibody synthesis in culture, the thymus did not appear to be a major site of anti-AChR production, probably contributing less than 5% of the total. This is consistent with the finding that anti-AChR antibody does not show an immediate and sustained fall following thymectomy.

7. THYMUS AND AUTOLOGOUS BLOOD LYMPHOCYTES IN ANTI-ACETYLCHOLINE RECEPTOR ANTIBODY PRODUCTION

We have found that thymus cells, as well as being able to produce antibody themselves in culture, also enhance anti-AChR production by autologous peripheral blood cells (Newsom-Davis et al., 1981). Myasthenic peripheral blood lymphocytes cultured alone typically make little or no anti-AChR. When co-cultured, however, with thymic cells which have been irradiated (1500 rads) to abro-

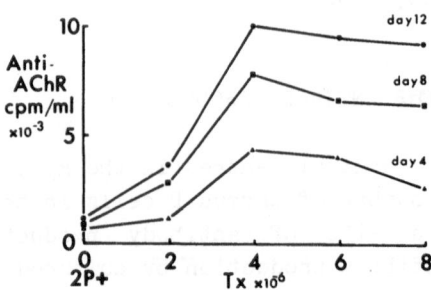

Fig. 1. Anti-acetylcholine receptor antibody production in culture by peripheral blood lymphocytes in a patient with myasthenia gravis. 2x10^6 peripheral blood cells (2P) were cultured in triplicate wells alone and with increasing numbers of irradiated (1500 rads) autologous thymic cells (Tx). Note optimal enhancement of anti-AChR production at thymic:peripheral blood lymphocyte ratio of 2:1.

gate antibody production, a striking enhancement of anti-AChR antibody production can be observed (Fig. 1).

The addition of an equal number of irradiated thymic cells could lead to a seven-fold increase in anti-AChR antibody production and in two cases the increase was 15-fold when the ratio of irradiated thymic cells to autologous blood lymphocytes was 2:1. The enhancing effect of thymic cells on anti-AChR production by autologous blood lymphocytes was significant and more consistent than that of pokeweed mitogen. The enhancing effect depended upon viable thymic cells. Thus if the cells were either repeatedly frozen and thawed, heated to 46° C for 20 minutes or sonicated, their ability to enhance anti-AChR production was lost.

The ability of thymic cells to enhance AChR antibody production by blood lymphocytes appeared to be selective in that neither total IgG nor anti-influenza antibody was increased.
The cell types involved in this response have not yet been determined. There appear to be two principal possibilities. First, the presence of antigen in the thymus, as mentioned above, together with the dependence of the response on viable celle, suggests that antigen (AChR)-presenting cells may be a component in the thymus. Alternatively, or additionally, there may be AChR-specific T-helper cells. Indirect support of this comes from the finding that the ratio of T-helper inducer (OKT4[+]) to T-suppressor cytotoxic (OKT8[+]) lymphocytes in thymus correlates with the ability of thymic cells to enhance the production of the specific antibody by autologous blood lymphocytes (Newsom-Davis et al., 1981). Were these cell populations to migrate from the thymus, they could enhance anti-AChR antibody production elsewhere, and since they are likely to be long-lived, this could account for the relatively slow time course for improvement following thymectomy that is usually observed.

8. SUMMARY AND CONCLUSIONS

Myasthenia gravis is a disorder of immunoregulation in which an autoantibody is produced, often in large amounts, to the self-antigen acetylcholine receptor. Clinical and experimental evidence for involvement of the thymus in the disease process is of particular interest in view of the recent evidence suggesting that developing T-cells may learn to recognize self-antigens there. The myasthenic thymus may contain AChR specific antigen presenting cells and/or T-helper cells. Faulty presentation or recognition of antigen within the thymus could lead to an autoimmune response. In some other autoimmune disorders, histological abnormalities of the thymus occur, raising the possibility that in these diseases too the thymus may be implicated.

REFERENCES

Abdou, N.I., Lisak, R.P., Zweiman, B., Abrahamsohn, I., and Penn, A.S., 1974, The thymus in myasthenic gravis. Evidence for altered cell populations, N. Engl. J. Med., 291:1271.

Barnes, E.W., and Irvine, W.J. 1973, Clinical syndromes associated with thymic disorders, Proc. Roy. Soc. Med., 66:151.

Buckingham, J.M., Howard, F.M., Bernatz, P.E., Spencer-Payne, W., Harrison, E.G., O'Brien, P.C., and Weiland, L.H., 1976, The value of thymectomy in myasthenia gravis, Ann. Surg., 184:453.

Compston, D.A.S., Vincent, A., Newsom-Davis, J. and Batchelor, J.R., 1980, Clinical, pathological, HLA antigen and immunological evidence for disease heterogeneity in myasthenia gravis, Brain, 103:579.

Drachman, D.B., Angus, C.W., Adams, R.N., Michelson, J.D. and Hofdfman, G.J., 1978, Myasthenic antibodies cross-link acetylcholine receptors to accelerate degradation, N. Engl. J. Med., 298:1116.

Engel, A.G., Lambert, E.H. and Howard, F. 1977, Immune complexes (IgG and C3) at the motor end plate in myasthenia gravis. Ultrastructural and light microscopic localization and electrophysiologic correlations, Mayo Clin. Proc., 53:267.

Engel, W.K., Trotter, J.L., McFarlin, D.E. and McIntosh, C.L. 1977, Thymic epithelial cell contains acetylcholine receptor, Lancet, i: 1310.

Fambrough, D., Drachman, D.B. and Satyamurti, S., 1973, Neuromuscular junction in myasthenia gravis. Decreased acetylcholine receptors, Science, 182:293.

Fuchs, S., Schmidt-Hopfield, I., Tridente, G. and Tarrab-Hazdai, R. 1980, Thymic lymphocytes bear a surface antigen which cross-reacts with acetylcholine receptor, Nature, 287:162.

Ito, Y., Miledi, R., Vincent, A., and Newsom-Davis, J., 1978, Acetylcholine receptors and end-plate electrophysiology in myasthenia gravis, Brain, 101:345.

Kao, I. and Drachman, D.B., 1977, Thymic muscle cells bear acetyl-

choline receptors: possible relation to myasthenia gravis,
    Science, 195:74.
Lennon, V.A. and Carnegie, P.R., 1971, Immunopharmacological disease
    a break in tolerance to receptor sites, Lancet, i:630.
Lindstrom, J.M., Lennon, V.A., Seybold, M.E. and Whittingham, S.,
    1976, Experimental autoimmune myasthenia gravis and myasthenia
    gravis: biochemical and immunochemical aspects, Ann. N.Y.
    Acad. Sci., 274:254.
Lindstrom, J.M., Seybold, M.E., Lennon, V.A., Whittingham, S. and
    Duane, D.D., 1976, Antibody to acetylcholine receptor in
    myasthenia gravis. Prevalence, clinical correlates and diag-
    nostic value, Neurology, 26:1065.
Lisak, R.PO., Zweiman, B. and Phillips, S.M. 1978, Thymic and
    peripheral blood T-cell and B-cell levels in myasthenia
    gravis, Neurology, 28:1298.
Mittag, T., Kornfeld, P., Tormay, A. and Woo, C., 1976, Detection
    of anti-acetylcholine receptor factors in serum and thymus
    from patients with myasthenia gravis, N. Engl. J. Med., 294:691.
Nakao, Y., Miyazaki, T., Ota, K., Matzumoto, H., Nishitani, H.,
    Fujita, T. and Tsuji, K., 1980, Gm allotypes in myasthenia
    gravis, Lancet, i:677.
Newsom-Davis, J., Willcox, N., Scadding,G., Calder, L. and Vincent,
    A., 1981, Anti-acetylcholine receptor antibody sythesis by
    cultured lymphocytes in myasthenia gravis: thymic and peripheral
    blood cell interactions, Ann. N.Y. Acad. Sci., (in press)
Opelz, G., Keesey, J., Glovsky, M. and Gale, R.P., 1978, Auto-
    reactivity between lymphocytes and thymus cells in myasthenia
    gravis, Arch. Neurol., 35:413.
Piantelli, P., Musiani, P., Lauriola, L., Carbone, A., Tonali, P.
    and Dina, M.A., 1980, Lymphocyte sub-populations in non-
    neoplastic thymus from myasthenia gravis patients, Clin. Exp.
    Immunol., 41:19.
Sahasi, K., Engel, A.G., Lambert, E.H. and Howard, F.M., 1980,
    Ultrastructural localisation of the terminal and lytic 9th
    complement component (C9) at the motor end-plate in myasthenia
    gravis, J. Neurol. Exp. Neuropathol., 39:160.
Scadding, G.K., Vincent, A., Newsom-Davis, J. and Henry, K.,
    Acetylcholine receptor antibody synthesis by thymic lympho-
    cytes "in vitro", Neurology Minneap., in press.
Simpson, J.A., 1958, An evaluation of thymectomy in myasthenia
    gravis, Brain, 81:1112.
Sloan, H.E., 1943, The thymus in myasthenia gravis. With observa-
    tion on the normal anatomy and histology of the thymus,

Surgery, 13:154.

Souadjian, J.V., Enriquez, P., Silverstein, M.N. and Pepin, J.M.,
    1974, The spectrum of diseases associated with thymoma, Arch.
    Intern. Med., 134:374.

Staber, F.G., Fink, U. and Sack, W., 1975, B lymphocytes in the
    thymus of patients with myasthenia gravis, N. Engl. J. Med.,
    292:1032.

Vincent, A., Scadding, G.K., Thomas, H.C. and Newsom-Davis, J.,
    1978, "In vitro" synthesis of anti-acetylcholine receptor
    antibody by thymic lymphocytes in myasthenia gravis, Lancet,
    i:305.

Weiger, V., 1901, Pathologisch-anatomischer Beitrag zur Erb'schen
    Krankheit Myasthenia gravis, Neurol. Zbl., 20:597.

MUSCULAR DYSTROPHIES AND THYMIC DEFICIENCY

David F. Horrobin

Efamol Research Institute, P.O. Box, 818, Kentville
Nova Scotia, Canada B4N 4H8

1. INTRODUCTION

The association between the thymus and the muscle has been intensively investigated in the case of "myasthenia gravis". The evidence that in some patients with "myasthenia gravis" there may be an excess of thymic function tended to point investigators in the direction of looking for excess thymic activity in muscular dystrophy also. However, in 1964, Walker demonstrated that neonatal thymectomy failed to influence the course of murine muscular dystrophy. This was thought to rule out the idea that excess thymus activity might be involved, at least in the mouse model of muscular dystrophy. It was a decade before interest was again aroused in the muscular dystrophy/thymus relationship.

In fact, the available evidence about the thymus and muscle should have made investigators think about the opposite possibility, namely that a lack of normal thymus function might be involved in the muscle disease. As early as 1906, Basch demonstrated that thymectomy in dogs was followed by muscle wasting. In 1938 Comsa demonstrated a similar thing in guinea pigs and in the 1950's and 1960's, muscle atrophy was found to follow thymectomy in rats, mice, frogs, tadpoles and guinea pigs again (Harms, 1952; Houssay et al., 1955; Pora et al., 1960; Jankovic, 1962; Miller, 1962; Parrot and East, 1962). Possibly this work failed to gain the attention of the world wide scientific community because almost all of the earlier papers were published in languages other than English!

In the mid-1970's, interest in the idea that a thymic deficiency might be involved in muscular dystrophy developed as a result of a change meeting in Canada between a group working in Australia and one in England. De Kretser and Livett (1976) in Melbourne and Karmali and Horrobin (1976) in Newcastle upon Tyne had both noticed that mice of the Bar Harbor ReJ 129 strain looked superficially very similar to mice which had been neonatally thymectomized. As a result of this chance meeting both groups decided to investigate the phenomenon further. At the same time Cosmos in Hamilton, doing muscle cross transplantation experiments between normal and dystrophy chicks, had noted that transplants into the dystrophic birds survived very much longer in a healthy state than transplants into the normal birds. These observations triggered a series of detailed investigations into the status of the thymus and the immune system in various forms of muscular dystrophy.

2. THE THYMUS IN DYSTROPHIC MICE

Homozygous dystrophic mice of the Bar Harbor ReJ 129 strain are very variable in size, have poor coat quality, have a very uncertain life span and are highly susceptible to infections. These characteristics are similar to those of mice which have been neonatally thymectomized. This superficial similarity led De Kretser and Livett (1976) and Kamali and Horrobin (1976) to wonder whether the Bar Harbor mice might have atrophied thymus tissue. Inspection of a few adult mice showed that this was indeed the case and led to a systematic investigation. De Kretser and Livett (1976) found that both the thymus and spleen were reduced in size in homozygous dystrophic animals as compared to phenotypically normal mice of the same strain. This reduction seemed to be particularly due to loss of the lymphoid elements of the thymus with the epithelial elements being unchanged or actually hypertrophied. Karmali and Horrobin (1976) investigated the time course of the changes in thymic size and found that the dystrophic animals had a normal thymic weight until the time of weaning. The thymus then atrophied very rapidly and at four weeks of age there was a dramatic difference between the normal and dystrophic animals. Between 4 and 12 weeks, however, when the gland in the normal animals was undergoing atrophy, the thymus in the dystrophics actually increased in size so that there was a significant rise in both thymus weight and thymus weight/body weight ratio.

Table 1. Allograft rejection time of skin grafts transplanted into
dystrophic mice and normal controls from the same strain.
Reproduced with permission from Colby-Germinario, et al.,
1981. Results are given as mean days to rejection $\pm$ SD.

Strain	Age (wks)	Recipient Normal	n	Genotype dy/dy	n	Significance P
C57B1	3	13.0 ± 0.6	6	17.2 ± 1.0	6	0.001
	6	31.3 ± 0.8	6	14.6 ± 0.5	6	0.05
	12	14.7 ± 1.5	6	14.7 ± 0.8	7	ns
129ReJ	3	13.3 ± 0.5	6	50	4	0.001
	6	12.5 ± 1.4	6	19.0 ± 5.1	6	0.05
	12	13.1 ± 1.6	6	14.7 ± 0.8	6	0.05

This pattern of rapid thymic atrophy after weaning is similar to that seen in certain other strains of mice such as "dwarf" and "lethargic" animals (Fabris et al., 1971; Dung, 1976). In the dwarf mice the thymus atrophy appears to be related to pituitary dysfunction since it can be at least partially corrected by injections of growth hormone or prolactin. Prolactin is secreted into milk and can be absorbed from the neonatal gut, so that it is possible that atrophy occurs at weaning because this exogenous source of prolactin is withdrawn. Karmali and Horrobin (1975) were able to show that prolactin injections could stimulate uptake of tritiated thymidine and partly prevent thymus atrophy in the Bar Harbor dystrophic animals.

Livett's group went on to conduct an intensive investigation of immunological function in dystrophic mice of the Bar Harbor 129 strain and also another dystrophic strain the C57B1 (Colby-Germinario et al., 1981; Livett et al., 1981). Skin grafts from normal mice of another strain were transplanted into either normal or dystrophic mice at 3 weeks (when thymus atrophy in the dystrophic animals is maximal as compared to the controls),and also at 6 and 12 weeks when the dystrophic thymus seems to be recovering. The results were clear cut (Table 1). At three weeks of age, graft survival was highly significantly prolonged in the dystrophic animals of both strains. In the C57B1, survival was still slightly prolonged at 6 weeks but at 12 weeks was normal. The differences in survival persisted throughout the experimental period in the 129 ReJ animals, but while they were dramatic at 3 weeks, they were reduced at 6 and still further reduced at 12 weeks. There is therefore a perhaps surprising parallelism between crude thymus size and the capacity for allograft rejection in both these strains. Interestingly blood counts showed no differences in the absolute numbers or proportions of any component of the white cell population between normal and dystrophic animals at any age (Livett et al., 1981). Only total lymphocytes were counted and it is possible that there could have been differences between lymphocyte subsets.

Szewcuk et al. (1980) reported that in mice of the C57B1 strain the number of antibody forming cells was reduced in the dystrophic animals. Although there initially appeared to be differences in Con A lymphocyte capping in the dystrophic animals, further studies could not confirm this observation (Livett et al., 1981). There is, therefore, a need for sophisticated immunological investigations to pinpoint the precise nature of the immunological deficit associated with thymus atrophy and the failure of allograft rejection. The crude relationship between thymus size and tolerance raises the possibility that a thymic hormonal factor whose rate of production is related to thymus bulk could be involved.

3. STUDIES IN THE CHICKEN

The idea that a thymic abnormality might be related to the development of muscular dystrophy in some rather fundamental way is supported by the finding of immunological deficits, not only in the two types of mouse dystrophy, but also in the dystrophy which occurs in chickens. Cosmos et al. (1977, 1980) were investigating the idea that dystrophic muscle becomes dystrophic because of a neurogenic factor. They, therefore, carried out transplantation experiments in which minced muscle from normal birds was transplanted into dystrophic birds and vice versa. They found that the normal muscle remained normal and the dystrophic muscle remained dystrophic suggesting that there was an endogenous muscle factor involved in the dystrophy. However, they did notice a dramatic difference in the fates of the transplants in the two host types. In the normal hosts the dystrophic muscle was rejected as expected. In contrast, in the dystrophic hosts, the survival of the grafts was quite remarkably prolonged. The group went on to test the effect of neonatal thymectomy in normal birds and were able to demonstrate that this led to the development of a syndrome very similar to the naturally occurring disease.

The effect of thymectomy on normal muscle suggests that not only is thymic atrophy associated with the natural muscular dystrophies, but it also contributes to the development of the diseases. My own view is that some fundamental metabolic error produces a widespread defect in biochemical function which affects thymus, muscle and other tissues as well. However this thymic damage produces functional deficits which further harm the defective muscle tissue (Horrobin et al., 1979).

4. HUMAN MUSCULAR DYSTROPHIES

Immunological function in the human dystrophies has been relatively little investigated. Most clinicians are aware that patients with muscular dystrophies have an increased susceptibility to infections. However, this is usually thought to be a secondary consequence of muscle damage leading, for example, to a failure of normally effective coughing. In myotonic dystrophy serum immunoglobulin levels are low and this is believed to be due to an increased rate of breakdown rather than to a defective synthesis (Wochner 1970; Wochner, et al., 1966). A surprising number of the abnormalities present in myotonic dystrophy are similar to those found in zinc deficiency (Horrobin and Morgan, 1980). These include the peculiarities of reproductive failure, the defects in metabolism, in gut function and in bone, and the congenital abnormalities which occur. In view of the recent evidence that zinc is crucial for immune function, a defect in zinc metabolism could lead to immunological defects. However there are important differences between myotonic dystrophy and zinc deficiency, notably with respect to the skin, and the immunological consequences appear quite different. We have therefore proposed that myotonic dystrophy may relate to the presence of an abnormal zinc binding ligand which restricts the access of zinc to some critical sites but not to others (Horrobin and Morgan, 1980).

In Duchenne dystrophy the evidence for an interaction between the thymus and the muscle disease is looking more promising.

Fabris (1980) investigated levels of serum thymic factor (measured by the technique of Bach) in boys with Duchenne dystrophy. In all five boys tested, the level of this factor was substantially reduced. Fabris has now extended this study to include 12 boys. In not one individual was there any overlapping with the age-matched normal range. It therefore seems that boys with Duchenne dystrophy, like dystrophic mice and chickens, have a serious thymic deficit. Duchenne dystrophy could therefore be a disease in which treatment with thymic factors is worthy of trial.

5. POSSIBLE BIOCHEMICAL BASES FOR THE THYMIC ATROPHY

My own research has deviated from direct investigation of the thymus in muscular dystrophy to an indirect attack in an attempt to find the possible biochemical defects which may be involved. I was intrigued by the effect of prolactin in both the dwarf mice and the dystrophic mice and decided to try to track down the mechanism of prolactin action at the second messenger level. Although indirect, this approach has led to a number of promising developments.

For a number of reasons, but most particularly its rapid responsiveness to prolactin, we chose to analyze the second messenger actions in arterial muscle. It appears that in this system, the effects of prolactin depend on its ability to mobilize the prostaglandin (PG) precursor, dihomogammalinolenic acid (DGLA) from its membrane stores. This leads to the formation of free DGLA which is then rapidly converted to PGE1 (Manku et al., 1979; Horrobin, 1979). This biochemical action of prolactin is interesting in an immunological context for several reasons:

1. In both animals and humans the thymus is unique in being exceptionally rich in PGE1 (Karim et al.,1968; Horrobin et al., 1979).

2. PGE1 in vitro is able to imitate the action of thymic hormone in inducing the appearance of theta antigen in immature mouse lymphocytes (Bach and Bach, 1974).

3. PGE1 has biphasic effects on antibody formation, enhancing it at low concentrations and inhibiting it at high concentrations (Ishizuka et al., 1974; Horrobin, 1980).

4. In NZB/W mice and in rats with adjuvant arthritis, PGE1 activates T suppressor cells and inhibits the development of the diseases (Zurier and Ballas, 1971; Zurier et al, 1977).

5. Glucocorticoids, which cause thymus atrophy , block the formation of both 1 and 2 series PGs (Horrobin, 1980).

6. Lithium, which also causes thymus atrophy (Perez-Cruet et al., 1977; Horrobin and Lieb, 1981) has a selective effect in blocking PGE1 formation. 2 series PG formation is inhibited only at much higher doses.

7. Zinc, which plays a critical role in thymus function, also activates PGE1 formation, partly by enhancing conversion of linoleic acid to gamma-linolenic acid and partly by mobilizing DGLA (Horrobin et al., 1979; Horrobin, 1980).

8. Ascorbic acid does not mobilize DGLA but enhances conversion of free DGLA to PGE1 (Manku et al., 1979). Phenytoin, which can precipitate auto-immune disease, has the opposite effect to vitamin C (Horrobin, 1980).

It thus seems possible that PGE1 is a key regulator of thymus and lymphocyte function and that the known effects of prolactin, zinc, glucocorticoids and phenytoin on immunological status may in part be mediated by their effects on PGE1. (Fig.1). If this is correct it raises the possibility that the thymic failure, and possibly the muscle damage, in dystrophic mice and chicks may relate to defective PGE1 formation or action. PGE1 action seems to

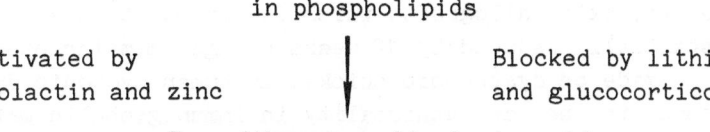

Dihomogammalinolenic acid
in phospholipids

Activated by   Blocked by lithium
prolactin and zinc   and glucocorticoids

Free dihomogammalinolenic acid

Activated by   Blocked by
ascorbic acid   phenytoin

Prostaglandin E1

Fig. 1. The factors involved in regulation of PGE1 formation.

depend in part on the presence of another product of PG metabolism, thromboxane A2, and so a defect there could also be involved
(Horrobin et al., 1979). There are, of course, many other possibilities which deserve following up because of the clinical importance of the subject.

6. CONCLUSIONS

The idea that there are immunological abnormalities in the
muscular dystrophies has now been firmly established by a variety
of experimental studies. Whether those abnormalities are merely
associated with the dystrophies or actually contribute to their
pathogenesis is at present unclear. It seems most likely that some
primary metabolic defect damages both muscle and thymus, but that
the muscle damage is then exacerbated by the immunological abnormality. The possible relationship of the defects to prostaglandin
metabolism may open up new therapeutic possibilities.

7. SUMMARY

The relationship between muscle and thymus has been tho-
roughly explored in the case of "myasthenia gravis" but until
recently little had been done on this relationship with regard to
the muscular dystrophies. A number of early studies reported that
thymectomy in several different species could lead to muscle
atrophy. In Bar Harbor 129 dystrophic mice, thymectomy failed to
prevent onset of the disease. In 1976 two groups reported that in
these mice, the thymus atrophied very rapidly after weaning and
then slowly recovered up to an age of 12 weeks. It has now been
shown that these mice also show a highly significantly increased
tolerance to skin allografts which is maximal soon after weaning
but substantially reduced by 12 weeks of age. Similar observations
have been made on dystrophic chicks. In human myotonic dystrophy,
there seems to be an abnormality in immunoglobulin metabolism.
Nothing was known about immunological abnormalities in boys with
Duchenne dystrophy until very recently. It has now been demonstrated that such boys have low circulating levels of serum thymic
factors. Thus, three different types of muscular dystrophy in the
mouse, the chick and the human have all been found to be associated with thymic deficiency. The relationship between the immune
system and the muscle in the human muscular dystrophies is worthy

of intensive investigation. It could lead to new therapeutic approaches involving immunostimulation rather than immunosuppression.

REFERENCES

Basch, K., 1906, Beitrage zur Physiologie und Pathologie der Thymus,
Jahrb, Kinderhilk, 64:285.

Colby-Germinario, S., Martial, E., and Livett, B.G., 1981, Delayed
graft rejection in murine muscular dystrophy: a hypothesis concerning the role of the thymus in neuromuscular disease, J. Ne-
uroimmunol., in press.

Comsa, J., 1938, Consequences de la thymectomie totale chez le co-
baye male, C.R. Soc. Biol., 27:903.

Cosmos, E., Butler, J., Mazliah, J., and Allard, E.P., 1980, Animal
models of muscle disease, Part 1., Avian dystrophy, Muscle and
Nerve, 3:252.

Cosmos, E., Perey, Y.E., Butler, J., and Allard, E.P., 1977, Thymic-
muscle interaction: a non-neural influence on metabolic differentiation of anaerobic muscle of normal and dystrophic genotype, Differentiation, 9:139.

DeKretser, T.A., and Livett, B.G., 1976, Evidence of a thymic abnormality in murine muscular dystrophy, Nature, 263:682.

Dung, H.C., 1976, Relationship between the adrenal cortex and thymic
involution in lethargic mutant mice, Amer. J. Anat., 147:255.

Fabris, N., 1980, Serum thymic factor determination in different human pathologies, Int. J. Immunopharmacol., 2:157.

Fabris, N., Pierpaoli, W., and Sorkin, E., 1971, Hormones and the immunological capacity. 3. The immunodeficiency disease of the hypopituitary Snell-Bagg dwarf mouse, Clin. Exp. Immunol., 9:209.

Harms, J.W., 1952, Experimentell-morphologische Untersuchungen uber
den Thymus von Xenopus leavis, Daudin. Gegemb. Morphol. Jahrb.,
92:256.

Horrobin, D.F., 1979, Cellular basis of prolactin action, Med. Hypotheses, 5:599.

Horrobin, D.F., 1980, The regulation of prostaglandin biosynthesis:
negative feedback mechanisms and the selective control of 1 and
2 series prostaglandins: relevance to inflammation and immunity, Med. Hypotheses, 6:687.

Horrobin, D.F., and Karmali, R.A., 1975, Effects of bromocriptine
and prolactin on thymus growth and thymus uptake of tritiated
thymidine in mice of the Swiss and Bar Harbor 129 strains, J.

Endocr., 67:58.

Horrobin, D.F., and Lieb, J., 1981, A biochemical basis for the actions of lithium on behaviour and on immunity, Med. Hypotheses, 7:899.

Horrobin, D.F., Manku, M.S., and Oka, M., 1979, The nutritional regulation of T lymphocyte function, Med. Hypotheses, 5:969.

Horrobin, D.F., Morgan, R.O., and Karmali, R.A., 1979, Thymic changes in muscular dystrophy and evidence for an abnormality related to prostaglandin synthesis or action, Ann. N.Y. Acad. Sci., 317:534.

Horrobin, D.F., and Morgan, R.O., 1980, Myotonic dystrophy: a disease caused by functional zinc deficiency due to an abnormal zinc-binding ligand? Med. Hypotheses, 6:375.

Houssay, B.A., Houssay, A.B., Cardeza, A.F. and Pinto, R.M., 1955, Tumeurs surrenales oestrogeniques and tumeurs hypophysaires chez les animaux castres, Schweiz. Med. Wochenschr., 85:291.

Ishizuka, M., Takeuchi, T., and Umezawa, H., 1974, Promotion of antibody formation by prostaglandin, Experientia, 30:1207.

Jankovic, B.D., Waksman, B.H., and Arnason, B.G., 1962, Role of the thymus in immune reactions in rats. I. Immunologic response to bovine serum albumin in rats thymectomized or splenectomized after birth, J. Exp. Med., 116:159.

Karim, S.M.M., Sandler, M., and Williams, E.D., 1967, Distribution of prostaglandis in human tissues, Br. J. Pharmacol., 31:340.

Karmali, R.A., and Horrobin, D.F., 1976, Abnormalities of thymus growth in dystrophic mice, Nature, 263:684.

Livett, B.G., Colby-Germinario, S.P., Mizobe, F., and Martial, E., 1981, Plasma membrane and immunocyte involvement in the muscular dystrophies: evidence for a developmental abnormality in cell mediated immunity, International Conference Series, Vol. 146, Excerpta Medica Foundation, Amsterdam, in press.

Manku, M.S., Horrobin, D.F., Karmazyn, M., and Cunnane, S.C., 1979, Prolactin and zinc effects on rats vascular reactivity: possible relationship to dihomogammalinolenic acid and to prostaglandin synthesis, Endocrinology, 104:774.

Manku, M.S., Oka, M., and Horrobin, D.F., 1979, Differential regulation of the formation of prostaglandins and related substances from arachidonic acid and from dihomogammalinolenic acid. II. Effects of vitamin C, Prostaglandins, 3:129.

Miller, J.F.A.P., 1962, Effect of thymic ablation and replacement, in: "The Thymus in Immunobiology," R.A. Good and A.E. Gabrielsen, eds., Hoeber, New York, p. 436.

Parrott, D.M.V., and East, J., 1962, Studies on a fatal wasting syndrome of mice thymectomized at birth, in: "The Thymus in Immubiology," R.A. Good and A.E. Gabrielsen, eds., Hoeber, New York, p. 523.

Perz-Cruet, J., and Dancey, J.T., 1977, Thymus gland involution induced by lithium cloride, Experientia, 33:646.

Pora, E., and Toma, V.V., 1960, Action des extraits de thymus sur le gastrocremien de grenouille intoxique aux acides lactiques our monoiodoacetiques ou par le fatigue, Stud. Cercet. Biol. Ser. Zool., 12:285.

Szewcuk, M.R., 1980, Abnormal age-associated immunoregulation in muscular dystrophic mice, Canad. J. Neurol. Sci., 7:124.

Walker, B.E., 1964, Mast cells, thymectomy and tumor rejection in dystrophic mice, Texas Rep. Biol. Med., 22:640.

Wochner, R.D., 1970, Hypercatabolism of normal IgG; an unexplained immunoglobulin abnormality in the connective tissue diseases, J. Clin. Invest., 49:454.

Wochner, R.D., Drews, G., Strober, W. and Waldmann, T.A., 1966, Accelerated breakdown of immunoglobulin G in myotonic dystrophy: a hereditary error of immunoglobulin catabolism, J. Clin. Invest., 45:321.

Zurier, R.B., and Ballas, M., 1973, Prostaglandin E suppression of adjuvant arthritis, Rheum., 20:723.

Zurier, R.B., Damjanov, I., Sayadoff, D.M., and Rothfield, N.F., 1977, Prostaglandin E1 treatment of NZB/W mice, II. Prevention of glomerulonephritis, Arthritis Rheum., 20:1449.

ATAXIA-TELANGIECTASIA: A NEURO-ENDOCRINE-IMMUNE DISEASE?

ALTERNATIVE MODELS OF PATHOGENESIS

Richard A. Gatti

Department of Pathology, UCLA School of Medicine
Los Angeles, Ca, 90024 U.S.A.

1. INTRODUCTION

Ataxia-telangiectasia (AT) is a disease characterized by early onset of a progressive cerebellar ataxia, sinopulmonary infections and dilated capillaries over the ears and eyes which are called "telangiectases". AT affects approximately 1 in 30,000, however, this incidence varies from one ethnic group to another. Patients seldom live beyond twenty years although this pattern has been gradually extended, perhaps due to better pulmonary hygiene and antibiotics. Despite an early demise, approximately 1 in 8 children with this disease develop a maligancy, usually lymphoid. Such children also show signs of premature aging (Boder and Sedgwick, 1958; Gatti and Walford, in press). There is no effective treatment to halt the steady deterioration.

AT was first noted as an entity by Syllaba and Henner (1926). It was again described by Louis-Barr (1941). In 1957, two pediatric neurologists in Los Angeles, E. Boder and R. Sedgwick, noticed a group of children within the public school system who shared the characteristic symptoms and described the syndrome for a third time (1958). These investigators later collected and studied post-mortem material on 150 cases (1964). These early reports noted most of what is known today of the clinical and histopathologic features, including abnormal thymic morphology.
Progress in AT research then awaited the support of the laboratory

Table 1. Landmark observations in Ataxia-Telangiectasia.

1926	described by Syllaba and Henner
1941	described by Louis-Barr
1954-64	150 post-mortem cases reviewed (Boder and Sedgwick)
1961	IgA deficiencies (Thieffry et al.)
1964	abnormal thymus and cellular immunity (Boder and Sedgwick)
1966	impaired lymphocyte transformation (Leikin et al.)
1967	8S IgM in serum (Stobo and Tomasi)
1967	untoward response to irradiation (Gotoff et al.)
1969	serum IgE deficiency (Ammann et al.)
1971	10-15% incidence of cancer (Gatti and Good)
1972	elevated serum alpha-fetoprotein(Waldmann and McIntire)
1975	non-random 14q+ translocation (McCaw et al.)
1978	T helper lymphocyte deficiency (Trompeter et al.)
1978	indentification of heterozygote by DNA repair? (Chen et al.)
1980	mitotic delay? (Painter and Young)
1982	cytoskeletal defect? (Gatti et al.)

to begin to unravel the pathogenesis.

Table 1 summarizes some of the landmark observations that have been made. They include evidence for both humoral and cellular immunodeficiencies, an unusual sensitivity to irradiation which is thought to be secondary to a defect in DNA repair, and a non-random chromosomal aberration characterized by a tandem translocation on the long arm of chromosome 14. Little progress has been made toward understanding the neurologic problem.
In addition, several reports document that AT patients often have endocrine abnormalities, such as diabetes or autoantibodies to endocrine organs (McFarlin et al., 1972).

It is difficult to propose a single hypothetical model for such a multisystem disease. A further constriction is that this model must acknowledge the autosomal recessive pattern of the disease. To propose a single gene/single enzyme is presently beyond our understanding of interactions between the neuro-
-endocrine and immune systems. There are, however, some inte-
resting "intermediate" models (i.e. they probe one system without offering an immediate explanation for the others).

2. A DEFECT OF IMMUNOREGULATION?

As early as 1961, it was noted that roughly 60 percent of AT patients have low serum Ig A levels (Table 1). This has been confirmed in virtually all ethnic groups where it occurs, although attempts to relate the IgA deficiency to increased pulmonary infections have been largely unsuccessful. IgE deficiencies have also been noted, often in the same patients with IgA deficiencies (Ammann et al., 1969). On the other hand, elevated IgE levels are found in some patients. We have noted decreased IgG_2 levels in 8 of 10 AT patients and in occasional parents and siblings (Oxelius et al., to be published). Low IgG_2 levels correlated quite well with IgA levels. IgM levels are usually normal or elevated in AT patients. They were normal in our patients. Elevated IgM levels should be further scrutinized for the presence of low molecular weight IgM which occurs in many AT patients and is known to diffuse in agar at a faster rate than 19S IgM. Thus, humoral immunodeficiencies are common in AT patients.

Defining cellular immune competence in this group of patients has been more difficult. Cellular methods are difficult to quantitate and often the amounts of blood necessary for serial investigations, with all appropriate controls, exceed the limits of what can be drawn from young patients. Further, age-matched controls are seldom used despite the young age of the AT study group and documented age-related changes of many immunological parameters (Pisciotta et al., 1967; Walford, 1970, 1976).

Once acquainted with the histopathology of the thymus from postmortem examinations of AT patients, it should come as no surprise that many parameters of cellular immunity are abnormal. What is surprising is that some patients have normal T cell numbers and functions to the extent that they have been tested.
In our recent studies, 7 of 12 patients had normal in vitro lymphocyte responses to phytohemagglutinin (PHA) stimulation, using three doses and a three-day incubation period. All but two patients had decreased (abolute and proportional) T cell levels: B cell levels were slightly increased. One patient consistently maintains 48% $SmIg^+$ cells which are polyclonal for light chain markers.

Hayward and coworkers reported proportions of T (helper) cells in 5 of 5 AT patients (Trompeter et al., 1978). Gupta et al.

noted a similar deficiency using the same marker (1978). We have
been unsuccessful in confirming this, using a monoclonal anti-T
(3A1 from dr. T. Fauci) which identifies primarily T helper cells.
We also attempted to utilize the alpha-naphthyl-acid-esterase
(ANAE) stain as a biomarker for T helper cells, based on a
suggestion by H.Peter (Peter et al. 1976; Peter and Pichler, 1980)
that this enzyme stains focally in T helper cells (as opposed to
no stain in about 38% of T cells and a diffuse stain in B cells
and monocytes) (Ranki and Hayry, 1979). We found decreased ANAE+/
/E+ cells in only 2 of 10 patients. Astaldi and coworkers have
also failed to confirm a T helper decrease in a group of AT patients, using monoclonal antisera (personal communication).
Waldmann, on the other hand, has found diminished T helper function in some patients (Bridges and Harnden ,1981). We evaluated
Con A-induced T suppressor function in 12 patients but found no
consistent pattern that differed significantly from normal; some
patients tended to have quite decreased T suppressor function, but
so did two of our normal donors (Gatti et al., to be publised).
Levis et al. (1979) and Nelson et al. (1980) have also reported
abnormal T cell killing in some patients. Thus, while it is clear
that patients with AT have cellular immunodeficiencies as well as
humoral, there is no uniformity as to the type of defect, even
among affected siblings.

To attempt to unify these observations under a single immunological and genetic model, one must consider the genes which govern immune responses. These map in essentially four areas: 1) the
so-called "immune response genes" of the Major Histocompatibility Complex (MHC) on chromosome 6p; 2) the genes for heavy chain
structure on chromosome 14q; 3) the genes for kappa light chain
structure on chromosome 2p; and 4) the genes for lambda light
chain structure on chromosome 22.

Our analysis of nine multiplex AT families for possible linkage to HLA-A and-B within the MHC showed no evidence for linkage
of an AT gene to this region (Hodge et al. 1980). How a single defect in either of the light chain genes could account for the myriad immunodeficiencies, is beyond our understanding of lymphoid
development at the moment. To this point, it is clear that, where
studied,patients with AT express both   and   chains. On the other
hand, since the functions of these two light chains is presently
unknown, it is difficult to argue convincingly that they could not
supply a common denominator for the immunodeficiencies in AT.

Chromosome 14q not only contains the genes for immunoglobulin heavy chain structure, it also has been implicated in this disease by virtue of the report by McCaw et al., (1975) of 14q tandem translocations in some AT patients and of earlier, less definitive, reports suggesting a similar kariotypic abnormality (Goodman et al., 1969; Sparkes et al., 1980). Alpha-1-antitrypsin (Pi) has also recently been mapped to 14q (Pearson et al., 1981) and the relationship of the pulmonary and liver disease in AT to this enzyme inhibitor is now being examined. Lastly, nucleoside phosphorylase (NP) is considered a genetic marker for 14q in comparative mapping (SRO:q 13-14). Deficiency of this enzyme is associated with a severe isolated T cell deficiency (Giblett et al., 1975) which in some ways resembles the immunologic profile of some AT patients. Other purine salvage pathway enzymes have important roles in lymphoid development and immunocompetence, such as adenosine deaminase (Giblett et al., 1972) and 5'-nucleotidase (Edwards et al., 1978). However, Pearson and coworkers have recently invoked some doubt as to whether NP maps to chromosome 15 instead to 14 (personal communication). So attempts to link an AT locus to Pi may be misplaced. Another reservation in this paradigm is that the 14q translocation is only detected in a minority of AT patients, perhaps as low as 10 percent (to be published).

From an immunological point of view the most intriguing model of all would be to propose that AT is an "Experiment of Nature" involving a defective gene for antibody structure or assembly. Let us consider which genetic defect(s) might lead to the typical immunologic profile of AT patients.
1. A defect in a structural gene for the constant portion of any particular heavy chain would be too restrictive since if, for example, the defect were to involve CH γ, only the IgG levels should be affected (unless IgG expression is a prerequisite for subsequent switching to IgA). Indeed, Waldmann et al., have evidence to suggest that the DNA sequences necessary for IgA production are present in AT patients (Bridges and Harnden, 1981).
2. Were a switching gene to be involved, this might explain the dysimmunoglobulinemias but would probably not impact heavily upon T cell function. It is intriguing, however, that if one looks at the order of CH genes in the CH region (Fig 1) the genes for IgG_2, IgE and IgA all appear to be adjacent to one another and these Ig classes are decreased most noticeably in AT patients.
3. A defective variable gene would be expected to express itself as an aberrant response to a particular antigen or antigen set

which involves all Ig classes. Thus, it would seem unlikely that a single VH gene defect could lower serum levels of several entire Ig classes.

4. On the other hand, it is assumed that T cell receptors must include some variable region gene products in order to manifest antigen specificity. It is also assumed that such "VHt" genes would map near to the other VH genes on 14q. A defect in such a basic immunological structure would lead to far-reaching consequences of cell-cell interactions and regulation within the immune system. Admittedly, however, such a model does not allow for any explanation of the neurological abnormalities or the chromosonal aberrations.

3. A HYPOPHYSEAL DEFECT?

In animal models, ablation of any of the endocrine organs results in a generalized immunodeficiency not unlike that seen in AT patients (Fabris 1977). Replacing growth hormone, thyroxine or insulin (or even giving brain-extracts to nude mice) reconstitutes immunocompetence (Pierpaoli, this volume). While some of these ablation models decrease the incidence of certain forms of malignancy, they increase that of others. Thus, that AT may be caused by a primary hormonal deficiency does not seem an unreasonable hypothesis. As noted previously, patients with AT demonstrate endocrine abnormalities.

The most consistent abnormality described among AT patients is one of glusose intolerance, elevated fasting plasma insulin levels, excessive insulin production following glucose challenge and failure of insulin to reduce blood glucose levels (McFarlin et al., 1972). Antibodies to insulin are not found. On the other hand, most other endocrine parameters are normal, including: pituitary function and growth hormone levels and thyroid function. Adrenal function remains questionable: whereas Ammann et al.,

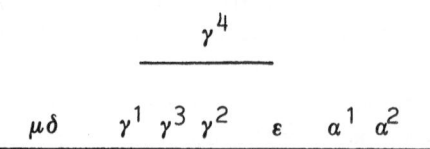

Fig. 1. Probable order of human CH genes on 14q.

(1970) reported normal 17-hydroxy steroid excretion in 5 of 5 patients, McFarlin et al. (1972) found low excretion levels in 3 of 16 patients. They found low 17-ketosteroid excretion in 10 of 15 patients, although several patients were pre-pubertal, making interpretation of these data difficult at the time. Dysgenesis and agenesis of gonadal tissue have been described in a significant number of AT patients. Aguilar et al. (1968) reported two patients with incomplete spermatogenesis and reduced numbers of Leydig cells. These findings take on more significance when coupled with the observations of Nishizuka and Sakakura (1969) and Besedovsky and Sorkin, (1974) that both neonatal thymectomy and the thymus-less nude mice show delayed sexual maturation.

Considering the marked changes that take place in the thymus and gonads around the time of puberty, it seems quite plausible that the gonadal changes seen in AT patients are mediated via a defective thymus. Such reasoning would implicate a basic AT defect at the level of the endocrine master gland -the pituitary- either via a direct genetic mechanism, such as a missing development enzyme or via a feedback mechanism from a defective thymus.

In a recent collaboration with A. Goldstein, we have found markedly low levels of thymosin-α_1 in our AT patients (to be published). What is most striking and unique to this group of patients is that this finding is uniform throughout all of the patients studied thus far. Parents and 3 of 4 siblings of patients also had very reduced levels, as measured by a new radio-immunoassay which promises to be more accurate than many previous attempts at measuring thymic factors. Using this same assay, Goldstein and coworkers (1981) now have data which show a diurnal cycle for thymosin-α_1 levels, with peaks in the afternoon and troughs during the early morning hours, approximately 180 out of phase with serum cortisol levels (Hall and Goldstein, this volume). This evidence of diurnal variation strongly suggests hypothalamic control. Taken together, these findings make a strong argument that AT can be considered a neuro-endocrine-immune model of disease and the common denominator that should be sought is a defective hormone-like substance. Perhaps a DNA probe for thymosin-α_1 would identify the chromosomal location of the AT gene.

4. A DEFECT OF DNA REPAIR AND/OR REPLICATION?

In 1967, an astute radiologist named Gotoff noted an unusual sensitivity to irradiation in the course of treating malignancy in a patient with AT. This finding was quickly confirmed by another radiologist (Morgan et al., 1968). Later, "in vitro" studies demonstrated that DNA repair is abnormal in fibroblasts and lymphoblastoid cell lines of these patients (Taylor et al., 1975; Chen et al., 1978; Bridges and Harnden, 1981). In collaboration with K. Hall and Walford, (1981), we have confirmed this in our own patients, using fresh lymphocytes, and have found a similar abnormality in many parents as well. However, measuring tritiated thymidine uptake by irradiated cells, in the presence of hydroxy-urea in order to block scheduled DNA synthesis, does not elucidate specific mechanisms of DNA repair. DNA repair, even of unscheduled synthesis, depends upon a variety of enzyme systems, such as liga-ses, polymerases, and endonucleases, which can now be evaluated directly (Van Lancker and Tomura, 1980). Thus, it is unclear at the present time whether or not DNA repair is defective in AT patients and if so, which mechanisms are involved. Further, in our own studies, we noted that age-matched controls reduced the diffe-rences between AT cells and controls, a point which virtually all other studies have ignored (to be published).

Painter and Young, (1980) suggest that another defect exists in AT cells. They found that the rate of DNA synthesis in fibroblasts from AT patients was hardly or not at all delayed by doses of irradiation which normally have a markedly inhibiting effect on such synthesis. This radioresistance was due primarily to much smaller inhibition of replicon initiation. They propose that such a shortened mitotic delay would not give AT cells sufficient time to repair single strand breaks caused by the irra-diation before they moved from G_2 into mitosis. This could explain the frequently observed chromatid aberrations of AT cells.
Another recent report by Edwards and Taylor (1980) also demon-strates that scheduled synthesis by lymphoblastoid cell lines from patients with AT has not typically been impaired by irradiation, nor were polymerase levels raised as in normal cells. Needless to say, any abnormality so basic as to effect DNA replication would be expected to have profound secondary effects on embryonic development and on lymphoproliferative responses.

Radiosensitivity experiments have produced another crucial piece of information. Complementarity between fibroblast stains has been noted by three groups of workers (Bridges and Harnden, 1981). Even more crucial is whether lack of complementarity holds true within families. Jasper and coworkers have demonstrated this between two siblings (personal communication). If this observation can be confirmed and expanded to other families, it would indicate that our models now must include either genetic subsets of disease or pleiotropic genes with multigene origins for the pathogenesis of AT. At present, there is no apparent clinical or laboratory evidence for heterogeneity. However, it would certainly seem appropriate to perform such complementation studies on any group of patients who will be used for further investigations and/or therapeutic trials.

One further observation links a common denominator to DNA repair and/or replication. We noted that virtually all of our patients have abnormal liver function tests, despite the lack of symptoms or signs of liver disease. McFarlin et al. (1972) made similar note of such changes. The elevated alkaline phosphatase, serum glutamic-pyruvic transaminase (SGPT) serum glutamic-oxalacetic transaminase (SGOT), and alphafetoprotein levels are all compatible with immature liver functions. Levels of carcinoembryonic antigen are also elevated in AT patients. A review of eight postmortem liver sections with B. Landing revealed a common finding which Aguilar et al. (1968) had reported previously: the nuclei of the hepatocytes vary markedly in size. Similar findings have been noted in the myocardium and central nervous system of such patients. They are also seen in advanced age of normal persons and occasionally in methotrexate toxicity. Although it is normally assumed that this variability, called "aneuploidy" by pathologists, represents chromosomal polyploidy, no studies of DNA content have been reported. This observation of AT cells represents another abnormality in the nucleus.

5. A CYTOSKELETAL DEFECT?

Microtubules and microfilaments are essential for cell replication, locomotion, and redistributing of cell surface macromolecules. Very recently our studies have revealed that the cell surface redistribution (i.e. capping) of receptors for Concanavalin A takes place in a greater proportion of the peripheral lymphocytes from AT patients than in normal or age-matched controls (Gatti et al. 1981). Neutrophil chemotaxis, another function which depends upon membrane motility and an intact cytoskeleton, is also generally diminished in these patients.

Walford and coworkers have shown that in patients with Down Syndrome, a disease associated with premature aging, both SmIg and Con A capping are decreased (Naeim and Walford, 1980). Lymphocytes from aged donors also show decreased proportions of capping lymphocytes in peripheral blood. The addition of colchicine, which inhibits microtubule formation, enhances capping in both DS patients and aged donors (Naeim et al. 1981). As discussed elsewhere in this volume (See Walford et al.) both of these groups of patients also exhibit marked biochemical changes, such as decreases in cAMP and increases in cGMP levels of resting T lymphocytes (Tam and Walford, 1980). cAMP/cGMP studies on AT patients were performed in collaboration with Walford and Tam and preliminary results suggest that cAMP levels are elevated while cGMP levels are decreased (to be published).

Taken together, these early observations herald still a fourth model of pathogenesis in AT, that of a cytoskeletal defect or a biochemical defect which impacts severely on the cytoskeletal system. Such a model could certainly effect the integrity of the neurological system as well and must be considered seriously.

The above four paradigms of disease in AT encompass most of the major clinical and laboratory findings in this group of patients. They are not intended to exclude other facts or models. They are advanced only as "working hypotheses" which may provoke further collaboration among immunologists, geneticists, endocrinologists, and molecular chemists interested in arresting this uniformly fatal disease of childhood.

6. SUMMARY

AT is an autosomal recessive disorder which effects approximately 1 in 30,000 persons. It is uniformly fatal after a slow progressive neurologic deterioration, accompanied by varying degrees of immunological impairment. Endocrine abnormalities are also commonly found. Because of the multisystem involvement of this disorder, it has been difficult to formulate a unifying hypothesis. Four alternative models of pathogenesis are discussed: a defect of immunoregulation, a hypophyseal defect, a defect of DNA repair and/or replication and a cytoskeletal defect. Recent evidence suggesting complimentarity of DNA repair abnormalities in this group of patients further complicates efforts to focus on a common   denominator   and may confound future genetic investigations and therapeutic trials.

REFERENCES

Aguilar, M.J., Kamoshita, S., Landing B.H., Boder, E., and Sedgwick, R.P., 1968, Pathological observations in ataxia-telangiectasia. A report on 5 cases, J. Neuropath. Exp. Neurol., 27:659.

Ammann, A.J., Cain, W.A., Ishizaka, K.,Hong, R., and Good, R.A.; 1969, Immunoglobulin E deficiency in ataxia-telangiectasia, New Engl. J. Med., 281:469.

Ammann, A.J., Duquesnoy, R.J., and Good,R.A., 1970, Endocrinological studies in ataxia-telangiectasia and other immunological deficiency diseases,   Clin. exp. Immunol,6:587.

Besedowsky, H.O. and Sorkin, E. 1974, Thymus involvement in female sexual maturation, Nature, 249:356.

Boder, E. and Sedgwick, R.P., 1954 Ataxia-telangiectasia, a familial syndrome of progressive cerebellar ataxia, oculocutaneous telangiectasia and frequent pulmonary infection. Pediatrics, 21:526.

Boder, E. and Sedgwick, R.P., 1964, Ataxia-telangiectasia. A review of 150, cases. Pro.Intnl., Copenhagen Congress on the Scientific Study of Mental Retardation, Aug., Denmark.

Bridges, B.A. and Harnden, D.G.; 1981 Untangling ataxia-telangiectasia, Nature, 289:223.

Chen, P.C., Lavin, M.F., and Kidson, C, 1978 Identification of ataxia telangiectasia heterozygotes, a cancer prone population, Nature, 274:484.

Edwards, M.J. and Taylor, A.M.R., 1980, Unusual levels of (ADP-ribose)n and DNA synthesis in ataxia telangiectasia cells following X-ray irradiation, Nature, 287:745.

Edwards, N.L., Magilavy, D.B., Cassidy, J.T., and Fox, I., 1978, lymphocyte ecto-5'-nucleotidase deficiency in agammaglobulinemia, Science, 201:628.

Fabris, N., 1977, Hormones and aging. in:"Immunology and Aging", Comprehensive Immunology, Vol. 1, T. Makinodan and E. Yunis., eds., Plenum Publ., New York, p. 73.

Gatti, R.A. and Good, R.A. 1971, Occurrence of malignancy in immunodeficiency disease, Cancer, 28:89.

Gatti, R.A., Bick, M., Boder, E., Medici, M.A., Naeim, F., Tam, C.F., and Walford, R.L., 1981, Evidence for a cytoskeletal lesion in ataxia telangiectasia, Clin. Res., 29:527.

Gatti, R.A. and Walford, R.L., 1981, Immune function and feature
    of aging in chromosomal instability syndromes, in: "Immuno-
    logic Aspect of Aging", D. Segre and L. Smith., eds., Marcel
    Dekker Inc., in press.
Giblett, E.R., Ammann, A.J., Wara, D.W.,Sandman, R., and Diamond,
    L.K., 1975, Nucleoside-phosphorylase deficiency in a child
    with severely defective T-cell immunity and normal B-cell immu-
    nity, Lancet, i:1010.
Giblett, E.R., Anderson, J.E., Cohen, F., Pollara, B., and Meuwissen,
    H.J., 1972, Adenosine deaminase deficiency in two patients
    with severely impaired cellular immunity, Lancet, ii:1067.
Goodman, W.N., Cooper, W.C., Kessler, G.B., Fischer, M.S., and
    Gardner, M.B., 1969, Ataxia telangiectasia a report of two
    cases in siblings presenting a picture of progressive spinal
    muscular atrophy, Bull. Los Angeles Neurol. Soc. 34:1.
Gotoff, S.P., Amirmokri, E., and Liebner, E.J., 1967 , Ataxia-
    telangiectasia: Neoplasia, untoward response to -irradiation
    and tuberous sclerosis, Amer. J. Dis. Child., 114:617.
Gupta, S. and Good, R.A., 1978 , Subpopulations of human T lympho-
    cytes. V. T lymphocytes with receptors for immunoglobulin M or
    G in patients with primary immunodeficiency disorders, Clin.
    Immunol. Immunopathol., 11:292.
Hall, K.y., Gatti, R.A., and Walford, R.L., 1981 , Repair of gamma-
    and bleomycin-induced DNA damage in ataxia-telangiectasia
    patients and families J. Supramol. Str. and Cell Biochem.,
    Suppl 5:200.
Hodge, S., Berkel, I., Gatti, R.S., Boder, E., and Spence, M.A.,
    1980 , Ataxia-telangiectasia and xeroderma pigmentosum: no
    evidence of linkage to HLA Tissue Antigens, 15: 313.
Leikin, S.L., Bazelon, M., and Hi Park, K., 1966 , In vitro lympho-
    cyte transformation in ataxia-telangiectasia, J. Pediat.,68:477.
Levis, W.R., Dattner, A.M., and Shaw, J.S. 1979 , Selective defects
    in T cell function in ataxia-telangiectasia, Clin. Exp.
    Immunol., 4:
Louis-Barr, D., 1941 , Sur un syndrome progressif comprenant des
    telangiectasies capillaires cutances et conjonctivales symme-
    triques, a disposition naevoide et de troubles cerebelleux,
    Confin. Neurol., (Basel) 4:32.
Mccaw, B., Hecht, F., Haenden, D.G., and Teplitz, R.L., 1975 ,
    Somatic rearrangment of chromosome 14 in human lymphocytes,
    Proc. Nat. Acad. Sci., (USA) 72:2071.
McFarlin, D.E., Strober, W., and Waldmann, T.A., 1972 , Ataxia-
    telangiectasia, Medicine, 51:281.

Morgan, J.l., Holcomb, T.M., and Morrissey, R.W., 1968 , Radia-
    tion reaction in ataxia telangiectasia, Amer. J. Dis. Child.,
    116:557.
Naeim, F., Bergmann, K., and Walford, R.L., 1981, Capping of Con-
    canavalin A receptors on lymphocytes of aged individuals and
    patients with Down's syndrome: enhancing effect of colchi-
    cine; possible relation to microtubular system, Age 4:5.
Naeim, F. and Walford, R.L. 1980, Disturbance of redistribution
    of surface membrane receptors on peripheral mononuclear cells
    of patients with Down's syndrome and of aged individuals,
    J. Gerontol., 35:650.
Nelson, D.L., Biddison, W.E., Bundy, B.M., and Shaw, S., 1980,
    Influenza virus specific HLA restricted cytotoxic T-cell
    responses in humans - heterogeneity of responsiveness in
    immunodeficiency patients, Proc. Fourth International
    Congress of Immunology, Abstract No. 14.2.20, (Paris, France).
Nishizuka, Y. and Sakakura, T., 1969, Thymus and reproduction:
    sex-linked dysgenesis of the gonad after neonatal thymectomy
    in mice, Science, 166:753.
Painter, R.b. and Young, B.R.; 1980, Radiosensitivity in ataxia-
    telangiectasia: a new explanation, Proc. Natl. Acad. Sci.
    (USA) 77:7315.
Pearson, S., Tetri, P., and Francke, U., 1981, Chromosome 14 codes
    for human alpha 1-antitrypsin (PI) expression in rat hepatoma
    x human fetal liver cell hybrids, Proc. Sixth International
    Workshop on Human Gene Mapping, Abstract No. 92, (Oslo, Norway).
Peter, H.H., Pavie-Fischer, J., Kalden, J.R., Roubin, R., Cesarini,
    J.P.,and Kourilsky, F.M., 1976, Isolation and immunological
    characterization of different lymphocyte populations from
    human peripheral blood with special emphasis on "null lympho-
    cytes", Semin. Technol. INSERM, 57:213.
Peter, H.H. and Pichler, W.J., 1980, The alpha-naphthyl esterase
    (ANAE) lymphocyte marker in common variable immunodeficiency
    (CVID), Proc. Fourth Internl. Congress of Immunology, Abstract
    No. 14.2.23, (Paris, France).
Pisciotta, A.V., Westring, D.W., De Prey, C., and Walsh, B., 1967,
    Mitogenic effect of phytohaemagglutinin at different ages,
    Nature, 215:193.
Ranki, A. and Hayry, P., 1979, Histochemical distinction between
    lymphocytic and monocytic acid alpha-naphthyl acetate (ANAE)
    esterases, J. Clin. Lab. Immunol, 1:333.
Sparkes, R.S., Como, R., and Golde, F.W., 1980, Cytogenetic abnor-
    malities in ataxia telangiectasia with T-cell chronic lympho-

cytic leukemia. <u>Cancer Genetics and Cytogenetics</u>, 1:329.

Stobo, J.D. and Tomasi, T.B., 1967, A low molecular weight immunoglobulin antigenically related to 19S IgM, <u>J. Clin. Invest.</u>,
46:1329.

Syllaba, L. and Henner, K., 1926, Contribution a l'independance
de l'athetose double idiopathique et congenital, <u>Rev. Neurol.</u>,
1:541.

Tam, C. and Walford, R.L., 1980, Alterations in cyclic nucleotides and cyclases specific activities in T lymphocytes of
aging normal humans and patients with Down's syndorme, <u>J.
Immunol.</u>, 125:1665.

Thieffrey, St., Arthuis, M., Aicard, J.,and Lyon, G., 1961,
L'ataxietelangiectasie (7 observation personnelles), <u>Rev.
Neurol.</u> 105:390.

Trompeter, R.S., Layward, L., and Hayward, A.R., 1978, Primary
and secondary abnormalities of T cell subpopulations, <u>Clin.
exp. Immunol.</u> 34:388.

Van Lancker, J.L. and Tomura, T., 1980, The action of a mammalian
endonuclease on psoralen-bound DNA, <u>Chem. Biol. Interactions</u>,
31:179.

Waldmann, T.A. and McIntire, K.R., 1972, Serum-alpha-feto-protein
levels in patients with ataxia-telangiectasia, <u>Lancet</u>,
ii:1112.

Walford, R.L., 1970, <u>The Immunologic Theory of Aging</u>, Munksgaard,
Copenhagen.

Walford, R.L., 1976, When is a mouse "old"?, <u>J. Immunol.</u>, 117:352.

ACCELERATED AGING IN DOWN'S SYNDROME: THE CONCEPT OF

HIERARCHICAL HOMEOSTASIS IN RELATION TO LOCAL AND GLOBAL FAILURE

Roy L. Walford, Faramarz Naeim, Kathleen Y. Hall,
C.F. Tam, Richard A. Gatti and Michael A. Medici

The Department of Pathology, UCLA Medical School
and Pediatric Oncology, Cedars-Saint Hospital
Los Angeles, Calif.

1. INTRODUCTION

A number of diseases are known to manifest various features of accelerated aging, including progeria, Werner's syndrome, most of the chromosomal instability syndromes (Gatti and Walford, 1981), various other maladies (Martin, 1978) and - reflecting our own particular interests - systemic lypus erythematosus (SLE) (Barnett et al., 1981) and Down's syndrome (DS) (Walford et al., 1981). Table 1 lists a number of the non-immune hallmarks of aging as seen normally and in various diseases characterized in part by accelerated aging. DS demonstrates many features of accelerated aging: premature greying of hair, degenerative vascular disease, amyloidosis, hypogonadism, senile dementia of the Alzheimer's type, immune dysfunction, possibly an increased susceptibility to diabetes, and decreased replicative capacity of fibroblasts, among others.

We shall here present those aspects of Down's syndrome which we have studied from the standpoint of gerontology, focusing upon the immune response, the behavior of lymphocyte surface receptors, DNA-repair of lymphocytes, and cyclic nucleotide metabolism of lymphocytes. Following that, we shall present a speculative analysis about how the diseases of accelerated aging, including

Table 1. Features of Aging in Selected Progeroid Syndromes

Parameters	Normal Aging	SLE	DS	Progeria	Werner's	Diabetes
Amyloidosis	+	+	+	−		±
Vascular disease	+	+	+	+		+
Atherosclerosis	+	+		+	+	+
Arteritis	+	+				
Hypertension	+	+				
Arthritis	+	+				
Disordered carbohydrate metabolism (diabetes or abnormal gluc. tolerance)	+	+	+	−	+	+
Dementia	±	+				
Cataracts	+	+	+	−	+	+
Increased lipofuscin pigment	+		+			
Loss of weight, and/or "shrivelling up" of body	+	+	+	+		
Collagen changes	+	+				
Solubility in weak acid	↓					
Alterations in chromatin	+					
Chromosomal aberrations	+		+			
Altered DNA repair capacity	+	+	+			
Increased susceptibility to cancer	+	±	+	−	+	+
Lymphoid	+	+	+			
Non-lymphoid	+					
Osteoporosis	+	+		+	+	
Characteristic skin changes	+	+		+	+	
Decreased fibroblast replicative life span	+		+	+	+	+
Premature graying or loss of hair	+	+	+	+	+	

DS, can be considered as representing various subgroups of normal aging, by reference to a principle that can best be described as "hierarchical homeostasis", and relating that to both local and global failures of subsystems.

2. IMMUNOLOGIC STATUS IN DOWN'S SYNDROME (DS) SUBJECTS

Many studies have been made in recent years to characterize the immunologic status of individuals with DS. Unfortunately, not all of these are comparable, since (1), some were performed on institutionalized subjects and on non-institutionalized subjects, and (2), age-matched controls were often overlooked, and the ages of individual patients often omitted. In any study relevant to aging, the youngest cohort should be young post-pubescent adults, rather than children (Walford, 1976). Despite these shortcomings, four essential features frequently recurr in these reports : dysgammaglobulinemias, reduced absolute numbers and proportions of T cell, decreased lymphoproliferactive activity of T cells, and autoantibodies to thyroid. How any of these relate to the chromosome 21 trisomy remains unclear, although a gene dosage effect with an increase in transcriptional products, such as superoxide dismutase and interferon, is probably involved (Kurnit, 1980).

Evaluating antibody formation in DS patients, Siegel (1948) found that both primary and secondary responses were markedly reduced. Immunization with tetanus toxoid and typhoid vaccine produced low titers of antibody which dissipated quickly. Two other groups used the same antigens and reported normal responses (Leibovitz and Yannel 1942; Griffiths and Sylvester, 1967). Lopez et al. (1975) measured antibody responses to bacteriophage OX174 in 17 patients and noted impaired primary and secondary responses.

Where immunoglobulin levels have been measured, reports also conflict. While most reports agree that IgG levels are elevated, especially in institutionalized patients, others note elevated IgD, IgE and IgA levels, reduced IgM and sometimes reduced IgG levels. Thom and McKay (1972) allotyped Gm markers on IgG in DS and recorded high levels of Gm 4,5,10, and 11. Despite reports of elevated IgE levels, severe allergic symptoms are uncommon among DS patients. Attempts to relate these various dysgammaglobulinemias quantitatively with the severity of infection have been

Table 2. PHA-response in lymphocytes of DS and age-matched
controls (adapted from Walford et al., 1981).

Group	$\underline{N}$	Cpm^3 H-Tdr uptake, 3.6 ug PHA/ml[a]
DS	39	4.60 ± 0.34[b]
Controls	21	4.88 ± 0.29[b]

[a] $\text{Log}_{10} \pm$ S.D.
[b] $p \leqslant 0.01$

unsuccessful, although respiratory infections are about 100 times
more common in DS than in age-matched healthy controls.

The aberrations of humoral immunity in DS patients suggests
that a cellular defect in antigen processing and/or T cell
regulation exists. Other considerations support this hypothesis.
As early as 1964, Kouvalainin noted abnormalities in the thymuses
of patients with DS. Dramatically enlarged Hassall's corpuscles
and marked lymphoid depletion have been described by several
groups of investigators (Kouvalainin, 1964; Bend and Strassman,
1965; Levin et al., 1979). Levin et al. (1979) studied thymuses of
12 patients, of which 11 had enlarged Hassall's corpuscles; eight
of these showed marked cystic changes; some were calcified. The
cystic changes in enlarged Hassall's corpuscles were seen even in
infants who had died within one week of birth. In some infants
Hassall's corpuscles were surrounded by a sheath of lymphocytes
which was clearly different from age-matched controls. Cortico-
medullary demarkation is absent in most DS thymuses. Such large
Hassall's corpuscles are also seen in systemic lupus erythematosus, myasthenia gravis and in preleukemic mice. Levin et al.
(1979) demonstrated poor responses of DS T-cells to mitogens. Interferon production by DS lymphocytes stimulated with either PHA
or Poly-IC was decreased by 80-90% (Epstein et al., 1980).

Our own studies included both institutionalized and non-
institutionalized young adult DS patients. As shown in Table 2,
T-cell proliferative responses to PHA were reduced in DS patients.
This deviation from normal responses seemed even more pronounced

Table 3. Proliferative response to allogenic stimulation (adapted from Walford et al., 1981).

Age group (yr)	Controls	DS	p-value
10-20	146 (4)	89	≤.05
20-30	130 (8)	106	n.s.
30	121 (11)	83	≤.05

Values are given as "percent of response", from normalization of response of all individuals in a given experiment. Number of subjects tested in each category are given in parenthesis.

when monocytes were present in the responding cell preparation. Spontaneous killer cell activity was not altered in DS. Comparative proliferative responses to alloantigens are shown in Table 3. In general, DS patients had a significantly lower response than the combined controls (p<.05). We noted a decrease in B-cells in our DS subjects (Walford et al., 1981). This has not been a common finding in earlier reports but was noted by Hann et al. (1979). Anti-thyroid antibodies were detected in 23% of our patients, and in 17% of controls. Autoimmune reactions are not in fact a major feature of DS.

3. SURFACE MEMBRANE RECEPTORS

We studied the per cent of B-cells showing capping of surface-membrane immunoglobulin (SmIg) receptors, and of T-cells showing capping of Concanavalin A (Con-A) receptor sites in young adult DS subjects, age-matched normal controls, and in aged humans. Results are shown in Tables 4 and 5. A larger study of Con-A capping yielded the same relative results as in Table 5 (Naeim and Walford, 1980). Both SmIg and Con-A capping were decreased to a statistically significant degree in both DS and aged persons compared to young adult controls. The effects of colchicine on Con-A capping in these three groups are also shown in Table 5. Addition of colchicine diminished Con-A capping in peripheral mononuclear cells of the young adult controls but enhanced capping in both DS and aged subjects.

Table 4. Capping of surface IgG in T-depleted peripheral lymphoid
         cells from DS subjects, age-matched controls, and aged
         persons (adapted from Naeim and Walford, 1980).

Group	No.of cases	Average age	Average % SmIg (+) cells showing capping at 37 °C
DS	19	27	6.5 ± 5.3
Age-matched controls	14	29	21.7 ± 9
Aged persons	11	88	5.2 ± 3.2

Capping involves a redistribution of cell membrane macromolecules and is controlled by membrane associated cytoskeletal
elements such as microtubules and microfilaments. These elements
may therefore be altered in the lymphocytes of DS and aged
subjects. Colchicine is an inhibitor of microtubule assembly. In
the steady state equilibrium between tubulin and microtubles
(microtubules are cylindrical structures consisting of polymerized
forms of tubulin), colchicine prevents microtubule assembly by
causing depolymerization. The enhancement of Con A capping by
colchicine in DS and aging may suggest the presence of an excess
of polymerized tubulin (microtubules) in these conditions, capping
being enhanced when colchicine decreases the excess.

4. DNA REPAIR

The ability of an organism to maintain the integrity of the
genetic material was first implicated as playing a role in aging
by the work of Hart and Setlow, (1974) who found a linear
relationship between the logarithm of species life span and the
amount of DNA repair of UV-induced DNA damage as measured by
unscheduled incorporation of tritiated thymidine into the DNA.
This correlation was subsequently found in several more closely
related groups, including the primates (Hall et al., 1981a), among
rodents using Mus musculus and Peromyscus leucopus (Sacher and
Hart, 1978), and among both embryonic fibroblasts (Paffenholz,

Table 5. Capping of Con-A receptor sites on unfractionated periphe-
         ral Mononuclear cells from DS subiects, age-matched con-
         trols, and aged persons, and the effect of colchicine the-
         reon (adapted from Naeim et al., 1981).

Groups	No.of cases	Average age	Colchicine	Average % capping at 37° C
DS	9	30	none 10^{-3}M	7 ± 4 15 ± 9
Age-matched controls	10	30.5	none 10^{-3}M	14 ± 3 9 ± 3
Aged persons	12	82	none 10^{-3}M	5.5 ± 3 9.8 ± 3

1978) and adult lymphocytes (Hall et al., 1981b) of different
inbred long-lived and short-lived strains of mice. The correlation
of repair and species life span potential would suggest that the
accumulation of genetic damage is determined, at least in one
aspect, by the degree of pre-determined genetic ability to repair
such damage.

There is some evidence of change of DNA repair activity with
age, including 1) a decrease of both scheduled and unscheduled DNA
synthesis in fibroblasts with increased donor age (Karran and
Ormerod, 1973) and passage number (Mattern and Cerulti, 1975); 2)
a correlation of chemical damage potentials with the age of
cultured human lymphocytes (Pero et al., 1978), and 3) an increased sensitivity to bleomycin, an inducer of strand breaks with age
in human lymphocytes (Seshadri et al., 1979) and between liver
nuclei of mature and old rats (Ove and Coelzu, 1978). However,
these repair defects associated with age might be secondary to
other effects of cellular senescence rather than directly related
to rates of senescence.

Many genetic syndromes are similarly deficient in one or more
facets of repair capacity, and many of these syndromes also
display some features of accelerated aging (Brown et al., 1976;
Rainbow and Howes, 1977; Hoar and Waghorne, 1978). Ataxia-telan-

giectasia, xeroderma pigmentosum, Fanconi's anemia, and systemic
lupus erythematosus,which are characterized by a high incidence of
chromosome breaks and neoplasms, are also defective in some forms
of DNA repair (Hall et al., 1977; 1981c; 1981d). Many of these
disease states also demonstrate altered immune responses (Gatti
and Walford, 1980) and at least two of them (ataxia-telangiectasia
and systemic lupus erythematosus) show signs of accelerated aging.

While fibroblasts from Down's patients have been reported to
be susceptible to an increased level of chromosome aberrations,
data on the ability of DS cells to perform excision repair is conflicting. While the susceptibility of DS chromosomes to 7,12-dime-
thylbenz-(α)-anthracene (DMBA) is greater than normal, lymphocytes
from DS patients were not found deficient in the ability to repair
either UV- or 4-nitroquinoline-1-oxide (4NQO) injury (O'Brien et
al., 1971). Although Lambert et al. (1976) reported evidence for
decreased UV-induced DNA repair synthesis in lymphocytes of Down's
syndrome patients, Yotti et al. (1980) failed to find altered
repair in DS fibroblasts. The latter study involved three fibroblast cell lines established from DS patients, whereas the work of
Lambert's group involved leucocytes from 12 DS patients and normal
controls. There is evidence that DNA repair capacities may vary
with the cell or organ source. DS lymphocytes display increased
numbers of sister chromatid exchanges following mitomycin C or
gamma irradiation, and sister chromatid exchanges are thought to
reflect unrepaired lesions in damaged DNA (Yotti et al, 1980).

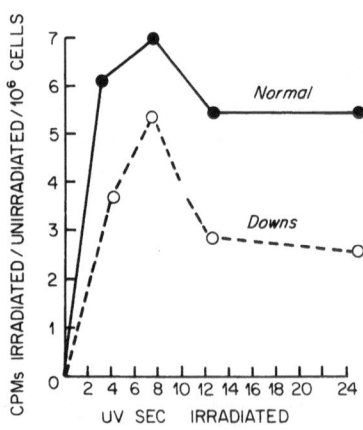

Fig. 1. Dose response curves for repair of UV-induced DNA damage
         in DS and normal lymphocytes (from Hall et al., 1982).

Table 6. Levels of cAMP and cGMP in T-lymphocytes from peripheral
blood of normal young adults, DS subjects and normal aged
controls (adapted from Tam and Walford, 1980)

Group	Average age	No. of subjects	cAMP[a]	cGMP[a]
young adults	35	23	18.4 ± 4	0.53 ± 0.2
DS	26,27[b]	11,26[b]	4.5 ± 0.4	6.4 ± 1.2
Aged adults	87	9	0.7 ± 0.3	4.7 ± 0.9

[a] Expressed as p. mol./10^7 cell
[b] First value refers to cAMP determination, second to cGMP

Preliminary evidence from our laboratory has indicated a
great deal of individual variation in repair of both UV-and
gamma-induced DNA damage in both DS subjects and normal controls,
suggesting the need of reasonable large samples for evaluating
repair function. When lymphocytes from fourteen Down's patients
were examined for excision repair of both UV and gamma induced DNA
damage, DNA repair, while showing inter-individual variation, was
approximately 45 to 50 per cent that of controls (Hall et al.,
1982). The repair level was consistently below that of normal
controls tested concurrently. Also, in dose-response experiments
for UV and gamma induced DNA damage, responses of lymphocytes from
Down's patients were approximately 50% those of controls (Fig.1).

5. CYCLIC NUCLEOTIDES, PURINE SALVAGE PATHWAYS, AND ENERGY CHARGE

Immune functional responses are generally detected by sub-
jecting an animal or cells "in vitro" to a stimulus, such as antigen or mitogen, and some days later measuring a product, such as
antibody production or uptake of tritiated thymidine. Most immune
responses decline with age. To the extent that this decline is
associated with intrinsic cellular lesions (Inkeles et al., 1977),
it would seem pertinent to look for possible metabolic or biochemical abnormalities in lymphocytes from old animals or humans.

Table 7. Specific activities of adenylate cyclase and guanylate cy-
         clase in T-lymphocytes from peripheral blood of normal
         young adults, DS subjects and normal aged controls (adap-
         ted from Tam and Walford, 1980).

Group	Average age	No. of subjects	Adenylate Cyclase[a]	Guanylate Cyclase[a]
young adults	32,31[b]	6,5[b]	385 $\pm$ 88	2997 $\pm$ 665
DS	22,23	13,8	1327 $\pm$ 229	965 $\pm$ 59
Aged adults	87	9,7	4147 $\pm$ 1334	316 $\pm$ 109

[a]Expressed as femtomoles cAMP or cGMP formed per mg protein per 15
minutes.
[b]First value refers to adenylate and second to guanylate cyclase
determinations.

    We have measured resting levels of cAMP, cGMP, and adenylate
and guanylate cyclases in isolated peripheral blood T-cells from
cohorts of humans in young adulthood, normal old humans (85-95
years of age), and adult DS subjects, as well as cAMP and cGMP
levels in T-cells from adult patients with systemic lupus erythematosus (SLE) (Tam and Walford 1980; Tam et al., 1980). Cyclic
nucleotide values relevant to DS and aging are given in Table 6,
and cyclase activities in Table 7. Values for DS parallel the
marked changes seen in aging.

    A number of factors affect the adenine nucleotide pool, and
accumulations of adenosine and/or deoxyadenosine with age, if such
occurs, it might well be expected to inhibit lymphocyte proliferation. Scholar et al., (1980) found a significant age-related
decrease in lymphocyte purine nucleoside phosphorylase by eight
months of age in mice, and pointed out that clinical states in man
characterized by a deficiency in this enzyme are accompanied by
impairment of T-cell but not B-cell function. It is known that
aging affects T-cell more that B-cell function, and it is noteworthy that T but not B lymphocytes are sensitive to the toxic ef-

fects of deoxyguanosine, one of the substrates which accumulate when purine nucleoside phosphorylase is deficient (Scholar et al., 1980). Recently Boss et al., (1980) measured the activity of lymphocyte ecto-5'-nucleotidase in relation to age in T-cells, T--cells subsets, and B-cells. In both T and B cells the activity was markedly reduced. Both T_G cells (suppressor cells) and T_{nonG} cells (helper cells) showed a decrease, which appeared to correlate with the age-related decline in immune system function. These aspects of purine salvage pathways have not yet been studied in DS.

Fig. 2 shows the relationships between the cyclic nucleotide system, purine salvage pathways, and energy charge. The cyclic nucleotides and purine salvage pathways enzymes might be expected to influence the energy charge within the lymphocyte. Energy charge is defined as $[(ATP) + 1/2 (ADP)] / [(ATP) + (ADP) + (AMP)]$ and reflects the utilizable metabolic energy available within the cell

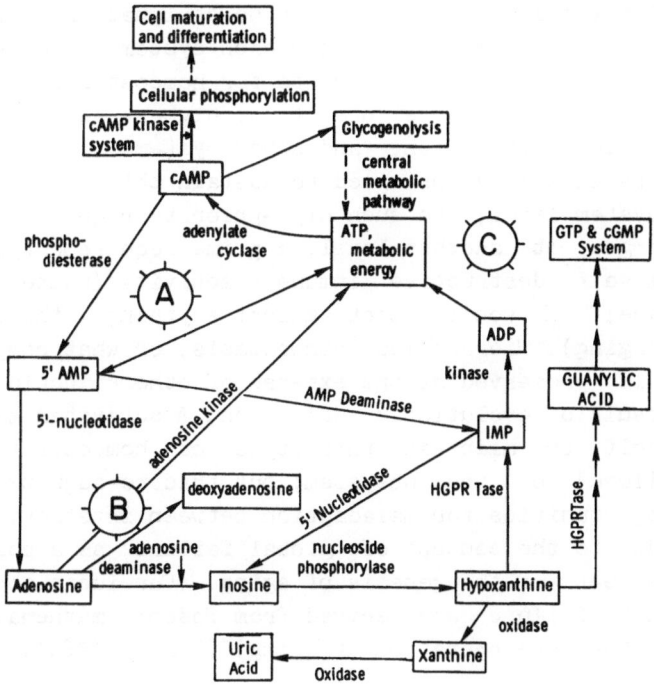

Fig. 2. Simplified version of interrelationships between cyclic nucleotide system (A), purine salvage pathway (B), and energy charge (C).

to do its work. Using the firefly bioluminescence method, we did
not find age-related changes in energy charge in resting peripheral blood T-cells from old compared to young adult humans but
Down's subjects had decreased values (Tam et al., 1980).

Compensating mechanisms may be operating to maintain this important parameter (Energy Charge) as constant as possible, despite
variability in related systems, or the variability in these others
might arise in order to maintain the energy charge as constant as
possible. Separate experiments from our laboratory (Weindruch et
al., 1980) have indicated a lower respiratory control index for
mitochondria from old mouse spleens and a diminished state 3
respiratory rate (maximum respiratory rate when excess ADP is
added), suggesting the possibility of a decreased rate of generation of ATP in mitochondria from lymphocytes of old animals.

6. DISCUSSION

     We shall attempt to relate some of the changes herein noted
for normal aging and DS to a concept we designate as "hierarchical
homeostasis". We assume that within each system or subsystem there
exists a hierarchy of requirements for homeostasis. For example:
at the whole organism level one of the highest requirements is to
maintain brain oxygenation, and other systems will re-adjust and
may even be largely compromised to sustain this. At the intracellular subsystem level, one such high-priority requirement might be
energy charge. At another level, a prime requirement might be to
avoid anti-self destructive immune reactivity (rather than react
against myself I won't react against anything = the immunodeficiency of aging). Hierarchical homeostasis, or what component of a
subsystem is preserved at the expense of others, could be assumed
to be a result of evolutionary selection. A subsystem may readjust
within itself to maintain this type of homeostasis and avoid
"local failure" of the subsystem; but this re-adjustment induces
greater opportunities for maladaption between interacting systems,
which leads to the concept of "global failure" as a possible fundamental aspect of the genesis of aging. (Our ideas about "local"
and "global" failure are derived from Rosen's mathematical model
approach to the interpretation of aging) (Rosen, 1981).

     There are two types of "failure":

     Local failure, i.e., in one key system. This approach accounts for most current theories of senescence : free radicals; somatic mutation or some form of chromatin change; cross-linking; failure of self/non-self descrimination; programmed senescence due to a "clock" mechanism, etc. The dilemma of the local failure approach is that there is sufficient flexibility both theoretically and experimentally that nearly every experimental observation can be made compatible with every theory.

The idea of local failure can be extended to include the concept of hierarchical homeostasis. Reference is made to Fig. 2, showing interrelations between the cyclic nucleotides, purine salvage pathways, and energy charge. The cyclic nucleotides and salvage pathway enzymes are altered with age, but the energy available for the cell is not, according to our experiments. Therefore, one might for illustrative purposes, assume energy charge to be at or near the top of the hierarchy, and the other subsystems will shift to maintain this most critical factor (Energy Charge = total utilizable metabolic energy for the cell to do its work). The system cannot be considered, on its own terms, to be undergoing substantial failure until it can no longer maintain energy charge, but considerable shifts in subcomponents may have to take place to preserve this pre-emptive homeostasis. These shifts, while maintaining a sort of homeostasis within the system, may be quite maladaptive for interactions with other systems, which situation involves a second and more complex category of failure, namely...

Global failure. A total system, such as an organism, can exhibit modes of failure which are global, involving subsystem interactions (Rosen, 1981). Global failure can occur before or without complete local failure, which may be why reductionist aging theories based on local failure of one sort or another have not been more successful. Our postulated relation between global

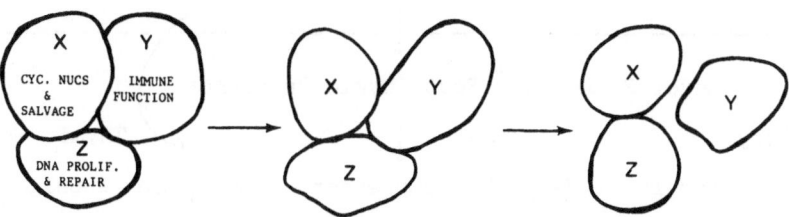

Fig. 3. Progression from local to global failure.

and local failure can best be explained by a heuristic diagram. (Fig 3). The lefthand side of the figure shows three subsystems all in perfect adjustment and interacting at their boundaries. If any of these requires re-adjustment in order to maintain its internal hierarchical homeostasis, this re-adjustment can be expressed as a change of shape of the set composing the elements of that subsystem. But this alteration disturbs the boundary relationships, i.e. the interactions between the subsystems, which situation defines a global failure. For example: alteration in purine salvage pathway enzymes needed to maintain energy charge within subsystem "X" may adversely affect the nucleotide precursor pool needed for adequate DNA synthesis and repair, i.e., subsystem "z". Subsystem "z" would then be forced to readjust and, according to our view of homeostasis, might sacrifice proliferative potential to maintain DNA repair. In "in vitro" senescence studies in diploid cell cultures, proliferative capacity diminishes well ahead of repair capacity.

Global failures can exist which do not in fact begin as local failures. These are generally characterized by feed forward controls, rather than feedback controls more familiar to biologists. In the equations

$$A_1 \to A_2 \to A_3 \to A_{n-1} \xrightarrow{E_{n-1}} A_n$$

the initial substrate A_1 may activate enzyme E_{n-1} which, however, is not required for use until later in the course of the reaction, as indicated. A discrepancy may develop between the actual final value of enzyme E_n-1 in relation to the amount of A_{n-1} substrate, and the value predicted by the initial level of A_1. Variations in intermediate substrates make such a feedforward

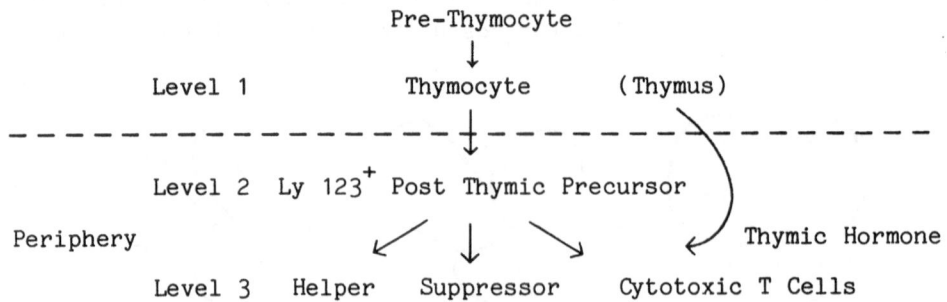

Fig. 4. Thymic hormone(s) as a feedforward control system.

control system less than fully adaptive. Figure 4 illustrates that the production and activity of thymic hormones may display some aspects of a feedforward control system. In an analysis of the disease of NZB/W mice Gottesman and I (1981) suggested that deregulation of thymic immunity probably occurs at levels 1 and 2 whereas most age-related functional tests have been confined to level 3, in which case the level of thymic hormone could be inappropriate for the 2 - 3 transition. The thymus is clearly abnormal in DS.

Our prior analysis of the disease of NZB/W mice, the animal counterpart of SLE, led us to conclude that such short-lived auto--immune mouse strains are legitimate models of accelerated aging, but they are models for a subgroup of the normally aging (Gottesman and Walford, 1981). DS may be a model of yet another subgroup. Along these lines, one recalls that even in inbred mouse strains a striking feature of aging is increasing variation. (A third of old C57B1/6J mice show an increase in suppressor cells for alloreactivity, the others a decrease. Some show auto-antibodies, others do not).

There may be not one process of "normal aging" but a collection of subgroups. The concept of hierarchical homeostasis may allow some insight into one approach as to how local and global failures arise and interact, and why the various progeroid syndromes emphasize certain but not all features of normal aging. The multiple defects of DS, as herein detailed, plus others, offer numerous possibilities for subsystem interactions. Most of these subsystems have been independently implicated in aging, which may be why DS is one of the best "experiments of nature" resembling aging. As an example of potential interactions: the increase in superoxide dismutase, known to occur in DS, may activate guanylate cyclase, leading to the observed increase in cGMP. cGMP activates cAMP phosphodiesterase, with a potential decrease in cAMP, and consequent disturbed immune function. On another level, the integrity of the nuclear material coding for cell growth and division, cellular differentiation and protein synthesis is a prerequisite for normal cellular and physiological function. Alterations to this genetic material in the form of misrepaired or unrepaired DNA damage may alter basic cellular function because of altered protein synthesis or altered states of differentiation. Such resultant changes in the cellular phenotype may lead to physiological expression of increased malignancy, cell death, and eventually physiological system malfunction, including altered immunological response. The local failure, therefore, of repair of DNA damage could conceivably produce a cascade effect subsequently involving other physiological parameters, producing alterations in internal homeostasis. Indeed most of the chromosomal instability syndromes present features (not necessarily the same features) of accelerated aging.

ACKNOWLEDGEMENTS

This study was supported by USPHS research grant AG-00790.

REFERENCES

Barnett, E.V., Chia, D., Knutson, D., Van Lancker, J., Cheney, K., Weindruch, R.and Walford, R.L., 1981, SLE an accelerated form of aging, in: "Immunological Aspects of Aging," Segre, D. and Smith, L., eds., Marcel Dekker Inc., New York.

Benda, C.E. and Strassman, G.S., 1965, The thymus in mongolism, J. Ment. Defic. Res., 9:109.

Boss, G.R., Thompson, L.F., Spiegelberg, H.L., Pichler, W.J. and Seegmiller, J.E., 1980, Age-dependency of lymphocyte 'Ecto-5'-nucleotidase activity, J. Immunol., 125:679.

Brown, W.T., Epstein, E.J., and Little, J.B, 1976, Progeria cells are stimulated to repair DNA by co-cultivation with normal cells, Exp. Cell. Res., 97:291-296.

Cox, D.R., Epstein, L.B. and Epstein, C.J., 1980, Gene coding for sensitivity to interferon (If Rec) and soluble superoxide dysmutase (SODI) are linked in mouse and man and map to mouse chromosome 16, Proc. Nat. Acad. Sci., 77:2168.

Epstein, L.B., Lee, S.H.S. and Epstein, C.J., 1980, Enhanced sensitivity of trisomy 21 monocytes to the maturation-inhibiting effect of interferon, Cell. Immunol., 50:191.

Gatti, R.A., and Walford, R.L., 1981, Immune function and features of aging in chromosomal instability syndrome, in: "Immunological Aspects of Aging", Segre, D.and Smith, L., eds., Marcel Dekker Inc., New York.

Gottesman, S., and Walford, R.L., 1980, Autoimmunity theories and aging, in: "Testing the Theories of Aging," V. XIV in the CRC Uniscience Series Methods in Aging Research, Adelman, R.C. and Roth, C.S., eds., CRC Press, in press.

Griffiths, A.W., and Sylvester, P.E., 1967, Monogols and non-
    mongols compared to their response to active tetanus immuni-
    sation, J. Ment. Defic. Res., 11:263.
Hall, K.Y., Hart, R.W., Benirschke, A.K., and Walford, R.L., 1981a,
    Correlation of repair of UV-induced DNA damage in primate
    lymphocytes and fibroblasts with maximum life span, Proc. Natl.
    Acad. Sci., in press.
Hall, K.Y., Bergmann, K. and Walford, R.L., 1981b, DNA repair,
    H-2, and aging in NZB and CBA mice, Tissue Antigens, 16:104.
Hall, K.Y., Gatti, R.A., and Walford, R.L., 1981c, Repair of gamma
    and bleomycin induced DNA damage in ataxia telangiectasia pa-
    tients and families. J. of Supramolecular Structure and Cellu-
    lar Biochemistry, Suppl. 5, C.F., Fox, Alan, ed., R. Liss Inc.,
    New York.
Hall, K.Y., Gatti, R.A., and Walford, R.L., 1981d, Excision repair
    of UV and gamma-induced DNA damage in Down's syndrome and syste-
    mic lupus erythematosus. Abst. Gerontological Society, Toronto,
    Canada.
Hann, H.W.., Deacon, J.C., and London, W.T., 1979, Lymphocyte surfa-
    ce markers and serum immunoglobulins in persons with Down's syn-
    drome. Am. J. Mental Deficiency, 85:245.
Hart, R.W., Hall, K.Y., and Daniel, F.B., 1978, DNA repair and muta-
    genesis in mammalian cells, Photochem Photobioo.
Hart, R.W. and Setlow, R.B., 1974, Correlation between deoxyribonu-
    cleic acid excision-repair and life-span in a number of mamma-
    lian species, Proc. Nat. Acad. Sci. U.S.A., 71:2169.
Hoar, D.I., and Waghorne, C., 1978, DNA repair in cockayne syndrome,
    Am. J. Hum. Genet., 30:590.
Inkeles, B., Innes, J.B., Kuntz, M.M., Kadish, A.S., and Weksler, M.
    E., 1977, Immunological studies of aging. III. Cytokinetic ba-
    sis for the impaired response of lymphocytes from aged humans
    to plant lectins, J. Exp. Med., 145:1176.
Karran, P., and Ormerod, M.G., 1973, Is the ability to repair dama-
    ged DNA related to the proliferative capacity of a cell? The re-
    joining of X-ray produced strand breaks, Biochem. Biophys.
    Acta, 299:54.
Kouvalainin, D., 1964, The pathology of the thymus, Ann. Med. Exp.
    Fenn., 42:177.
Kurnet, D.M., 1980, A molecular approach to Down's syndrome, Down's
    Syndrome, 3:1-2.
Lambert, B., Hansson, K., Bui, T.H., Funes-Cravioto, F. and Lindsten,
    J., 1976, DNA repair and frequency of X-ray and UV-light induced
    chromosome aberrations in leukocytes from patients with Down's

Syndrome, Ann. Hum. Genet., 39:293.

Leibovitz, A., and Yannet, H., 1942, The production of humoral anti-
    bodies by the mongolian, Amer. J. Ment. Defic., 46:304.

Levin, S., Schlesinger, M., Handzel, Z., Hahn, T., Altman, T., Czer-
    nobilshy, B. and Boss, J., 1979, Thymic deficiency in Down's
    syndrome, Pediatr., 63:80.

Lopez, V., Ochs, H.D., Thuline, H.C., Davis, S.D., and Wedgwood, J.R.
    J., 1975, Defective antibody response to bacteriophage OX 174
    in Down's syndrome, J. Pediatr., 86:207.

Martin, G.M., 1978, Genetic syndromes in man with potential relevan-
    ce to the pathobiology of aging in: "Genetic Effects on Aging,"
    D. Bergsma and D.E. Harrison, eds., Alan Liss Inc., N.Y.,
    p. 5-40.

Mattern, M.R., and Cerutti, P.A., 1975, Age-dependent excision re-
    pair of damaged thymine from gamma-irradiated DNA by isolated
    nuclei from human fibroblasts, Nature, London, 254:450.

Naeim, F., and Walford, R.L., 1980, Disturbance of redistribution of
    surface membrane receptors on peripheral mononuclear cells of
    patients with Down's syndrome and of aged individuals, J. Geron-
    tol., 35:640.

Naeim, F., Bergmann, K. and Walford, R.L., 1981, Capping and concana-
    valin A receptors on lymphocytes of aged individuals and pa-
    tients with Down's syndrome: enhancing effect of colchicine;
    possible relation to microtubular system, Age, 4:5.

O'Brien, R.L., Poon, P., Kline, E., and Parker, J.W., 1971, Suscepti-
    bility of chromosomes from patients with Down's syndrome to 7,
    12-dimethyl-benz (a)anthracene-induced aberrations in vitro,
    Int. J. Cancer, 8:202.

Ove, P., and Coetzee, M.L., 1978, A difference in bleomycin-induced
    DNA synthesis between liver nuclei from mature and old rats,
    Mech. Age. Develop., 8:363.

Paffenhalz, V., 1978, Correlation between DNA repair of embryonic
    fibroblasts and different life span of 3 inbred mouse strains,
    Mech. Age. Develop., 7:131.

Pero, R.W., Bryngelsson, C., Mitelman, F., Kornfalt, R., Thulin, T.,
    and Norden, A.,1979, Interindividual variation in the respon-
    ses of cultured human lymphocytes to exposure from DNA damaging
    chemical agents, Interindividual variation to carcinogen expo-
    sure, Mutation Res., 53:327.

Rainbow, A.J., and Howes, M., 1977, Decreased repair of gamma ray
    damaged DNA in progeria, Biochem. Biophys. Res. Commun., 74:714.

Rosen, E., 1981, Dynamical aspects of senescence, in: "Biological
    Mechanisms in Aging, "Conference," Bethesda, Md., in press.

Sacher, G.A., and Hart, R.W., 1978, Longevity, aging and comparati-
    ve cellular and molecular biology of the house mouse, Mus mu-
    sculus, and the white-footed mouse, Peromyscus leucopus. in:
    "Genetic effects on Aging", D. Bergsma and Harrison, D.E.,
    Alan R. Liss, Inc, New York.

Scholar, E.M., Rashidian, M., and Heidrick, M.L., 1980, Adenosine
    deaminase and purine nucleoside phosphorylase activity in
    spleen cells of aged mice, Mech. Age. Develop., 12:323.

Sechadri, R.S., Morley, A.A., Trainor, K.J., and Sorrell, J., 1979,
    Sensitivity of human lymphocytes to bleomycin increases with
    age, Experientia, 35:233.

Siegel, M., 1948, Susceptibility of mongoloids to infection. I. In-
    cidence of pneumonia, influenza A and shigella dysenteriae (Son-
    ne), Amer. J. Hyg., 48-53.

Tam, C.F., and Walford, R.L., 1980, Alterations in cyclic nucleoti-
    des and cyclase specific activities in T-lymphocytes of aging
    normal humans and patients with Down's syndrome, J. Immunol.,
    125:1665.

Tam, C.F., Cheung, M., Mock, D.C., Verity, A.M., and Walford, R.L.,
    1980, Energy charge values and adenine nucleotides in resting
    peripheral T-cells from young, normal aged, SLE and Down's sub-
    jects, The Gerontologist 20, Part 2:211, abstr.

Tam, C.F., Mock, D.C. and Walford, R.L., 1980, Alterations in cyclic
    nucleotide metabolism in resting peripheral T-cells from young
    and old, Down's and SLE subjects, Human Immunology, 1:291, abstr.

Thom, H., and McKay, E., 1972, Gm antigenic titres in adults with
    Down's syndrome (mongolism), non-mongoloid mental defectives
    and healthy blood donors, Clin. Exp. Immunol., 12:515.

Walford, R.L., 1976, When is a mouse "old"? J. Immunol., 117:352.

Walford, R.L., Barnett, E.V., Chia, D., Fahey, J.L., Gatti, R.A.,
    Gossett, T.C., Grossman, H., Medici, M.A., Motola, M., Naeim, F.,
    Sparkes, R.S., Spina, C., Tam, C.F., Tomura, T. and Van Lancker,
    J., 1981, Immunological and biochemical studies of Down's syn-
    drome as a model for accelerated aging, in: "Immunological A-
    spects of Aging," Segre, D., and Smith, L., eds., Marcel Dek-
    ker, Inc., p.

Weindruch, R., Cheung, M.K., Verity, M.A., and Walford, R.L. 1980,
    Modification of mitochondrial respiration by aging and dietary
    restriction, Mech. Age. and Develop., 12:375.

Yotti, L.P., Glover, T.W., Trosko, J.E. and Segel, D.J., 1980, Com-
    parative study of X-ray and UV induced cytotoxicity, DNA repair,
    and mutagenesis in Down's syndrome and normal fibroblasts, Pe-
    diatric Res., 2:88.

NATURAL RESISTANCE AGAINST TUMORS "IN VIVO"

Anna Maria Iorio", Franca Campanile*, Mariela Neri",
Abraham Goldin**, Enzo Bonmassar*

" Chair of Virology, University of
  Perugia, 06100 Perugia, Italy
* Institute of Pharmacology, University
  of Perugia, 06100 Perugia, Italy
** National Cancer Institute, National Institute
   of Health, Bethesda, Maryland 20205, USA

1. INTRODUCTION

Host's immunity against tumor cells can be classified according to two distinct functions, i.e. elicitable responses, evoked
by tumor-associated antigens, and natural resistance (NR) not
requiring previous exposure to antigenic determinants.

In the recent years, great attention has been paid to various
NR-associated phenomena, studied either "in vivo" or "in vitro" in
view of their possible role in the first-line of defence against
cancer. Various NR-type systems have been described in the
literature. It is reasonable to assume that they are mediated by
different populations of effector cells. Some of them have been
well characterized "in vitro", such as the (a) natural killer
lymphocytes directed mainly against lymphoma cells, (NK, Herberman
and Holden, 1978; Herberman et al., 1979; Roder et al., 1981); (b)
the natural cytotoxic effectors, lytic for solid tumors (Stutman
et al., 1978); (c) the activated macrophages cytotoxic or cytostatic for a large variety of neoplastic cells (Hibbs, 1976;
Keller, 1976, 1979, 1980); (d) the promonocytes showing NK-like
activity "in vitro" (Lohmann-Matthes and Domzig, 1979, 1980); and
(e) the polymorphonucleates capable of producing cytostatic (Korec

419

et al., 1980) or cytotoxic (Clark and Klebanoff, 1975; Dvorak et al., 1978) effects against tumor cells of various origin.

The role played by these effector immunocytes in the "in vivo" NR against tumors has not been fully elucidated. A number of studies has been performed to correlate the cytostatic and/or cytolytic effects "in vitro" with the "in vivo" antitumor activity of macrophages (Keller, 1979; Puccetti and Holden, 1979; Adam and Snyderman, 1979) or of NK cells (Carlson and Wegman, 1977; Riccardi et al., 1979 a, 1980; Herberman and Holden, 1979; Carlson et al., 1980). However, the "in vivo" NR phenomena appear to be rather complex, being presumably the result of combined subpopulations of immunocytes, including effector systems not presently detectable or fully characterized "in vitro".

One of the most classical "in vivo" NR directed against normal or malignant hematopoietic grafts has been described by Cudkowicz (1964 and 1968) in the sixties. Lethally-irradiated F1 hybrid mice were shown to be able to reject parental bone marrow cells (Cudkowicz and Bennet, 1971b). In addition, similar phenomenon was detected using hematopoietic tissue inoculated into allogeneic irradiated recipients, incapable of mounting classical elicitable graft responses (Cudkowicz and Bennet, 1971a). This type of NR "in vivo" has been found to be genetically regulated by histocompatibility loci called Hh (Hematopoietic histocompatibility, Cudkowicz and Lotzova, 1973; Cudkowicz, 1975a). Immunobiological studies concerning the Hh system revealed peculiar properties, distinguishable from those associated with the "classical" immune apparatus involved in tissue graft rejection. In particular, the Hh system, as previously mentioned, is relatively radioresistant and breaks the rule of codominance of histocompatibility loci in F1 hybrids, promoting rejection of parental bone marrow cells in F1 heterozygous recipients.

Additional properties of the Hh-mediated immunity can be summarized as follows: (a) graft rejection neither requires an antigen-induced sensitization phase, nor is enhanced by previous contact with the relevant antigen (Cudkowicz and Lotzova, 1973), thus showing the characteristics of natural immunity; (b) transplantation resistance is thymus independent, as shown by the studies performed in neonatally thymectomized mice (Cudkowicz and Bennet, 1971a) or in genetically athymic "nude" mice (Cudkowicz, 1975b); (c) the onset of resistance is age dependent, not being

detectable in mice younger than 21 days (Cudkowicz and Bennet, 1971a; Cudkowicz and Bennet, 1971b); (d) the genetic pattern of the Hh system shows that at least 2 separate sets of genes, the Hh and Ir-like genes, are involved in its regulation. The Hh genes code for Hh products acting as target antigens for tissue rejection. Among them, the strongest locus has been found to be linked with the D-region of the H-2 complex (i.e. the Hh-1 locus, Cudkowicz and Lotzova, 1973; Cudkowicz, 1975a), whereas "minor" Hh loci have been identified within the H-2K region (Cudkowicz and Lotzova, 1973) or outside the H-2 complex (Cudkowicz and Rossi, 1972). Donor-recipient incompatibility at one or more Hh loci is a necessary but not sufficient requirement for bone marrow rejection. It has been shown that Ir-like genes, located mainly outside the H-2 complex (Cudkowicz and Bennet, 1971a; Cudkowicz, 1971; Cudkowicz and Bennet, 1971b), regulate host's recognition of Hh products, or activate suppressor mechanisms, thus modulating the strength of resistance against a Hh-incompatible marrow graft.
It follows that successful bone marrow take can be found in selected strains of lethally-irradiated H-2-incompatible mice, in spite of Hh difference between donor and recipient (Cudkowicz and Lotzova, 1973; Cudkowicz, 1975a).

The relevance of the Hh system in the "in vivo" NR against a variety of malignant cells of hematopoietic origin has been confirmed more recently by a number of studies performed mainly in lethally-irradiated mice. In particular, evidence has been obtained that strong transplantation resistance occurs in the spleen of irradiated recipients challenged with H-2D-Hh-1-incompatible lymphomas (Bonmassar and Cudkowicz, 1976).
However, further investigations showed that anti-lymphoma NR can occur also in lethally-irradiated mice susceptible to the graft of bone marrow cells of the same host of origin of the tumor used for challenge (Iorio et al., 1978).

These findings point out that natural graft resistance against lymphoma and possibly other tumor cells is a rather complex phenomenon. As previously mentioned, it can be the result of various natural immune functions, some of them underlying the Hh system itself, such as the NK activity, which has been hypothesized to share common cellular effector pathways with the "in vivo" killing of hematopoietic grafts (Kiessling et al., 1977; Cudkowicz and Hochman, 1979).

Table 1. Genetic patterns of the animal used.

Strain	H-2 haplotype	H-2 regions								
		K	IA	IB	IJ	IE	IC	S	G	D
C57Bl/6 (B6)[a]	b	b	b	b	b	b	b	b	b	b
C57Bl/10 Sn Cr (B10)	b	b	b	b	b	b	b	b	b	b
B10.129(5M) (5M)	b	b	b	b	b	b	b	b	b	b
C57Bl/6-nu/nu (B6-nu/nu)	b	b	b	b	b	b	b	b	b	b
C57Bl/6-nu/+ (B6-nu/+)	b	b	b	b	b	b	b	b	b	b
B10.D2	d	d	d	d	d	d	d	d	d	d
DBA/2	d	d	d	d	d	d	d	d	d	d
BALB/c	d	d	d	d	d	d	d	d	d	d
BALB/c-nu/nu	d	d	d	d	d	d	d	d	d	d
BALB/c-nu/+	d	d	d	d	d	d	d	d	d	d
AKR	k	k	k	k	k	k	k	k	k	k
CBA	k	k	k	k	k	k	k	k	k	k
C3H	k	k	k	k	k	k	k	k	k	k
SJL	s	s	s	s	s	s	s	s	s	s
B10.A(5R) (5R)	i5	b	b	b	k	k	d	d	d	d
(C57Bl/6xDBA/2)F1 (BD2F1)	b/d	b/d	b/d	b/d	b/d	b/d	b/d	b/d	b/d	b/d
(BALB/c x DBA/2)F1 (CD2F1)	d/d	d/d	d/d	d/d	d/d	d/d	d/d	d/d	d/d	d/d
(B10.A(5R) x B10)F1	i5/b	b/b	b/b	b/b	k/b	k/b	d/b	d/b	d/b	d/b
NIH-nu/nu	non-inbred mice derived from NIH-Swiss mice									

[a] abbreviations in parenthesis

On the basis of these considerations, we elected to use the general term NR throughout the present paper to indicate the non-elicitable immunity directed against tumor cells "in vivo". In particular NR has been classified as graft resistance in hybrid (NRh), allogeneic (NRa) or syngeneic (NRs) recipients. It is conceivable that the various types of natural immune functions play a differential role in determining these 3 distinct classes of NR "in vivo".

The present paper will describe the patterns of natural immunity against murine lymphomas in a number of tumor-host combinations, using either Hh-resistant or Hh-susceptible recipient strains. The term "susceptible" has been applied to either Hh--compatible recipients, or to Hh-incompatible hosts with genetic background containing Ir-like gene(s) for non-responsiveness to Hh antigens.

2. DETAILS ON THE GENETIC PATTERN OF MICE
   AND ON THE ORIGIN OF THE TUMORS USED

Euthymic, 2-3 months old, inbred or hybrid mice of both sexes, or congenitally athymic mice, used in the present study, were obtained from the Mammalian Genetics and Animal Production, National Cancer Institute (NCI), National Institutes of Health (NIH) Bethesda, Md, U.S.A. The genetic patterns of the animals are reported in Table 1. The designation of transplantable tumors used, the strain of origin and other pertinent information are listed in Table 2.

3. ASSAY FOR NR

3.1. In Intact Mice

Transplantation resistance in intact mice was evaluated in terms of survival times of mice challenged with test tumors. Lymphoma cells were injected subcutaneously (s.c.) or intravenously (i.v.) into recipient mice of different strains. The animals were checked daily for mortality within 60 days after tumor inoculation and the presence of local or generalized tumor in dead mice was confirmed grossly at autopsy. For each group of recipient mice results were expressed in terms of median survival

Table 2. Origin and characteristics of the transplantable mouse tumors used.

Tumor designation	Strain of origin	Characteristics	Reference
L5MF-22	B10.129(5M)	Radiation-induced lymphoma	Bonmassar et al.,1970
RBL-5	C57 Bl/6	Rauscher-virus-induced lymphoma, ascites	Mc Coy et al., 1967
EL-4	C57 Bl/6	Benzopyrene-induced lymphoma	Gorer, 1950
P388	DBA/2	Chemically-induced lymphoma, ascites	Dawe and Potter, 1957
L1210-Ha	DBA/2	Chemically-induced lymphoma, ascites	Bonmassar et al.,1973
L1210-Cr	DBA/2	Chemically-induced lymphoma, ascites	Bonmassar et al.,1973
LSTRA	BALB/C	Moloney-virus-induced lymphoma, ascites	Glynn et al., 1964
K36	AKR	Spontaneous leukemia of Gross-Leukemia virus origin, ascites	Old et al., 1965

times (MST) and dead over total mice tested (D/T) or percent of survivors over total number of animals challenged.

3.2. In lethally-Irradiated or Drug-Treated Mice

Transplantation resistance was also tested in mice subjected to treatments capable of inhibiting most of the elicitable responses and endogenous cell proliferation. In these conditions relatively radioresistant or drug-resistant NR is selectively tested, measuring the extent of tumor cell proliferation in mouse organs.

Total body irradiation of mice: mice were exposed to a single treatment of total body irradiation, 4 or 5 hrs before tumor challenge, using a ^{60}Co irradiator (Hot Spot, MKIV, Harwell, England) delivering γ-rays at the rate of 1000 R/minute.

Drugs: 5(3,3'-dimethyl-1-triazeno)-imidazole-4-carboxamide (DTIC) was dissolved in distilled water mixed with citric acid and mannitol (Carlo Erba, Milan). The ratio of DTIC : citric acid : mannitol was 1:1:0.375 wt/wt. Cyclophosphamide (Cy) was dissolved in 0.85% NaCl solution. Both drugs were supplied by Dr. V.L. Narayanan of the Drug Synthesis and Chemistry Branch, Division of Cancer Treatment, NCI, NIH, Bethesda, Md. DTIC (250 mg/kg i.p.) and Cy (200 mg/kg i.p.) were administered on day -5 and 0, respectively before tumor challenge.

Evaluation of ^{125}I-labeled-5-iodo-deoxyuridine (^{125}IUdR) uptake by spleen, liver and lung "in vivo": lethally-irradiated or drug-treated mice were inoculated with lymphoma cells into the lateral tail vein. Tumor graft proliferation were assessed 4 days later by measuring the uptake of ^{125}IUdR, a radioactive analog of thymidine, incorporated into DNA (Hofer and Hughes, 1970; Bonmassar and Cudkowicz, 1976). The animals were treated with a single i.p. dose of 5-fluoro-2'-deoxyuridine (FUdr, 25 μg/ mouse) to decrease the availability of endogenous thymidine (Hofer and Hughes, 1970). One hr later they were inoculated with 0.5 μCi of IUdR in 0.25 ml of 0.85% NaCl solution. From 16 to 24 hrs later the animals were killed, the organs were removed and their radioactivity was measured in a well-type-crystal scintillation counter (Packard model 5110). Alternatively, the organs were removed 3 or 4 hrs after ^{125}IUdR injection. The ^{125}IUdR not incorporated into DNA was eluted by soaking the organs in 70% ethanol for 3 days

Table 3. Growth of lymphoma cells of different lines into Hh-resistant lethally-irradiated hybrid mice.

Recipient mice(No.)	H-2 haplotype	Lymphoma line	H-2 haplotype	Inoculum size (i.v.) (day 0)	% ^{125}IUdR uptake (day+4)			
					Spleen Mean (SE)^a	p^b	Liver Mean (SE)	p
B6^c (9)	b	L5MF-22	b	5×10^5	2.13(2.38–1.90)	–	7.13(8.00–6.35)	–
BD2F$_1$ (5)	b/d	L5MF-22	b	5×10^5	0.07(0.09–0.07)	A	4.85(5.28–4.25)	B
B6 (5)	b	RBL-5	b	1×10^6	0.58(0.76–0.44)	–	1.45(1.61–1.31)	–
BD2F$_1$ (7)	b/d	RBL-5	b	1×10^6	0.08(0.09–0.06)	A	0.24(0.28–0.21)	A
B6 (8)	b	EL-4	b	5×10^6	2.52(3.40–1.86)	–	5.30(5.52–5.08)	–
BD2F$_1$ (8)	b/d	EL-4	b	5×10^6	0.02(0.03–0.02)	A	0.96(1.11–0.82)	A

^{a}Geometric mean (GM), SE, standard error. In parenthesis GM+SE, GM-SE.
^{b}p was calculated comparing the uptake values of compatible mice with respect to those of Hh-resistant hybrid mice. A, p 0.01; B, p< 0.005.
^{c}Splenic and hepatic ^{125}IUdR uptake of B10.129 (5M) mice bearing L5MF-22 leukemia was not significantly different from that of C57Bl/6 mice as tested in a separate experiment (data not shown).

(Bennett, 1972). The results were expressed as the geometric mean and the upper and lower limit of the mean, ranging within its standard error, of the percentage of ^{125}IUdR incorporated into the test organs.

3.3. Statistical Evaluation

The statistical analysis for % ^{125}IUdR uptake was performed according to Student's test, calculated on the logs of the original counts per minute. The analysis of mortality data of mice was performed according to the Mann-Whitney-"V" test.

4. NR IN F1 HYBRID MICE (NRh)

4.1. NRh in Hh-Resistant Recipients

Three different lines of H-2 lymphomas were inoculated i.v. into lethally-irradiated H-2-compatible homozygous B6 or F1 hybrid BD2Fl recipients. Marked inhibition of lymphoma growth as evidenced by the ^{125}IUdR uptake values, was observed particularly in the spleen of hybrid hosts, as shown by the data illustrated in Table 3.

It is reasonable to assume that the "localized" resistance detected in the spleen and liver of irradiated hybrid recipients, could be relevant to anti-lymphoma NR in terms of survival times. Studies performed with L5MF-22 lymphoma cells inoculated by the s.c. or i.v. route into non-irradiated B6 or BD2F1 mice pointed out that hybrid recipients survived significantly longer than hosts homozygous for the H-2 haplotype, when tumor inocula did not exceed 10^4- 10^5 cells (Fig. 1). These results are in agreement with those described by Klein et al. (1978), who showed NRh against RBL-5 leukemia, by Gallagher et al. (1976) and Schimitt-Verhulst (1977), who used spontaneous AKR leukemias, by Harmon et al. (1977) and Clark et al. (1977) who utilized EL-4 lymphoma inoculated into Hh-1-incompatible F1 hybrid mice.
However, in the studies described by Harmon and Clark all recipient mice were incompatible for minor histocompatibility loci (MHL) with the tumor. Therefore, elicitable graft response (EGR) against MHL-coded tumor-associated alloantigens could have not been entirely ruled out. Since the same criticism holds true for

Table 4. Growth of L5MF-22 (H-2^b) (6x10^5 cells i.v. at day 0) lymphoma cells into Hh- resistant lethally-irradiated hybrid mice not treated or pretreated with IDF.

Recipient mice (No)	H-2 haplotype	Pretreatment[a] (day -3)	%^{125}IUdR uptake (day + 4)			
			Spleen Mean (SE)[b]	p[c]	Liver Mean (SE)	p
B6 (6)	b	None	2.04(2.35-1.77)	-	3.47(4.28-2.81)	-
B6 (8)	b	IDF	2.15(2.51-1.84)	NS	4.55(5.00-4.07)	NS
BD2F1 (8)	b/d	None	0.013(0.018-0.009)	A	1.38(1.49-1.27)	A
BD2F1 (10)	b/d	IDF	0.008(0.011-0.007)	A	1.76(1.91-1.62)	B

[a]IDF was obtained from sera of infected BD2F1 donors (Iorio et al., 1976).
[b]Geometric mean (GM), SE, standard error. In parenthesis GM + SE, GM - SE.
[c]p was calculated comparing the uptake values of compatible mice with respect to those of hybrid mice. A, p < 0.01; B, p < 0.05; NS, not significant.

L5MF-22 lymphoma inoculated into BD2F1 mice (Table 6). Significant growth inhibition of the tumor occurred in the spleen of F1 recipients with impaired EGR.

Transplantation immunity of EGR type was inhibited in BD2F1

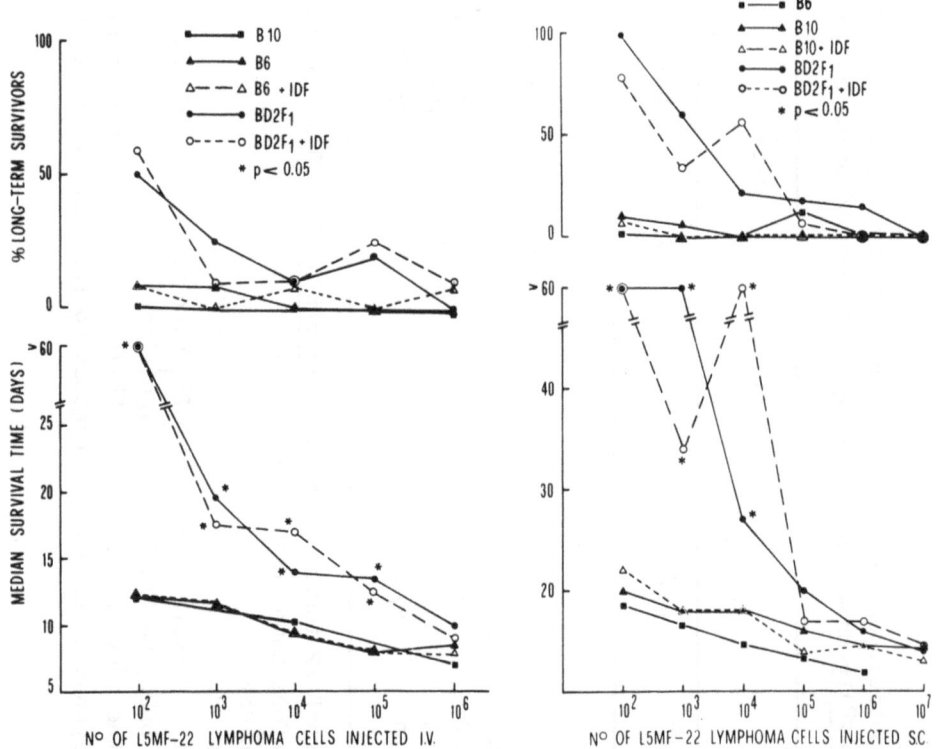

Fig. 1. Median survival time and percentage of long term survivors (>60) of B10, B6 and BD2FI mice inoculated with graded numbers of L5MF-22 lyphoma cells. Groups of B6 or B10 and BD2F1 mice were pretreated with IDF obtained from sera of infected BD2F1 donors (Iorio et al., 1976); 15-20 animals per point. The activity of IDF was tested in CD2F1 mice challenged with 10^7 cells i.v. of allogenic L5MF-22 lymphoma: all untreated recipients rejected the tumor, whereas 100% of the mice pretreated with the IDF preparation died with generalized lymphoma, with an MST of 7 days. (B10.A(5R)xB10) F1 mice were given 10^2 cells i.v. and the mortality was 100% with a MST of 22 days (p < 0.05 when compared with the mortality of B10 hosts).

Table 5. Mortality of histocompatible or $\underline{Hh}$-resistant hybrid mice non-pretreated or presensitized against L2MF-22($\underline{H-2^b}$)lymphoma and challenged with graded doses of the same tumor.

Pretreatment[a]	Inoculum size	Recipient mice B6 ($\underline{H-2^b}$)			Recipient mice BD2F$_1$ ($\underline{H-2^b/H-2^d}$)			
		MST[b]	D/T[c]	P$_1$[d]	MST	D/T	P$_1$	P$_2$[e]
None	10^4	15.0	17/17	–	27.0	11/19	–	A
Irr-L5MF-22	10^4	15.0	8/8	NS	32.0	9/17	NS	A
None	10^5	13.0	18/18	–	23.0	14/19	–	A
Irr-L5MF-22	10^5	12.0	8/8	NS	25.0	17/18	NS	A
None	10^6	12.0	17/17	–	15.5	18/18	–	A
Irr-L5MF-22	10^6	12.0	8/8	NS	14.5	17/18	NS	A

[a]Irr-L5MF-22, 3×10^7 cells of L5MF-22 tumor, irradiated $\underline{in\ vitro}$ (10,000 R) and inoculated ip into recipient mice 14 days before tumor challenge.
[b]MST, median survival time in day.
[c]D/T, dead over total mice tested.
[d]P$_1$ was calculated comparing the survival times of BD2F$_1$ mice presensitized against L5MF-22 with those of non-sensitized BD2F$_1$ hosts. NS, not significant.
[e]P$_2$ was calculated comparing the survival times of C57Bl/6 hosts with those of BD2F$_1$ challenged with the same number of lymphoma cells and subjected to the same pretreatment. [1]A, p<0.01; B, p<0.05.

mice by pretreatment with a tumor-associated factor of viral origin, IDF (Bonmassar et al., 1973; Iorio et al., 1976), capable of impairing EGR immunity (Bonmassar et al., 1973). The results (Fig. 1 and legend of Fig. 1) confirmed that anti-lymphoma transplantation resistance was detectable in B10xB10.A(5R) F1 and in IDF-pretreated BD2F1 recipients. Suppression of EGR mediated by the IDF preparation used in these studies, was also confirmed by the successful take of L5MF-22 lymphoma cells into 1DF -pretreated CD2F1 mice incompatible for the entire H-2 complex (see legend of Fig. 1).

It should be noted also that no difference in survival times was found between fully histocompatible B10 and MHL-incompatible B6 recipients challenged with 10^2 - 10^6 cells, nor between non--treated or IDF-pretreated B6 mice (Fig. 1). These data provide further support to the hypothesis that MHL-incompatibility does not play a significant role in transplantation resistance detectable in hybrid recipients differing for MHL with lymphoma cells. The experiments conducted in mice pretreated with IDF relied on the assumption that the factor was capable of depressing EGR without impairing NR, as suggested by previous studies conducted in non-irradiated nude mice (Bonmassar et al., 1975) or in lethally-irradiated euthymic hosts (Bonmassar et al., 1979).

In order to confirm that IDF does not depress NR in the present host-tumor model, B6 or BD2F1 mice were pretreated with IDF, subjected to lethal total-body irradiation, inoculated with L5MF-22 lymphoma cells, and tested for tumor cell proliferation on day +4 after challenge. The results (Table 4) are in agreement with those of previous studies mentioned before (Bonmassar et al., 1979) since NRh levels were comparable in either non-treated or IDF-treated BD2F1 hosts.

A distinct feature of NR is the absence of second-set responses following sensitization with the relevant antigen (Bonmassar et al., 1975; Campanile et al., 1977; Iorio et al., 1978; Riccardi et al., 1979, 1980). Therefore additional studies were performed in B6 or BD2F1 hosts presensitized with irradiated L5MF-22 cells and challenged with the same lymphoma 14 days after immunization. The results (Table 5) showed that presensitization neither affected significantly transplantation resistance in hybrid mice, nor produced detectable graft immunity in B6 recipients. Therefore these results add further support to the hypo-

Table 6. Growth of lymphoma cells of different lines into Hh-susceptible lethally-irradiated hybrid mice.

Recipient mice(No)	H-2 haplotype	Lymphoma line	H-2 haplotype	Inoculum size(i.v.) (day 0)	% ^{125}IUdR uptake (day+4)			
					Spleen Mean (SE)[a]	p[b]	Liver Mean (SE)	p
CD2F$_1$ (7)	d/d	P388	d	1×10^6	0.81(0.93-0.71)	-	2.64(2.81-2.48)	-
BD2F$_1$ (7)	b/d	P388	d	1×10^6	0.09(0.10-0.09)	A	1.40(1.62-1.20)	A
CD2F$_1$ (7)	d/d	L1210Ha	d	2×10^5	0.60(0.66-0.54)	-	3.33(3.68-3.02)	-
BD2F$_1$ (7)	b/d	L1210Ha	d	2×10^5	0.23(0.30-0.17)	A	2.64(2.90-2.40)	NS
CD2F$_1$ (8)	d/d	L1210Cr	d	2×10^5	0.82(0.88-0.77)	-	4.38(4.75-4.03)	-
BD2F$_1$ (5)	b/d	L1210Cr	d	2×10^5	0.28(0.42-0.19)	A	2.81(3.66-2.16)	NS

[a] Geometric mean (GM), SE, standard error. In parenthesis GM+SE, GM-SE.
[b] p was calculated comparing the uptake values of compatible mice with respect to those of Hh-susceptible hybrid mice. A, p < 0.01; NS, not siginificant.

thesis that NRh of presumable Hh type would play a substantial
role in antilymphoma resistance of BD2F1 mice.

4.2. NRh in Hh - Susceptible Mice

    It has been shown that irradiated BD2F1 mice obtained from
C57Bl/6xDBA/Cr2 substrain are essentially non-responder against

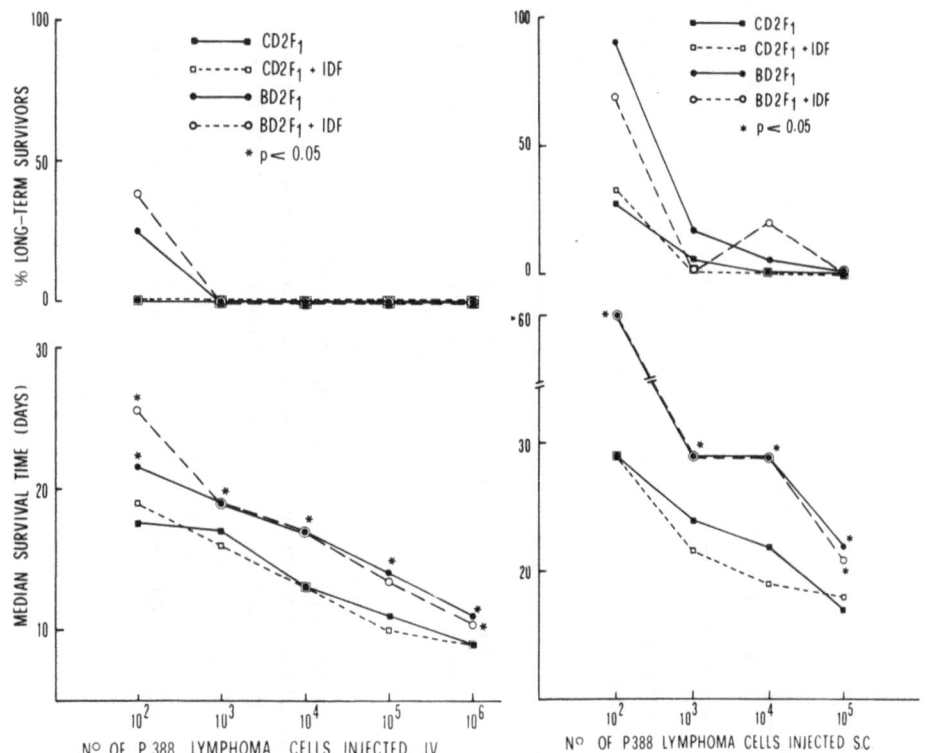

Fig. 2. Median survival time and percentage of long term survivors
        (>60) of CD2F1 and BD2F1 mice inoculated with graded doses
        of P388 lymphoma, pretreated or non-pretreated with IDF ob-
        tained from sera of infected BD2F1 mice (Iorio et al., 1976).
        8 animals per point. In DBA/2 mice given 10^2 P388 lymphoma
        cells i.v. the mortality was 100% with a MST of 21.0 days
        (p < 0.05, when compared with the mortality of CD2F1 hosts).
        In DBA/2 mice given 10^2 P388 lymphoma cells s.c., the mor-
        tality was 75% with a MST of 28.5 days (p 0.05, when com-
        pared with the mortality of CD2F1 hosts).

Table 7. Growth of P388(H-2^d) (6 x 10^5 cells i.v. at day 0) lymphoma cells into Hh-susceptible lethally-irradiated hybrid mice not treated or pretreated with IDF.

Recipient mice(No.)	H-2 haplotype	Pretreatment[a] (day -3)	%^{125}IUdR uptake (day + 4)			
			Spleen Mean (SE)[b]	P[c]	Liver Mean (SE)	P
CD2F1[d] (8)	d/d	None	0.18(0.21-0.16)	-	0.92(1.05-0.82)	-
BD2F1 (8)	b/d	None	0.03(0.04-0.02)	A	0.56(0.65-0.48)	B
BD2F1 (8)	b/d	IDF	0.03(0.04-0.02)	A	0.38(0.44-0.33)	A

[a]IDF was obtained from sera of infected BD2F1 donors (Iorio et al., 1976).
[b]Geometric mean (GM), SE, standard error. In parenthesis GM + SE, GM - SE.
[c]p was calculated comparing the uptake values of compatible mice with respect to those of
hybrid mice. A, p < 0.01; B, p < 0.05.
[d]Splenic and hepatic ^{125}IUdR uptake of DBA/2 mice bearing P388 leukemia was not significantly different from that of CD2F1 mice as tested in a separate experiment (data not shown).

DBA/2Cr bone marrow cells (Cudkowicz and Rossi, 1972). Therefore BD2F1 mice have been considered Hh-susceptible for hematopoietic tissues of DBA/2 origin. Two DBA/2 lymphomas, the P388 and the L1210 Cr and its L1210 Ha subline were inoculated i.v. into lethally-irradiated histocompatible CD2F1 mice homozygous for the H-2^d complex and into hybrid BD2F1 mice (Table 6). Significant growth inhibition of the tumor occurred in the spleen of F1 recipients inoculated with all lymphoma lines, whereas limited tumor impairment was detectable in the liver of BD2F1 mice inoculated with P388 leukemia, but not with the other two lymphoma lines.

Studies parallel to those described for lethally-irradiated Hh-resistant mice, were performed in order to test the possible role of NRh on host's survival after leukemia challenge. The results of these investigation, illustrated in Fig. 2, confirmed that limited but significant increase in survival times occurred in hybrid recipients with respect to those detectable in H-2^d homozygous mice. Again resistance in the hybrids was not affected by host's pretreatment with IDF. In this model it should be remembered that no histoincompatibility for MHL occurs between host and tumor. In addition, the survival times of syngeneic DBA/2 mice inoculated with as low as 10^2 P388 lymphoma cells did not differ significantly from those of CD2F1 recipients, used as homozygous controls (see legend of Fig.2). NRh in Hh-susceptible mice was also non-affected by pretreatment of hybrid recipients with IDF. This was confirmed in lethally-irradiated mice, as shown by the results illustrated in Table 7.
Presensitization studies carried out with P388 lymphoma, similar to those described for the Hh-resistant model, confirm that BD2F1 mice did not mount a second-set response against P388 lymphoma cells (Table 8), thus providing support to the hypothesis of NR-nature of their resistance to parental lymphoma challenge.

5. NR IN ALLOGENEIC MICE (NRa)

5.1. NRa in Hh-Resistant Recipients

Previous studies conducted with a number of tumor-host combinations pointed out that graft resistance against allogeneic lymphoma can be detected in lethally-irradiated mice. This has been found always with tumor cells of the same genotype of bone

Table 8. Mortality of histocompatible H-2 homozygous CD2F mice ($\underline{H-2^d/H-2^d}$) or of H-2 heterozygous hybrid BD2F$_1$ mice ($\underline{H-2^b/H-2^d}$) not pretreated or presensitized against P388 ($\underline{H-2^d}$) lymphoma, and challenged with graded doses of the same tumor s.c.

Pretreatment[a]	Inoculum size	Recipient mice						
		CD2F$_1$			BD2F$_1$			
		MST[b]	D/T[c]	P$_1$[d]	MST	D/T	P$_1$	P$_2$[e]
None	10^3	25.0	8/8	–	60.0	3/10	–	A
Irr-P388	10^3	22.5	8/8	B	46.5	6/10	NS	A
None	10^4	22.5	8/8	–	30.0	10/10	–	A
Irr-P388	10^4	20.0	8/8	NS	27.5	10/10	B	A
None	10^5	20.0	9/9	–	25.0	10/10	–	A
Irr-P388	10^5	20.0	8/8	NS	22.5	10/10	NS	A

[a] Irr-P388, 3×10^7 cells of P388 tumor, irradiated $\underline{in\ vitro}$ (10,000 R) and inoculated ip into recipient mice 14 days before tumor challenge.

[b] MST, median survival time in days.

[c] D/T, dead over total mice tested.

[d] P$_1$ was calculated comparing the survival times of mice presensitized with P388 lymphoma with those of non-sensitized hosts. B, p < 0.05; NS, not significant.

[e] P$_2$ was calculated comparing the survival times of CD2F$_1$ hosts with those of BD2F$_1$ recipients challenged with the same number of lymphoma cells and subject to the same pretreatment.
A, p < 0.01.

Table 9. Growth of different lymphoma cell lines into <u>Hh-resistant</u> lethally-irradiated allogeneic mice.

Recipient mice(No.)	H-2 haplotype	Lymphoma line	H-2 haplotype	Inoculum size(i.v.) (day 0)	% [125]IUdR uptake (day+4)			
					Spleen Mean (SE)[a]	p[b]	Liver Mean (SE)	p
CD2F$_1$ (10)	d/d	P388	d	6x10^6	2.06(2.32-1.83)	-	9.40(9.86-8.95)	-
CBA (5)	k	P388	d	6x10^6	0.27(0.35-0.21)	A	2.00(2.43-1.64)	A
CD2F$_1$ (8)	d/d	P388	d	6x10^5	0.49(0.54-0.46)	-	2.27(2.51-2.05)	-
B6 (8)	b	P388	d	6x10^5	0.08(0.10-0.06)	A	1.86(2.41-1.44)	NS
B10 (3)	b	P388	d	6x10^5	0.12(0.15-0.09)	A	2.78(3.03-2.55)	NS
BALB/c(7)	d	LSTRA	d	2x10^5	1.56(1.74-1.39)	-	5.89(6.62-5.24)	-
B6 (8)	b	LSTRA	d	2x10^5	0.08(0.14-0.05)	A	6.14(7.32-5.14)	NS
CBA (7)	k	LSTRA	d	2x10^5	0.01(0.014-0.008)	A	0.29(0.41-0.21)	A

[a] Geometric mean (GM), SE, standard error. In parenthesis GM+SE, GM-SE.
[b] p was calculated comparing the uptake values of syngeneic or compatible mice with those of allo-geneic mice. A, p< 0.01. NS, not significant.

Table 10. Growth of 2×10^6 L5MF-22 (H-2^b) lymphoma cells inoculated i.v. into lethally-irradiated conventional or nude mice.

Recipient mice(No.)	H-2 haplotype	Hh[a]	%[125]IUdR uptake (day + 4)			
			Spleen Mean (SE)[b]	P[c]	Liver Mean (SE)	P
5M (8)	b	S	1.54(1.64-1.46)	-	2.78(3.15-2.46)	-
NIH-nu/nu (11)	random-bred	NT	1.40(1.71-1.15)	NS	3.80(4.58-3.15)	NS
BAMB/c-nu/nu (4)	d	R	0.09(0.10-0.08)	A	1.22(1.44-1.04)	A
BALB/c-nu/+ (6)	d	R	1.56(1.80-1.40)	NS	2.96(3.23-2.68)	NS
BALB/c (10)	d	R	0.28(0.38-0.22)	A	2.74(3.45-2.18)	NS

[a] Susceptibility to transplantation of bone marrow cells of the host of origin of the lymphoma. S=Susceptible; R=Resistant; NT= Not tested.

[b] Geometric mean (GM), SE, standard error. In parenthesis GM + SE, GM - SE.

[c] p was calculated comparing the uptake values of syngeneic mice with respect to those of allo-geneic, nu/+ or nu/nu hosts. A, $p < 0.01$; NS, not significant.

marrow which would undergo Hh-dependent rejection by the irradiated recipients (Houchens et al., 1975; Bonmassar and Cudkowicz,
1976; Iorio et al., 1978; Bonmassar et al., 1979). The results of
additional investigation, illustrated in Table 9, confirm that
strong resistance against H-2^d lymphomas (i.e. P388 and LSTRA
lines) is detectable in the spleen of Hh-resistant B6, B10 or CBA
recipients. Localized resistance in the liver provides a more
complicated picture being detectable in CBA but not in B6 or B10
hosts.

The independency of NRa from thymus influence has been
repeatedly observed in the course of studies carried out in
irradiated "nude" mice as recipients of allogeneic lymphoma cells
(Bonmassar et al., 1975, 1978; Campanile et al., 1977). This has
been confirmed in the present investigation (Table 10). In particular, significant resistance against L5MF-22 (H-2^b) lymphoma
cells was detected in the spleen of either conventional BALB/c
mice or nu/nu hosts carrying the BALB/c (H-2^d) background,
Hh-incompatible for bone marrow cells of H-2^b donors (Cudkowicz
and Bennett, 1971a; Cudkowicz, 1975b). Notably localized NRa of
BALB/c-nu/nu recipients was not only greater than that found in
euthymic BALB/c mice, but was also detectable in the liver.

Worthy of further comments are the data pointing out that no
NRa could be demonstrated in either athymic NIH-nu/nu recipients
or in euthymic heterozygous BALB/c-nu/+ carrying the same genetic
background of resistant BALB/c-nu/nu hosts (Table 10). It can be
hypothesized that the NIH-nu/nu mouse population contains high
percentage of individuals sharing common genetic traits for low Hh
responsiveness. In this context it must be emphazized that these
mice show high NK reactivity similar, if not greater than that of
BALB/c-nu/nu mice (Herberman et al., 1975).

The finding that euthymic BALB/c-nu/+ are essentially non-
responder against L5MF-22 lymphoma is more difficult to explain.
It can be suggested that heterozygousity would activate a thymus-
dependent Ir-like genetic function for unresponsiveness, not
operating in homozygous BALB/c-nu/nu recipients. It should be also
stressed that BALB/c-nu/+ and BALB/c Cr strains might differ for
the non-H-2 genetic background. Survival times of "nude" mice
inoculated with L5MF-22 (H-2^b) or LSTRA (H-2^d) lymphomas (Table
11) show that significant transplantation resistance can be
detected not only in allogeneic recipients incompatible for the

Table 11. Survival of conventional or inbred or random-bred nude mice inoculated with H-2-compatible or H-2-incompatible lymphoma lines.

Recipient mice	H-2 haplotype	Hh[a]	Lymphoma line	H-2 haplotype	Inoculum size(i.v.)	MST[b]	D/T[c]	P[d]
5M	b	S	L5MF-22	b	1×10^7	6.0	6/6	—
B6-nu/+	b	S	L5MF-22	b	1×10^7	6.0	6/6	NS
B6-nu/nu	b	S	L5MF-22	b	1×10^7	9.0	6/6	A
BALB/c-nu/nu	d	R	L5MF-22	b	1×10^7	11.5	10/10	A
BALB/c	d	S	LSTRA	d	1×10^5	7.0	12/12	—
NIH-nu/nu	d	NT	LSTRA	d	1×10^5	11.5	8/8	A
BALB/c-nu/nu	d	S	LSTRA	d	1×10^5	10.0	8/8	A
BALB/c	d	S	LSTRA	d	1×10^3	10.0	6/6	—
NIH-nu/nu	d	NT	LSTRA	d	1×10^3	14.5	7/8	A

[a] Susceptibility to transplantation of bone marrow cells of the host of origin of the lymphoma. S=susceptible; R=resistant; NT=not tested.
[b] MST, median survival time in days.
[c] D/T, dead over total mice tested.
[d] p, probability values calculated comparing the survival times of syngeneic mice with those of allogeneic, nu/+ or nu/nu hosts. A, $p < 0.01$; NS, not significant.

major histocompatibility complex, but also in mice homozygous for the H-2 haplotype indentical to that of the tumor line used (i.e. L5MF-22 and LSTRA lymphomas inoculated into B6-nu/nu or BALB/c -nu/nu respectively).

Moreover transplantation resistance against LSTRA cells was detected in NIH-nu/nu hosts. Growth inhibition of subcutaneous tumors in histocompatible nude mice was also found by Warner et al (1977) who tested a number of different lymphoid tumor lines of BALB/c origin in either euthymic or nu/nu BALB/c recipient mice.

5.2. NRa in Hh-Susceptible Recipients

Two H-2^d lymphoma lines, namely P388 of DBA/2 origin and LSTRA of BALB/c origin, were inoculated i.v. into lethally-irradiated histocompatible or allogeneic recipients, susceptible for H-2^d bone marrow cells. In all, cases significant resistance against tumor growth (Table 12) was detectable either in the spleen or in the liver of allogeneic hosts. Worthy of consideration is also the finding that resistance against P388 lymphoma cells could have been demonstrated in H-2^d compatible homozygous BIO.D2 mice.

All these results are in agreement with preceeding observations conducted in a number of tumour-host models (Iorio et al., 1978; Bonmassar et al., 1979). Of particular interest appears to be the finding that no correlation is detectable between spleen and liver resistance. Actually highly resistant H-2-incompatible B6 mice did not show liver impairment of P388 lymphoma growth (Table 9), whereas the weakly resistant BIO.D2 strain or the more resistant C3H hosts both susceptible for the Hh system, produced significant inhibition of P388 lymphoma proliferation (Table 12) in the liver with respect to that found in histocompatible mice. These data are difficult to interpret and might be the result of differential distribution of effector cells responsible of NRa in spleen and liver, according to the host-tumor system used, independently from the Hh patterns of responsivity.

Additional studies were carried out in the C3H-LSTRA model, using drug-treated instead of lethally-irradiated recipients. Previous investigations showed that the sequential treatment of mice with DTIC and Cr impairs severely most of T-dependent immuno-

Table 12. Growth of different lymphoma cell lines into Hh-suceptible lethally-irradiated allogeneic mice.

Recipient mice(No.)	H-2 haplotype	Lymphoma line	H-2 haplotype	Inoculum size(i.v.) (day 0)	% ^{125}IUdR uptake (day + 4)			
					Spleen Mean (SE)[a]	p[b]	Liver Mean (SE)	p
CD2F$_1$ (10)	d/d	P388	d	6x10^6	2.06(2.32-1.83)	–	9.40(9.86-8.95)	–
B10.D2 (5)	d	P388	d	6x10^6	1.00(1.06-0.95)	A	6.23(6.74-5.76)	A
CD2F$_1$ (9)	d/d	P388	d	6x10^5	0.48(0.53-0.43)	–	2.03(2.18-1.89)	–
C3H (8)	k	P388	d	6x10^5	0.08(0.09-0.07)	A	0.43(0.57-0.32)	A
BALB/c (8)	d	LSTRA	d	5x10^5	1.96(2.15-1.79)	–	8.62(9.45-7.86)	–
C3H (8)	K	LSTRA	d	5x10^5	0.26(0.30-0.22)	B	2.51(3.29-1.92)	A

[a]Geometric mean (GM), SE, standard error. In parenthesis GM+SE, GM-SE.
[b]p was calculated comparing the uptake values of syngeneic or compatible mice with respect to those of allogeneic mice. A, $p < 0.01$; B, $p < 0.05$.

Table 13. Growth of 10^5 LSTRA (H-2$\underline{d}$) lymphoma cells inoculated iv into Hh-susceptible drug-pretreated mice.

Recipient mice(No.)	H-2 haplotype	Pretreatment[a]	% ^{125}IUdR uptake (day + 4)			
			Spleen Mean (SE)[b]	P[c]	Liver Mean (SE)	P
CD2F$_1$ (7)	d/d	DTIC+ Cy	3.43(3.80-3.09)	-	15.7(16.52- 14.93)	-
C3H (6)	k	DTIC+ Cy	0.24(0.34-0.17)	A	5.3(7.89-3.59)	A

[a] DTIC, 250 mg/kg ip, day -5; Cy, 200 mg/kg ip, day 0.
[b] Geometric mean (GM), SE standard error. In parenthesis GM + SE, GM - SE.
[c] p was calculated comparing the uptake values of compatible mice with respect to those of allogeneic hosts. A, p< 0.01.

Table 14. Preferential growth of lymphoma cells of two different lines in lethally-irradiated allogeneic recipients with respect to that detectable in irradiated syngeneic mice.

Recipient mice(No)	H-2 hapl.	Lymphoma line	H-2 hapl.	Inoculum size(iv) (day 0)	% ^{125}IUdR uptake (day + 4)					
					Spleen Mean (SE)[a]	P[b]	Liver Mean (SE)	P	Lung Mean (SE)	P
B6 (8)	b	EL-4	b	2x10^5	0.04(0.04-0.03)	–	0.29(0.32-0.26)	–	0.14(0.15-0.12)	–
SJL (8)	s	EL-4	b	2x10^5	0.23(0.28-0.18)	A	0.24(0.30-0.19)	NS	0.10(0.14-0.08)	NS
B6 (8)	h	EL-4	b	1x10^6	0.14(0.15-0.12)	–	1.65(2.00-1.33)	–	1.24(1.61-0.95)	–
SJL (8)	s	EL-4	b	1x10^6	0.53(0.74-0.37)	A	0.55(1.00-0.30)	NS	0.96(1.18-0.77)	NS
B6 (8)	b	EL-4	b	5x10^6	2.04(2.28-1.82)	–	5.25(5.37-5.14)	–	5.67(6.45-4.97)	–
SJL (8)	s	EL-4	b	5x10^6	3.30(3.52-3.09)	A	4.60(4.99-4.25)	NS	4.40(4.59-4.22)	NS
AKR (4)	k	K36	k	2x10^5	0.39(0.43-0.36)	–	2.67(2.85-2.50)	–	1.79(1.88-1.61)	–
BALB/c (7)	d	K36	k	2x10^5	1.06(1.14-0.99)	A	3.38(3.94-2.89)	NS	2.45(2.88-2.09)	NS
SJL (5)	s	K36	k	2x10^5	1.19(1.36-1.03)	A	4.70(5.60-3.93)	B	3.06(3.38-2.76)	A
CBA (8)	k	K36	k	2x10^5	1.15(1.24-1.07)	A	3.87(4.48-3.34)	NS	1.97(2.59-1.50)	NS
AKR (4)	k	K36	k	6x10^5	0.75(0.88-0.64)	–	11.14(11.80-10.50)	–	8.41(9.26-7.63)	–
BALB/c (8)	d	K36	k	6x10^5	2.00(2.17-1.85)	A	9.70(10.40-9.03)	NS	7.20(7.71-6.74)	NS
SJL (4)	s	K36	k	6x10^5	1.70(1.99-1.47)	A	9.28(11.32-7.60)	NS	6.92(7.92-6.05)	NS

[a] Geometric mean (GM), SE, standard error. In parenthesis GM + SE, GM - SE.
[b] p was calculated comparing the uptake values of syngeneic mice with respect to those of allogeneic hosts. A, p<0.01; B, p<0.05; NS, not significant.

logical functions, producing effects similar to those of total
body irradiation (Giampieri et al., 1978; Campanile and Bonmassar,
1980; Bonmassar et al., 1980, 1981).
In the present study, recipient drug-treated mice were inoculated
with 10^5 LSTRA cells i.v. and organ ^{125}IUdR uptake was evaluated
on day +4 after tumor challenge. The results (Table 13) show that
localized resistance against lymphoma cells occurs also in drug-
-treated Hh-susceptible C3H recipients, both in the spleen and in
the liver. These data, in agreement with those of previous investigations (Campanile and Bonmassar, 1980), point out that NRa
could be present in the host, even after treatment with extremely
high doses of antineoplastic agents.

6. NR IN SYNGENEIC MICE (NRs)

A number of studies have been performed to demonstrate a
certain degree of resistance in mice syngeneic with the tumor line
used for challenge. In order to detect NRs, several experimental
tools can be utilized. It is possible to compare tumor growth in
mice following drug-induced modulation of NR with respect to that
detectable in non-treated controls. Alternatively, tumor cell
proliferation can be evaluated in histocompatible hosts in comparison with that occurring in allogeneic recipients non responsive
for NR systems. Differential lymphoma growth in intact versus Cy-
pretreated (i.e. NR-depressed) histocompatible hosts has been
described for a drug-treated tumor line (Ricciardi et al., 1978).

Moreover, lymphoma growth was found to be severely impaired
in histocompatible recipients pretreated with Adriamicin (ADM), as
a result of drug-induced enhancement of NRs responsiveness (Ricciardi, 1979b). This interpretation was supported by the finding
that no lymphoma graft impairment occurred in ADM-pretreated
histocompatible mice when the host was treated with two NR-abro-
gating agents such as silica particles or carrageenan (Lotzova and
Cudkowicz, 1974; Cudkowicz and Jung, 1977; Cudkowicz and Hochman,
1979) before tumor challenge. The present studies (see Table 14)
show that differential lymphoma growth can be detected in lethally-irradiated histocompatible mice with respect to allogeneic
recipients susceptible for the Hh system. In particular graded
numbers of EL-4 lymphoma cells grew better in the spleen of allogeneic SJL mice than in the same organ of syngeneic B6 hosts.
Similarly, the growth of K36 lymphoma was greater in the spleen of

allogeneic BALB/c and CBA mice or in the spleen, liver and lung of allogeneic SJL recipients than in the organs of syngeneic AKR mice. All these data are compatible with the hypothesis that antilymphoma NR is more pronounced in syngeneic recipients than in Hh-susceptible allogeneic mice, in these particular tumor-host combinations. Therefore the experimental design, adopted in the present study, appears to reinforce the evidence for the existence of NRs at least for some murine lymphoma lines.

7. CONCLUDING REMARKS

The pattern of "in vivo" anti-lymphoma NR in mice appears to be rather complex. Any type of classification seems to be inadequate to provide a well defined picture of the entire immune system underlying NR phenomena. This is due to the limited information available at the present time concerning the cellular and possibly humoral mechanisms involved in "in vivo" non-elicitable resistance. In any case a preliminary classification based on the Hh system, as we proposed in the present study can be outlined as follows:
(a) Hh-type resistance, i.e. resistance detectable in lethally--irradiated mice showing genetic patterns parallel to those regulating rejection of normal bone marrow cells;
(b) non-Hh-type resistance, i.e. resitance detectable in lethally--irradiated mice, under a genetic control different from that involved in the Hh system;
(c) resistance in non-irradiated hosts, showing genetic patterns of regulation similar or different from those associated with the Hh system.

According to the host-tumor system under investigation, NR has been classified also as NRa, and NRs, i.e. non-elicitable tumor graft resistance detectable in hybrid, allogeneic or syngeneic hosts, respectively.

Little is known, at the present time, on the antigenic determinants involved in the "in vivo" NR. In the case of Hh-type NR, it is conceivable that lymphoma cells express Hh-like antigen(s) similar to those present on normal bone marrow cells.
In non-Hh-type NR, it can be hypothesized that Hh-like antigen(s) restrictively expressed on lymphoma cells, but undetectable on normal hematopoietic tissues, could be the target of NR effector

immunocytes   acting through a mechanism similar to that involved in
Hh immunity.

In   non-irradiated   recipients it is reasonable to assume that
a   relatively   large   number of effector immunocytes susceptible to
lethal   irradiation   and   capable   of   recognizing   lymphoma   cell
surface   antigens   would   contribute   to   the entire NR phenomenon.
Therefore,   in   intact   hosts   it is likely that a wider variety of
tumor-associated   antigenic   determinants   would   be involved in NR
mechanisms.   In   any   case,   there   is   little   doubt that effector
systems,   well   defined   in   "in vitro" studies (e.g. NK, activated
macrophages, promonocytes etc), would participate to "in vivo" NR.
They   could   be   involved   both   in   intact   or irradiated or drug-
treated   hosts,   being   their   role conditioned by degree of radiosensitivity   or   chemosensitivity   of   the relevant immunocompetent
cells.

ACKNOWLEDGEMENT

This   work   was   supported by a C.N.R. (Rome, Italy) contract,
Progetto Finalizzato Virus, No 81.00263.84.

The   authors   wish to thank Dr. J. Mayo and Mr. C.R. Reeder of
the   Mammalian   Genetics   and   Animals   Production   Section,   Drug
Research   and   Development   Division   of Cancer Treatment, National
Cancer   Institute,   NIH,   Bethesda,   Maryland,   20014,   U.S.A.,   for
having   provided   the   inbred,   hybrid   and "nude" mice used in our
studies,   and   also   Dr.   V.L.   Narayanan of the Drug Synthesis and
Chemistry   Branch,   Division   of   Cancer   Treatment,   NCI,   NIH,
Bethesda,   Md,   for   his   courtesy   in supplying us with drugs. The
authors   are   also   grateful for the expert technical assistance of
Mr. Mario Andrielli and Mr. Robert De Filippi.

REFERENCES

Adam, D.O., and Snyderman, R., 1979, Do macrophages destroy nascent
      Tumors?, J. Natl. Cancer Inst., 62:1341.
Bennett, M., 1972, Rejection of marrow allografts. Importance of H-2
      homozygosity of donor cells, Transplantation, 14:289.
Bonmassar, A., Riccardi, C., Rivosecchi-Merletti, P., Goldin, A.,
      and Bonmassar E., 1980, Transplantation resistance of drug-

-treated hybrid or allogeneic mice againsty murine lymphomas.
I. Immuno-pharmacology studies, Int. J. Cancer, 26:819.

Bonmassar, A., Rivosecchi-Merleti, P., Barzi, A., Goldin, A., and
Bonmassar, E., 1981, Transplantation resistance of drug-treated
allogeneic mice against murine lymphomas. II. Studies with
various tumor-host combinations, Int. J. Immunopharmac., 3,
in press.

Bonmassar, E., Cudkowicz, G.,Vadlamudi, S., and Goldin, A., 1970,
Influence of tumor-host differences at a single Histocompatibility Locus (H-1) on the antileukemic effect of 1,3-Bis (2-
cloroethyl)-1-nitrosurea, Cancer Res., 30:2538.

Bonmassar, E., Bonmassar, A., Goldin, A., and Cudkowicz, G., 1973,
Depression of antilymphoma allograft reactivity by tumor-associated factors, Cancer Res., 33:1054.

Bonmassar, E., Campanile, F., Houchens, D., Crino', L., and Goldin,
A., 1975, Impaired growth of a radiation-induced lymphoma in
intact or lethally irradiated allogeneic athymic (nude) mice,
Transplantation, 20:343.

Bonmassar, E., Campanile, F., Houchens, D., Goldin, A., and Herber-
mann, R.B., 1978, Growth inhibition of allogeneic lymphoma
cells in lethally irradiated nude mice, in: "Proceeding of Symposium on the Use of Athymic (nude) mice in Cancer Research,
Houchens, D., and Ovejera, A. eds., Gustav Fisher, New York,
p. 73-80.

Bonmassar, E., Riccardi, C., Campanile, F., Iorio, A.M., Puccetti,
and P., Herberman, R.B., 1979, Radioresistant inhibition of
tumors (RIT): biological and pharmacological studies, in:
"Current Trends in Tumor Immunology," S., Ferrone, S., Gorini,
R.B., Herberman, R.A., and Reisfeld, eds., Garland Press, New
York, p. 49.

Campanile, F., and Bonmassar, E., 1980, Differential graft resistance of C3H mice pretreated with antitumor drugs against
BALB/c bone marrow or lymphoma cells, J. of Immunopharmac.,
2:527.

Campanile, F., Crino, L., Bonmassar, E., Houchens, D., and Goldin,
A., 1977, Radioresistant inhibition of lymphoma growth in congenitally athymic (nude) mice, Cancer Res., 37:394.

Carlson, G.A., and Wegman, T.G., 1977, Rapid "in vivo" destruction
of semi-syngeneic and allogeneic cells by non immunized mice
as a consequence of non identity at H-2, J. Immunol., 118:2130.

Carlson, G.A., Melnychuk, D., and Meeker, M.J., 1980, H-2 associated
resistance to leukemia transplantation natural killing "in
vivo," Int. J. Cancer, 25:111.

Clark, E.A., Harmon, R.C., and Wicker, L.S., 1977, Resistance of H-2 heterozygous mice to parental tumors. II. Characterization of Hh-1 controlled hybrid resistance to syngeneic fibrosarcomas and EL -4 lymphoma, J. Immunol., 119:648.

Clark, R.A., and Klebanoff, S.J., 1975, Neutrophil-mediated tumor cell cytotoxicity: role of the peroxidase system, J. Exp. Med., 141:1442.

Cudkowicz, G., 1968, Hybrid resistance to parental grafts on hematopoietic and lymphoma cells, in: "The Proliferation and Spread of Neoplastic Cell," XXI Annual M.D. Anderson Symposium on Fundamental Cancer Research, Baltimore, Williams and Wilkins Co., p. 661.

Cudkowicz, G., 1971, Genetic control of bone marrow graft rejection. I. Determinant specific difference of reacting in two pairs of inbred mouse strains, J. Exp. Med., 134:281.

Cudkowicz, G., 1975a, Genetic control of resistance to allogeneic and xenogeneic bone marrow grafts in mice, Transplant. Proc., 7:155.

Cudkowicz, G., 1975b, Rejection of bone marrow allografts by irradiated athymic mice, Proc. Am. Assoc. Cancer Res., 16:170.

Cudkowicz, G., and Bennett, M., 1971a, Peculiar immunobiology of bone marrow allografts. I. Graft rejection by irradiated responder mice, J. Exp. Med., 134:83.

Cudkowicz, G., and Bennett, M., 1971b, Peculiar immunobiology of bone marrow allografts. II. Rejection of parental grafts by resistant F1 hybrid mice, J. Exp. Med., 134:1513.

Cudkowicz, G., and Hochman, P.S., 1979, Do natural killer cells engaged in regulated reactions against self to ensure homeostasis?, Immunol. Rev., 44:13.

Cudkowicz, G., and Lotzova, E., 1973, Hemopoietic cell-defined components of the major histocompatibility complex of mice: identification of responsive and unresponsive recipients for bone marrow transplants, Transplant. Proc., 4:1399.

Cudkowicz, G., and Rossi, G.B., 1972, Hybrid resistance to parental DBA/2 grafts: indipendence from H-2 locus. I. Studies with normal hematopoietic cells, J. Nat. Cancer Inst., 48:131.

Cudkowicz, G., and Stimpfling, J.H., 1964, Deficient growth of C57B1 marrow cells transplanted in F1 hybrid mice. Association with the histocompatibility-2 locus, Immunology, 7:291.

Cudkowicz, G., and Yung, Y.P., 1977, Abrogation of resistance to foreign bone marrow grafts by carrageenans. I. Studies with the antimacrophage agent seakem carrageenan, J. of Immunol., 119:483.

Dawe, C.J., and Potter, M., 1957, Morphologic and biologic progres-
    sion of a lymphoid neoplasm of the mouse "in vivo" and "in
    vitro", Am. J. Pathol., 33:603.

Dvorak, A.M., Connel, A.B., Proppe, K., and Dvorak, H.F., 1978, Im-
    munologic rejection of mammary adenocarcinoma (TA3-St) in
    C57B1/6 mice: participation of neutrophiles and activated ma-
    crophages with fibrin formation, J. Immunol., 120:1240.

Gallagher, M.T., Lotzova, E., and Trentin, J.J., 1976, Genetic resi-
    stance to marrow transplantation as a leukemia defence mecha-
    nism, in: "Immuno-aspects of the Spleen," J.R. Battisto, J.W.,
    Streilein eds., Elsevier-North-Holland Biomedical Press,
    Amsterdam, The Netherlands, p. 359.

Giampietri, A., Bonmassar, E., and Goldin, A., 1978, Drug induced
    modulation of immune response in mice: effects of 5-(3,3'-di-
    methyl-1-triazeno)-imidazole-4-carboxamide (DTIC) and cyclopho-
    sphamide, J. of Immunopharmac., 1:61.

Glynn, J.P., Bianco, A.R., Goldin, and A., 1964, Studies on induced
    resistance against iso-transplants of virus induced leukemia,
    Cancer Res., 24:502.

Gorer, P.A., 1950, Studies in antibody response of mice to tumor ino-
    culation, Br. J. Cancer, 4:372.

Harmon, R.C., Clark, E.A., O'Toole, C., and Wicker, L.S., 1977, Re-
    sistance of H-2 heterozygous mice to parental tumors. I. Hybrid
    resistance and natural cytotoxicity to EL-4 are controlled by
    the H-2D Hh-1 region, Immunogenetics, 4:601.

Herberman, R.B., nd Holden, H.T., 1979, Natural killer cells as an-
    titumor effector cells, J. Natl. Cancer Inst., 62:441.

Herberman, R.B., Nunn, M.E., and Lavrin, B.H., 1975, Natural cyto-
    toxic reactivity of mouse lymphoma cells against syngeneic and
    allogeneic tumors, I Distribution of reactivity and specificity,
    Int. J. Cancer, 16:216.

Herberman, R.B., Djeu, J.Y., Kay, H.D., Ortaldo, J.R., Riccardi, C.,
    Bonnard, G.D.,Holden, H.T., Fagnani, R., Santoni, A., and Puc-
    cetti, P., 1979, Natural killer cells: characteristics and re
    gulation of activity, Immunol. Rev., 44:43.

Hibbs, J.B., 1976, The macrophage as tumoricidal effector cell: a
    review of "in vivo" and in vitro studies of the mechanism of
    the activated macrophage non-specific cytotoxic reaction, in:
    "The Macrophage in Neoplasia," M.A., Fink, ed., Academic Press,
    New York, p. 83.

Hofer, K.G., and Hughes, L., 1970, Incorporation of Iodo-deoxyuri-
    dine-125, into the DNA of L1210 leukemia cells during tumor de-
    velopment, Cancer Res., 30:236.

Houchens, D., Iorio, A.M., Barzi, A., Goldin, A., and Bonmassar, E.,
     1975, Inhibition of antilymphoma allograft response in normal
     and lethally irradiated mice by cyclophosphamide (NSC-26271)
     and isophosphamide (NSC-109724), Cancer Chemioter. Rep., 59:967.
Iorio, A.M., Barzi, A., Merletti, P., Goldin, A., and Bonmassar, E.,
     1976, A viral immunodepressive factor (IDF) associated with
     experimental mouse tumors, Cancer Res., 36:3851.
Iorio, A.M., Campanile, F., Neri, M., Spreafico, F., Goldin, A., and
     Bonmassar, E., 1978, Inhibition of lymphoma growth in the spleen
     and liver of lethally irradiated mice, J. Immunol., 120:1679.
Keller, R., 1976, Susceptibility of normal and transformed cell li-
     nes to cytostatic and cytocidal effects exerted by macrophages,
     J. Natl. Cancer Inst., 56:369.
Keller, R., 1979, Suppression by radioactive strontium of the spon-
     taneous cytotoxicity expressed by adherent, predominantly phago-
     citic cells, from various mouse tissues, Immunolology., 37:333.
Keller, R., 1979, A consideration of the involvement of mononuclear
     phagocytes in tumor resistance, in: "Current trends in tumor
     immunology," S. Ferrone, S. Gorini, R.B. Herberman, and R.A.
     Reisfeld, eds., Garland Press, New York, p. 121.
Keller, R., 1980, Regulatory capacities of mononuclear phagocytes
     with particular reference to natural immunity against tumors,
     in: "Natural cell-mediated immunity against tumors," R.B. Her-
     berman ed., Accademic Press, New York, p. 1219.
Kiessling, R., Hochman, P.S., Haller, O., Shearer, G.M., Wigzell, H.,
     and Cudkowicz, G., 1977, Evidence for a similar or common me-
     chanism for natural killer cell activity and resistance to
     hemopoietic grafts, Eur. J. Immunol., 7:655.
Klein, G.O., Klein, G., Kiessling, R., and Karre Klas, 1978, H-2
     associated control of natural cytotoxicity and hybrid resi-
     stance against RBL-5 Immunogenetics, 6:561.
Korec, S., Herberman, R.B., Dean, J.H., and Cannon, G.B., 1980,
     Cytostasis of tumor cell lines by human granulocytes, Cell.
     Immunol., 53:104.
Lohmann-Matthes, M.L., and Doxzig, W., 1979, Promonocytes have the
     functional characteristics of natural killer cells, J. Immunol.,
     123:1883.
Lohmann-Matthes, M.L., and Domzig, W., 1980, Natural cytotoxicity of
     macrophage precursor cells and of mature macrophages, in:
     "Natural Cell-mediated Immunity against Tumors," R.B. Herberman,
     ed., Academic Press, New York, p. 117.
Lotzova, E., and Cudkowicz, G., 1974, Abrogation of resistance to
     bone marrow grafts by silica particles. Prevention of the silica

effects by the macrophage stabilizer poly-2-vinylpyridine N-oxide, J. of Immunol., 113:798.

McCoy, J.L., Fefer, A., and Glynn, J.P., 1967, Comparative studies on the induction of transplantation resistance in BALB/c and C57B1/6 mice in three murine leukemia systems, Cancer Res., 27:1743.

Old, L.J., Boyse, E.A., and Stockert, E., 1965, The G (Gross) leukemia antigen, Cancer Res., 25:813.

Puccetti, P., and Holden, H.T., 1979, Cytolitic and Cytostatic anti-tumor activities of macrophages from mice injected with murine sarcoma virus, Int. J. Cancer, 23:123.

Riccardi, C., Fioreti, M.C., Giampietri,A., Puccetti, P., Goldin, A., and Bonmassar, E., 1978, Growth inhibition of normal or drug-treated lymphoma cells in lethally irradiated mice, J. Natl. Cancer Inst., 60:1083.

Riccardi, C., Puccetti, P., Santoni, A., and Herberman, R.B., 1979a, Rapid "in vivo" assay of mouse natural killer cell activity, J. Natl. Cancer. Inst., 63:1041.

Riccardi, C., Puccetti, P., Santoni, A., Herberman, R.B., and Bonmassar, E., 1979b, Adriamycin-induced antitumor response in lethally irradiated mice, Immunopharmac., 1:211.

Riccardi, C., Santoni, A., Barlozzari, T., Puccetti, P., and Herberman, R.B., 1980, "In vivo" natural reactivity of mice against tumor cells, Int. J. Cancer, 25:475.

Roder, J.C., Karre, K., and Kiessling, R., 1981, Natural Killer cells, Prog. Allergy, 28:66.

Schimitt-Verhulst, A.M., and Zatz, M.M., 1977, F1 Resistance to AKR lymphoma cells "in vivo" and "in vitro," J. Immunol., 118:33.

Stutman, O., Paige, C.G., and FeoFigarella, E., 1978, Natural Cyto-toxic cells against solid tumors in mice. I Strain and age distribution on target cell susceptibility, J. Immunol., 121:1819.

Warner, N.L., Woodruff, M.F.A., and Burton, R.C., 1977, Inhibition of growth of lymphoid tumors in syngeneic athymic (nude) mice, Int. J. Cancer, 20:146.

IMMUNOGENETIC DETERMINANTS CONTROLLING

THE METASTATIC PROPERTIES OF TUMOR CELLS

S. Katzav, P. De Baetselier, B. Tartakovsky,
E. Gorelik, S. Segal and M. Feldman

Department of Cell Biology, The Weizmann Institute of
Science Rehovot 76100, Israel

1. INTRODUCTION

The generation of metastases by tumor cells is preceeded by a sequence of processes, each of which is controlled by different properties of the invading cells. Thus, the detachment of tumor cells from its local population might be associated with alterations in cell-to-cell recognition patterns, its metastatic penetration through the basement membrane of blood capillaries might require the synthesis of specific enzymes capable of degrading membrane proteins (Liotta et al., 1977; Strauli and Weiss, 1977), its "homing" to specific organs might be determined by specific adherance to the normal cells of the target organ (Kramer and Nicolson, 1979), whereas its growth at its new site might require the secretion of angiogenic factors (Folkman and Hochberg, 1973; Folkman and Handeschild, 1981).

In addition, the invasiveness, circulation, survival and growth of the tumor cell may depend on its capacity to resist host immune responses. Such properties might in fact characterize only a fraction of the local tumor cell population which would then be

P. De Baetselier is a fellow of the Belgian N.F.W.O. Present address: Dienst Algemene Biologie, Vrije, Universitait Brussels.

programmed to generate metastases. In this case the primary tumor would constitute a heterogeneous population with regard to the metastatogenic potential of the cells. In fact, studies performed by Fidler and Kripke (1977) and Kripke et al., (1978) demonstrated that the local tumor cell population is indeed heterogeneous with regard to the capacity of individual cells to generate experimental lung metastases.

In our previous studies on the 3LL Lewis lung carcinoma, a transplantable C57BL/6-originated lung carcinoma, we demonstrated that the cell surface antigens of the local tumor, differ from those which characterize the metastatic cells (Fogel et al., 1979; Gorelik et al., 1980). Immunoselective processes might then be involved in the control of cell dissemination. An immune response against antigens of the local tumor would select antigenic variants for metastatic spread. Since the effector phase of cell mediated immune reactions against cell surface associated antigens seems to be restricted by gene products of the MHC, it seemed of interest to investigate the expression of the H-2 encoded antigens on tumor cells of the local growth as distinct from tumor cells of the metastatic population. Aiming at mouse tumor models which will be closer to the human situation than tumors originated in animals of homozygous inbred strains, we have chosen a tumor which was induced by Dr. J. Gordon of Montreal by methylcholanthrene in a (C3H/eb x C57BL/6) F_1, the Sarcoma T10 (Brodt and Gordon, 1978). The tumor was maintained in syngeneic animals by subcutaneous transplantations. Animals carrying s.c. solid tumor (L-T10), show the appearance of metastatic nodules in the lungs (M-T10). Our main aims were to investigate whether (a) cells of the local tumor (L-T10) differ from cells obtained from lung metastases (M-T10), in the expression of MHC encoded antigens; (b) whether such differences are related to the metastatogenic potential of the tumor cells; (c) whether cells of diverse expression of MHC determinants pre-exist within the local tumor cell population and (d) whether a state of diversity with regard to MHC expression and metastatogenic properties is generated within cloned tumor cell populations.

2. CELLS OF THE LOCAL T10 TUMOR DIFFER FROM CELLS OF LUNG METASTASIS IN THE EXPRESSION OF H-2 GENE PRODUCTS

The first set of experiments aimed at testing whether the H-2^k

Table 1. Parental H-2 haplotype expression on L-T10 and
M-T10 tumor cells.

| Tumor cells | Percentage of cells brightly stained with | | | |
	$H-2^b$	$H-2^k$	$H-2D^k$	$H-2K^k$
L-T10	87	13	4	4
M-T10$_1$[a]	55	85	74	42
M-T10$_2$[a]	50	82	83	44
M-T10$_3$[a]	40	81	66	49

[a]M-T10$_1$, M-T10$_2$, M-T10$_3$ - refers to cells of different metastatic nodules.

and the $H-2^b$ haplotypes, which characterized the tumor's strain of
origin, are expressed on L-T10 differently than on cells of M-T10.
The expression of H-2 antigens was analyzed using fluorescent
serology carried out by means of the fluorescence-activated cell
sorter (FACS II). Cells of T10 were transplanted subcutaneously
into syngeneic recipients and cells of the local growth thus
developed (L-T10), and cells from a lung metastases (M-T10), were
then grafted to secondary recipients. The tumors originating from
such transplants of L-T10 and M-T10 in (C3Heb x C57BL/)F_1 mice
were trypsinized, and the single cell suspension were analyzed for
the binding of anti $H-2^k$ or of anti $H-2^b$ antisera. The results,
expressed either by the relative number of tumor cells expressing
$H-2^k$ and $H-2^b$ antigens (Table 1), or by the fluorescence
distribution of M-T10 or L-T10 cells stained with antisera
directed against $H-2^k$ or $H-2^b$ (Fig. 1), indicated a striking
difference between the membrane expression of the parental H-2
haplotypes on cells of the local tumor (L10) and their expression
on cells from lung metastases (M-T10): L-T10 cells expressed
mainly or exclusively the $H-2^b$ haplotype, whereas M-T10 cells
expressed both the $H-2^b$ (although at a lower density than L-T10)
and the $H-2^k$ haplotypes. The expression of the two haplotypes by
the M-T10 cells was a stable property; it was retained following
successive transplantations. Individual nodules of lung metastases
were identical in their staining patterns, implying that with
regard to the expression of the parental haplotypes the M-T10

cells constitute a homogeneous population.

To test whether the entire H-2^k haplotype is expressed on M-T10 cells, we stained the cells with antisera directed against the products of the H-2D and H-2K subregions of the H-2^k haplotype. Table 1 indicates that both were expressed on the M-T10 cells, whereas the L-T10 cells were negative when stained with these antisera.

3. METASTATOGENIC H-2^k POSITIVE T10 CELLS PRE-EXIST WITHIN THE LOCAL TUMOR CELL POPULATION

We then studied whether the M-T10 cells characterized by the expression of the H-2^k haplotype derived from H-2^k positive cell variants pre-existing within the local tumor cell population. To approach this question, we cloned L-T10 cells in semi-solid agar, and individual clones were passaged in F_1 recipients, then analyzed for the presence of H-2^k or H-2^b antigens on their cell surface. Out of 10 randomly chosen clones, 2 clones (IE7 and IB9) expressed both H-2^k and the H-2^b haplotyes, whereas the other 8 clones were essentially H-2^k negative, expressing predominantly

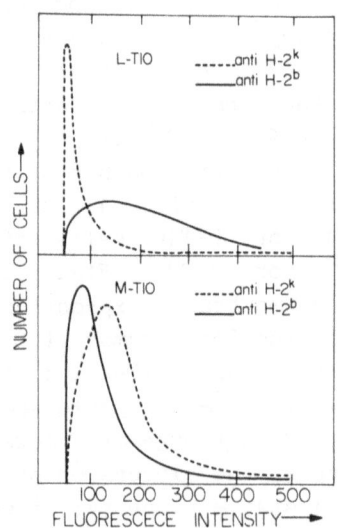

Fig. 1. Fluorescence distribution of L-T10 and M-T10 cells stained with anti H-2^k or anti H-2^b antisera.

Table 2. Parental H-2 haplotype expression on L-T10 and T10 cloned
tumor cells and their ability to produce experimental pulmonary metastasis.

Tumor cells	Percentage of cells brightly stained with		Experimental pulmonary metastasis after i.v. inoculation
	Anti H-2^b	Anti H-2^k	weight of lungs (mg + S.E.[a])
L - T10	84	23	300 + 25
Clone IC9	66	14	212 + 20
IG2	67	16	214 + 25
IIF3	73	8	241 + 50
IG3	81	11	243 + 15
IB9	73	75	607 + 75
IE7	91	93	947 + 78
IF7	93	17	271 + 27
IID6	77	14	214 + 5
IID9	82	15	n.d
IB7	85	14	n.d

[a]S.E - standard error

the H-2^b haplotypes (Table 2). We then tested whether the H-2
positive clones differed from the H-2^k negative clones in their
capacity to generate experimental lung metastases. Cells of
individual clones were injected intravenously at doses of 1×10^6
per recipient, and two weeks later the animals were tested for
lung metastases. The results (Table 2) were that the 2 clones
which were H-2^k positive (IB9 and IE7) were the only clones which
produced lung metastasis when injected into syngeneic animals.
Cells of the 8 H-2^k negative clones did not generate experimental
pulmonary metastases. They did, however, generate metastases when
injected to animals immuno-suppressed by total body irradiation
(Katzav et al., 1981).
It thus appeared that the local T10 tumor constituted a mixture of
H-2^k positive and H-2^k negative tumor cells. The H-2^k positive
cells seem to represent the metastatogenic variants within the
local tumor cell population. The pre-existance of variants mani-
festing different metastatic potentials was demonstrated previous-

Table 3. Serial transfers of H-2^k negative clones resulted in the appearance of H-2^k positive cells concomitantly with the acquisition of metastatic capacity.

T10 tumor cells	Genera- tion[a]	Percentage of cells brightly stained with		Experimental metastases after i.v. inoculation	
		anti- H-2^b	anti- H-2^k	presence of nodules in lung[b]	weight of lung (mg) $\pm$ S.E.
L-T10	1	57	6	$\pm$	235 $\pm$ 12
	5	46	9	$\pm$	228 $\pm$ 12
	25	62	58	+++	599 $\pm$ 81
Clone IC9	1	66	14	–	212 $\pm$ 20
	5	21	0	–	223 $\pm$ 16
	15	8	14	n.d	n.d
	25	6	8	–	249 $\pm$ 14
	35	58	45	+++	398 $\pm$ 80
Clone IID6	1	77	14	n.d	n.d
	5	77	10	–	214 $\pm$ 5
	15	58	39	+++	559 $\pm$ 55
	25	86	90	++	409 $\pm$ 42
Clone IE7	1	97	73	+++	759 $\pm$ 59
	5	91	93	+++	947 $\pm$ 78
	15	87	95	+++	1031 $\pm$ 123
	25	82	90	+++	1202 $\pm$ 70
Clone IB9	1	93	65	+++	704 $\pm$ 72
	5	73	75	+++	607 $\pm$ 75
	15	82	95	+++	800 $\pm$ 90
	25	81	95	n.d	n.d
Clone IG3	1	81	11	–	243 $\pm$ 15
	27	79	94	n.d	n.d
Clone IF7	1	93	17	–	271 $\pm$ 27
	27	79	94	++	436 $\pm$ 65

[a] generation refers to number of in vivo passages in syngeneic F1 mice.
[b] refers to tumor development in lungs: – = no metastases; ++ = moderate involvement (multiple nodules); +++ = extensive involvement (numerous, confluent nodules).
[c] S.E. – Standard error.

ly by Fidler and Kripke (1977) and Kripke et al., (1978). Yet the association between the expression of the $H-2^k$ haplotype and the metastatogenic properties of the cells is an intriguing observation.

4. METASTATOGENIC $H-2^k$ POSITIVE CELLS ARE GENERATED "IN VIVO" AND SELECTED FROM $H-2^k$ NEGATIVE TUMOR CELLS

We then aimed at further substantiating the relationship between the differential expression of the two haplotypes and the capacity to generate lung metastases. We also aimed at testing whether $H-2^k$ positive variants are generated from $H-2^k$ negative cells, and if so whether such variants have a selective advantage "in vivo" over the less malignant $H-2^k$ negative cells.

To achieve this, the cloned population were passaged by subcutaneous transplantations in syngeneic $(C3HebxC57BL/6)F_1$ and at various transplant generations the tumor cells were assayed for the expression of the $H-2^b$ and $H-2^k$ haplotypes.

Cells of clones IC9, IID6, IG3 and IF7 which were $H-2^b$ positive and $H-2^k$ negative, and of clones IB9 and IE7 which were $H-2^k$ positive, and cells of the uncloned L-T10 tumor, were subjected to serial transplantations in syngeneic recipients, and were tested at every fifth transfer for the expression of the parental haplotypes and for their capacity to generate experimental lung meta-stasis. The results (Table 3) were that the IB9 and IE7 clones, retained both the co-expression of the two haplotypes and the metastatogenic properties throughout 25 serial passages in syngeneic F_1 hybrid recipients. On the other hand, the $H-2^k$ negative clones, IID6, IC9, IG3 and F7 clones, and the uncloned L-T10 did change: the cells acquired, at different passages, the expression of the $H-2^k$ haplotype and concomittantly, the capacity to generate metastasis. It is of interest to note that the IC9 clone has on the third transfer, lost the expressed $H-2^b$ products, and thus remained $H-2^k$ negative for quite a number of transfers. It still remained non-metastatic. Only at the 35th transfer, its cells manifested $H-2^k$ haplotypes coincidentally with the $H-2^b$, and concomittantly it acquired metastatogenic properties.

It   thus appears that (a) the expression of the $H-2^k$ haplotype in cells deriving from $H-2^k$ negative precursors is associated with the   acquisition of metastatogenic properties; (b) the generation of such variants took place in every clone tested as well as in the uncloned T10 tumor population, and seems therefore to be a general process and (c) the metastatogenic $H-2^k$ variants have a selective   advantage   even   within   the   local   subcutaneous   tumor growth. Thus, tumor progression towards increased malignancy seem to take place within the local population.

5. IMMUNE FUNCTION OF PRODUCED $H-2^k$ HAPLOTYPES

The   very   fact that an $H-2^b$ positive, $H-2^k$ negative IC9 clone which has lost after the first passages its $H-2^b$ expression, and appeared   essentially   H-2   negative did not acquire metastatogenic capacity   until   it   expressed $H-2^k$, suggests that gene products of the H-2 haplotype have an active function in enabling metastatic growth. At this stage any suggestion of such function may not be more than a guess. So, then, will be the notion that the $H-2^k$ products on tumor cells are linked, on its cell surface, to some tumor-associated determinants, and thus function in preventing the syngeneic hosts from reacting against such determinants. That such a suppression of response evoked by products of the $H-2^k$ haplotype on the T10 tumor is feasible, gains support from experiments we carried out testing the growth of M-T10 and L-T10 cells, following transplantation in mice of parental strains. We found that cells of L-T10 ($H-2^b$ positive and $H-2^k$ negative) did grow in $H-2^b$ recipients but, as expected, were rejected by $H-2^k$ mice. On the other hand, cells of M-T10 origin expressing both the $H-2^k$ and the $H-2^b$, showed progressive growth in both parental recipients (De Baetselier et al., 1980; Katzav et al., 1981).
Thus, the existence of the $H-2^k$ on the M-T10 tumor cells prevented the $H-2^b$ mice from responding by graft rejection against the $H-2^k$ products of the tumor and likewise it prevented $H-2^k$ mice from responding against the $H-2^b$ products on the M-T10 cells. Whether or not the effects of the $H-2^k$ haplotype in allowing growth in allogeneic recipients is relevant to its effect in allowing metastasis formation in syngeneic mice is, as, yet, an open question.

6. HOW DO H-2^k NEGATIVE T-10 CELLS ACQUIRE METASTATOGENIC PROPERTIES?

The mechanism associated with the conversion of non-metastatic H-2^k negative to metastatogenic H-2^k positive cells are unknown. Two distinct categories of mechanisms for the acquisition of expressed H-2^k could be postulated: (a) a repressed H-2 locus within the H-2^k negative cells was switched to express its own H-2^k gene products thus acquiring malignancy and a selective advantage; (b) a T10 H-2^k negative cell following transfers in syngeneic mice has acquired an expressable H-2^k haplotype by somatic hybridization with a normal cell of the H-2^k positive host. Its H-2^k haplotype was then donated by a host's normal cell and thus was associated by the acquisition of metastatic potency.

Although we have no reason, at this phase of our work, to prefer one mechanism over the other for the shifts within T10 clones, we do have evidence that in principal somatic hybridization between a non-metastatic tumor cell and a normal cell may result in a metastatic hybridome. In our laboratory we carried out studies with the plasmocytoma NSI, which, upon transplantation to syngeneic Balb/c recipients, grows locally, but does not produce spontaneous metases. When, however, such plasmocytoma cells, were hybridized with spleen B-cells of C57BL/6 origin, we obtained hybridomas which produce spontaneous metases of distinct organ specificities (De Baetselier et al., 1981). Some hybridomas produced, following transplantation to syngeneic recipients, spontaneous metastases in the spleen and in the liver. Other produced only liver metastases. Tumor cells from liver metastases of hybridomas which generated both spleen and liver metastases when transplanted to normal animals, grew locally, and again showed metastases formation in the spleen and liver. Metastatic cells from livers of hybridomas which generated only liver metastasies, metastasized only to the liver when grafted to normal recipients (De Baetselier et al., 1981). Thus, somatic hybrization, "in vitro", resulted in the acquisition of metastatogenic properties.

If this is relevant to our case of "in vivo" shifts in properties of the T10 tumor, then it implies that somatic hybridization between a neoplastic and a normal cell can take

place "in vivo". In fact, studies carried out in Klein's laboratory suggest that this, in fact, is the case. Whether or not such
"in vivo" hybridization may result in increased malignancy as suggested by Goldenberg (1974) and whether the changes of our $H-2^k$
negative clones to $H-2^k$ positive and the acquisition of metastatogenic properties are indeed due to "in vivo" hybridization is an
attractive, yet so far, a hypothetical possibility.

ACKNOWLEDGMENT

We thank Mr. Ezra Varay for his excellent technical assistance
and Mr. Avigdor Petrank for useful advice and help with FACS analysis. This work was supported by grant number CA-28139-02 awarded by
the National Cancer Institute DHHS.

REFERENCES

Brodt, P., and Gordon, J., 1978, Anti tumor immunity in B lymphocyte deprived mice, I. Immunity to chemically induced tumor, J.
Immunol., 121:359.

De Baetselier, P., Gorelik, e., Eshar, Z., Ron, Y., Katzav, S., Feldman, M., and Segal, S., 1981, Hybridization between plasmacy-
toma cells and B lymphocytes confers metastatic properties on
a non-metastatic tumor, J. Nat. Cancer Inst., in press.

De Baetselier, P., Katzav, S., Gorelik, E., Feldman, M., and Segal,
S., 1980, Differential expression of H-2 gene products in tumor
cells is associated with their metastatogenic properties, Nature, 288:179.

Fidler, I.J., and Kripke, M.L., 1977, Metastasis results from pre-
existing variant cells within a malignant tumor, Science, 197:
893.

Fogel, M., Gorelik, E., Segal, S., and Feldman, M., 1979, Differences in cell surface antigens of tumor metastases and those of
the local tumor, J. Natl. Cancer Inst., 62:585.

Folkman, J., and Handeschild, C., 1981, Angiogenesis in vitro, Nature, 288:551.

Folkman, J., and Hochberg, M., 1973, Self-regulation in three dimen-
sions, J. Exp. Med., 138:745.

Goldenberg, D.N., Pavia, R.A., and Tsao, M.C., 1974, In vivo hybridization of human tumor and normal hamster cells, Nature, 250:
649.

Gorelik, E., Fogel, M., Segal, S., and Feldman, M., 1980, Tumor associated antigenic differences between the primary and the descendant metastatic tumor cell population, J. Supramolecular Structure, 12383.

Liotta, L.A., Kleinerman, J., Catanzaro, P., and Rynbrandt, D.J., 1977, Degradation of basement membrane by murine tumor cells, J. Nat. Cancer Inst., 58:1427.

Katzav, S., De Baetselier, P., Gorelik, E., Feldman, M., and Segal, S., 1981, Immunogenetic control of metastasis formation by a methylcholanthrene induced tumor, (T10) in mice: Differential expression of H-2 gene products, Transpant. Proc., 13:742.

Kramer, R.H., and Nicolson, G.L., 1979, Interactions of tumor cells with vascular endothelial cell monolayers: A model for metastatic invasion, Proc. Natl. Acad. Sci., U.S.A., 76:5704.

Kripke, M.L., Gruys, E., and Fidler, I.J., 1978, Metastatic heterogeneity of cells from an ultraviolet light-induced murine fibrosarcoma of recent origin, Cancer Res., 38:2962.

Strauli, P., and Weiss, L., 1977, Cell locomotion and tumor penetration, Eur. J. Cancer., 13:1.

CONTRIBUTORS

R. ABE,Department of Immunology, Faculty of Medicine, University of
   Tokyo, Tokyo, Japan.
T. ABO, The Cellular Immunobiology Unit of the Tumor Inst.,Depts. of
   Pediatrics, Surgery and Microbiology, and the Comprehensive Cancer
   Center, University of Alabama in Birmingham, Alabama 35294, U.S.A.
R. ADER,Department of psychiatry, University of Rochester, School of
   Medicine and Dentistry Rochester, New York, 14642.
L. ADORINI, CNEN-Euratom Immunogenetics Group, Laboratory of Radio-
   pathology, C.S.N. Casaccia, Rome, Italy.
G. AGAROSSI, CNEN-Euratom Immunogenetics Group, Laboratory of Radio-
   pathology, C.S.N. Casaccia, Rome, Italy.
F. ALMERIGOGNA, Clinical Immunology, University of Florence, Policli-
   nico di Careggi, Viale Morgagni, 50134 Firenze, Italy.
G.C. ANDRIGHETTO, Chair of Immunopathology, University of Padova,
   Borgo Rome Hospitals, 37100, Verona, Italy
C.M. BALCH, The Cellular Immunobiology Unit of the Tumor Inst., Depts.
   of Pediatrics, Surgery and Microbiology and The Comprehensive
   Cancer Center, University of Alabama in Birmingham, Alabama 35294
   U.S.A..
B. BENATO, Chair of Immunopathology, University of Padova, Borgo Rome
   Hospitals, 37100, Verona, Italy.
H.O. BESEDOVSKY, Swiss Research Institute, Medical Department, CH-
   7270 Davos, Switzerland.
R. BIAGIOTTI, Clinical Immunology, University of Florence, Policlini-
   co di Careggi, Viale Morgagni, 50134 Firenze, Italy.
F. BISTONI, Institute of Microbiology, University of Perugia, Italy.
E. BONMASSAR, Institute of Pharmacology, University of Perugia, 06100
   Perugia, Italy.
F. CAMPANILE, Institute of Pharmacology, University of Perugia, 06100
   Perugia, Italy.
M. CECKA, Imperial Cancer Research Fund, Tumor Immunology Unit, Depart-
   ment of Zoology, University College London, Gower Street London

WC1E 6BT.

M.D. COOPER,The Cellular Immunobiology Unit of the Tumor Inst. Depts.
  of Pediatrics, Surgery and Microbiology and The Comprehensive
  Cancer Center, University of Alabama in Birmingham, Alabama 35294·
  U.S.A..

E. CULBERT,Imperial Cancer Research Fund, Tumor Immunology Unit,
  Department of Zoology, University College London, Gower Street
  London WC1E 6BT.

P. DE BAETSELIER,Department of Cell Biology, The Weizmann Institute
  of Science Rehovot 76100, Israel.

V. DEL GOBBO,Institutes of Microbiology, University of Rome, Italy

G.F. DEL PRETE,Clinical Immunology, University of Florence, Policlinico di Careggi, Viale Morgagni, 50134 Firenze, Italy.

A. DEL REY,Swiss Research Institute, Medical Department, CH-7270
  Davos, Switzerland.

G. DORIA,CNEN-Euratom Immunogenetics Group, Laboratory of Radiopathology, C.S.N. Casaccia, Rome, Italy.

D.C. DUMONDE,Department of Immunology, St Thomas's Hospital and
  Medical School, London SE1 7EH, United Kingdom.

N. FABRIS,Immunological Centre, Gerontological Research Dept.,
  I.N.R.C.A., Ancona, and Chair of Immunology, University of Pavia,
  Italy.

C. FAVALLI,Institutes of Microbiology, University of Rome, Italy.

M. FELDMAN,Department of Cell Biology, The Weizmann Institute of
  Science,Rehovot 76100, Israel.

M. FELDMANN,Imperial Cancer Research Fund., Tumor Immunology Unit
  Department of Zoology, University College, London.

D. FIORAVANTI,CNEN-Euratom Immunogenetics Group, Laboratory of Radio-
  pathology, C.S.N. Casaccia, Rome, Italy.

A. FISCHER,Imperial Cancer Research Fund, Tumor Immunology Unit,
  Department of Zoology, University College London, Gower Street
  London WC1E 6BT.

E. GARACI,Institutes of Microbiology, University of Rome, Italy.

R.A. GATTI,Department of Pathology, UCLA School of Medicine,Los Angeles, Ca, 90024 U.S.A.

G.M. GIUDIZI,Clinical Immunology, University of Florence, Policlinico di Careggi, Viale Morgagni, 50134 Firenze, Italy.

A. GOLDIN,National Cancer Institute, National Institute of Health,
  Bethesda, Maryland 20205, U.S.A.

A.L. GOLDSTEIN,Dept. of Biochemistry, The George Washington University, School of Medicine and Health Sciences, Washington D.C.,
  20037, U.S.A.

E. GORELIK,Department of Cell Biology, The Weizmann Institute of

Science Rehovot 76100, Israel.

P.L. HABER, The Cellular Immunobiology Unit of the Tumor Inst. Depts.
of Pediatrics, Surgery and Microbiology, and The Comprehensive
Cancer Center, University of Alabama in Birmingham, Alabama 35294
U.S.A..

J.W. HADDEN, Laboratory of Immunopharmacology Memorial Sloan Kettering
Cancer Center, New York, NY 10021, U.S.A.,

K.Y. HALL, The Department of Pathology, UCLA Medical School, and Pediatric Oncology, Cedars-Saint Hospital, Los Angeles, Calif..

N.R. HALL, Dept. of Biochemistry, The George Washington University,
School of Medicine and Health Sciences, Washington D.C., 20037,
U.S.A..

A.S. HAMBLIN, Department of Immunology, St Thomas's Hospital and Medical School, London SE1 7EH, United Kingdom.

D. HOFER, The Department of Surgery, S.U.N.Y. Downstate Medical Center
Brooklyn, New York,.

D.F. HORROBIN, Efamol Research Institute, P.O. Box, 818, Kentville,
Nova Scotia, Canada B4N 4H8.

Y. HIRAMATSU, Department of Immunology, Faculty of Medicine, University of Tokyo, Tokyo, Japan.

A.M. IORIO, Chair of Virology, University of Perugia, 06100 Perugia,
Italy.

B.M. JAFFE, The Department of Surgery, S.U.N.Y., Brooklyn, New York,
U.S.A..

R. JAMES, Imperial Cancer Research Fund, Tumor Immunology Unit, Department of Zoology, University College London, Gower Street London
WC1E 6BT.

W.A. KAMPS, The Cellular Immunobiology Unit of The Tumor Inst. Depts.
of Pediatrics, Surgery and Microbiology, and The Comprehensive
Cancer Center, University of Alabama in Birmingham, Alabama 35294
U.S.A..

E. KASP-GROCHOWSKA, Department of Immunology, St Thomas's Hospital
and Medical School, London SE1 7EH, United Kingdom.

D. KATZ, Imperial Cancer Research Fund, Tumor Immunology Unit, Department of Zoology, University College London, Gower Street London
WC1E 6BT.

S. KATZAV, Department of Cell Biology, The Weizmann Institute of
Science, Rehovot 76100, Israel.

S. KONTIAINEN, Department of Bacteriology and Immunology, University
of Helsinki Haartmaninkatu, 00290 Helsinki, 29 Finland.

Y. KUMAGAI, Department of Immunology, Faculty of Medicine, University
of Tokyo, Tokyo, Japan.

P. LE PORT, The Department of Surgery, S.U.N.Y. Downstate Medical.

Center, Brooklyn, New York, U.S.A..

J.M. MAESTRONI,Institute for Integrative Biomedical Research, Lohwisstrasse 50,8123 Ebmatingen, Switzerland.

E. MAGGI,Clinical Immunology, University of Florence, Policlinico di Careggi, Viale Morgagni, 50134 Firenze, Italy.

C. MANCINI,CNEN-Euratom Immunogenetics Group, Laboratory of Radio-pathology, C.S.N. Casaccia, Rome, Italy.

P. MARCONI,Institute of Microbiology, University of Perugia, Italy.

M.A. MEDICI,The Department of Pathology, UCLA Medical Scool, and Pediatric Oncology, Cedars-Saint Hospital, Los Angeles, Calif..

S. MIYATANI,Department of Immunology, Faculty of Medicine, University of Tokyo, Tokyo, Japan.

N.A. MITCHISON,Imperial Cancer Research Fund, Tumor Immunol. Unit, Department of Zoology, University College, London Gower Street, London WC1E 6BT, U.K..

E. MOCCHEGIANI,Immunological Centre, Gerontological Research Dept., I.N.R.C.A., Ancona, Italy.

M. MUZZIOLI,Immunological Centre, Gerontological Research Dept., I.N.R.C.A., Ancona, Italy.

F. NAEIM,The Department of Pathology, UCLA Medical School, and Pediatric Oncology, Cedars-Saint Hospital, Los Angeles, Calif..

M. NERI,Chair of Virology, University of Perugia, 06100 Perugia, Italy.

J. NEWSOM-DAVIS,Department of Neurological Science, Royal Free Hospital Scool of Medicine, Pond Street, London NW3 2QG, England.

W. PIERPAOLI,Institute for Integrative Biomedical Research Lohwis-strasse 50,8123 Ebmatingen, Switzerland.

C. PINI,Laboratory of Cell Biology and Immunology, Istituto Superiore di Sanità, 00100, Roma, Italy.

M.S. PULLEY,Department of Immunology, St Thomas's Hospital and Medical Scool, London SE1 7EH, United Kingdom.

M. RICCI,Clinical Immunology, University of Florence, Policlinico di Careggi, Viale Morgagni, 50134 Firenze Italy.

P. RICCIARDI-CASTAGNOLI,CNR Center of Cytopharmacology, Department of Pharmacology, University of Milano, 20129 Milano, Italy.

C. RINALDI,Institute of Microbiology, UNiversity of Rome, Italy.

S. ROMAGNANI,Clinical Immunology, University of Florence, Policli-nico di Careggi, Viale Morgagni, 50134 Firenze,Italy.

M.G. SANTORO,The Institute of Microbiology, University of Rome, Rome, Italy.

S. SEGAL,Department of Cell Biology, The Weizmann Institute of Science,Rehovot 76100, Israel.

E. SORKIN,Swiss Research Institute, Medical Department, CH-7270

Davos, Switzerland .

N.H. SPECTOR,The Neurosciences Program, School of Medicine, University of Alabama in Birmingham, Birmingham, Alabama 35295, U.S.A..

G. SUNSHINE,Imperial Cancer Research Fund, Tumor Immunology Unit,
Department of Zoology, University College London, Gower Street,
London WC1E 6BT.

G. SUZUKI,Department of Immunology, Faculty of Medicine, University
of Tokyo, Tokyo, Japan .

T. TADA,Department of Immunology, Faculty of Medicine, University
of Tokyo, Tokyo, Japan .

N. TALAL,Medical Centre, Clinical Division, Immunology, 151-T.,
San Francisco, California .

C.F. TAM,The Department of Pathology, UCLA Medical School, and Pediatric Oncology, Cedars-Saint Hospital, Los Angeles, California .

B. TARTAKOVSKY,Department of Cell Biology, The Weizmann Institute
of Science,Rehovot 76100, Israel .

I. TODD,Imperial Cancer Research Fund, Tumor Immunology Unit, Department of Zoology, University College London, Gower Street,London
WC1E 6BT.

G. TRIDENTE,Chair of Immunopathology, University of Padova, Borgo
Rome Hospitals, 37100, Verona, Italy .

J. URBAIN,Université Libre de Bruxelles, Lab. of Animal Physiology
67, rue des Chevaux, B 1640 Rhode-St-Gènese, Belgium .

S. VIETRI,CNEN-Euratom Immunogenetics Group, Laboratory of Radio-
pathology, C.S.N. Casaccia, Rome, Italy .

E. ZANDERS,Imperial Cancer Research Fund, Tumor Immunology Unit,
Department of Zoology, University College London, Gower Street,
London WC1E 6BT.

R.L. WALFORD,The Department of Pathology, UCLA Medical School, and
Pediatric Oncology, Cedars-Saint Hospital, Los Angeles, California.

R.A. WOLSTENCROFT,Department of Immunology, St Thomas's Hospital
and Medical School, London SE1 7EH, United Kingdom.

INDEX